NATIONAL GEOGRAPHIC GUIDE TO

Medicinal Herbs

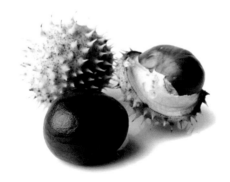

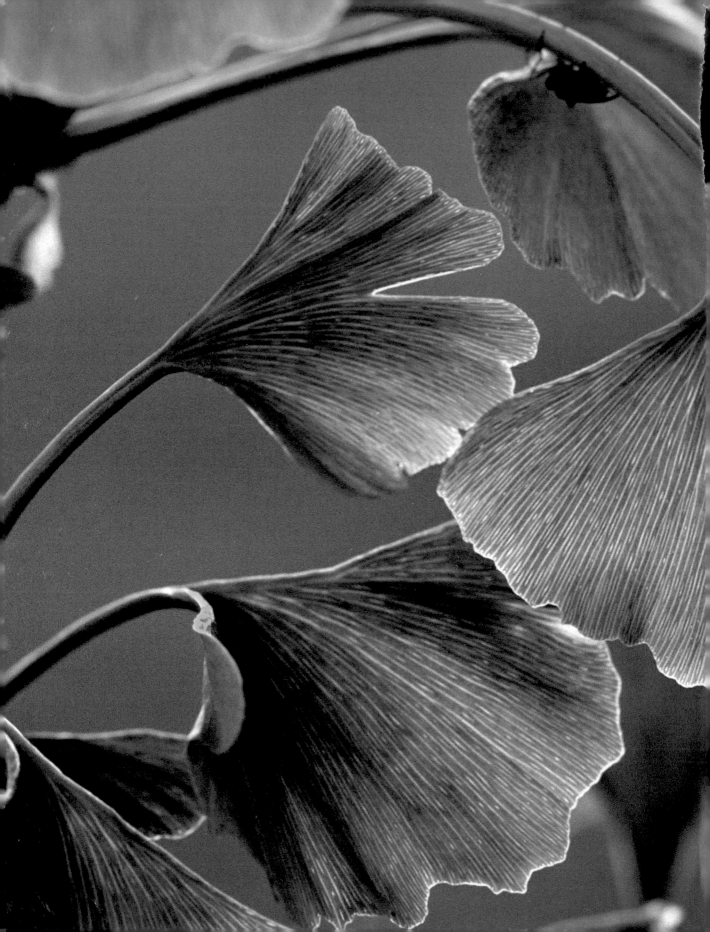

NATIONAL GEOGRAPHIC GUIDE TO

Medicinal Herbs

THE WORLD'S MOST EFFECTIVE HEALING PLANTS

Rebecca L. Johnson & Steven Foster
Tieraona Low Dog, M.D. & David Kiefer, M.D.
Photography by Steven Foster

Foreword by
Andrew Weil, M.D.

NATIONAL GEOGRAPHIC
WASHINGTON, D.C.

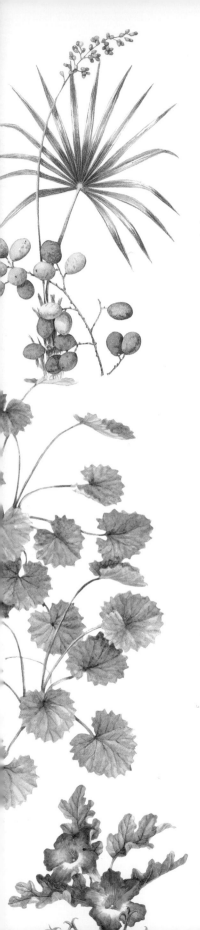
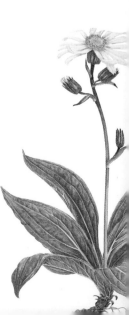

Contents

CHAPTER ONE

Mental Health *and the* Nervous System   14

CHAPTER TWO

Respiratory System   56

CHAPTER THREE

Heart *and* Circulation   98

CHAPTER FOUR

Digestive System   140

CHAPTER FIVE

Joints, Muscles, *and* Skin   186

CHAPTER SIX

Urinary *and* Male Health   236

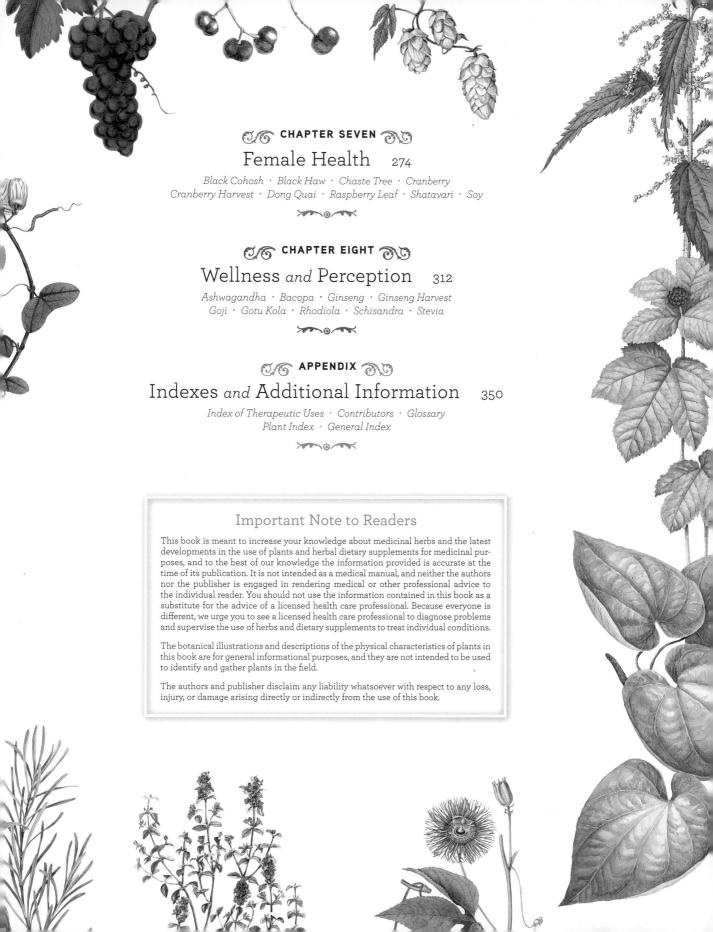

Important Note to Readers

This book is meant to increase your knowledge about medicinal herbs and the latest developments in the use of plants and herbal dietary supplements for medicinal purposes, and to the best of our knowledge the information provided is accurate at the time of its publication. It is not intended as a medical manual, and neither the authors nor the publisher is engaged in rendering medical or other professional advice to the individual reader. You should not use the information contained in this book as a substitute for the advice of a licensed health care professional. Because everyone is different, we urge you to see a licensed health care professional to diagnose problems and supervise the use of herbs and dietary supplements to treat individual conditions.

The botanical illustrations and descriptions of the physical characteristics of plants in this book are for general informational purposes, and they are not intended to be used to identify and gather plants in the field.

The authors and publisher disclaim any liability whatsoever with respect to any loss, injury, or damage arising directly or indirectly from the use of this book.

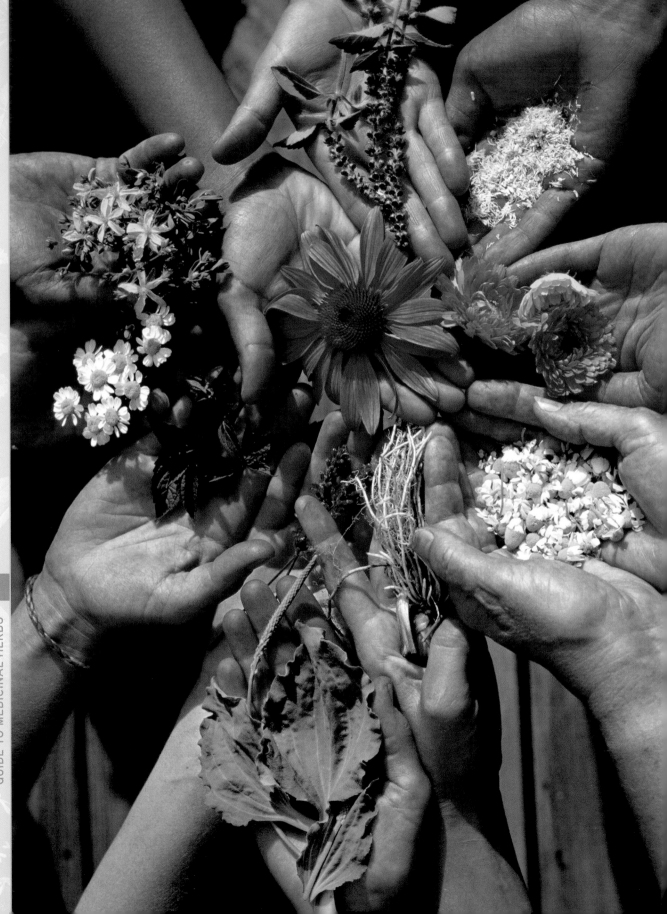

Foreword

Andrew Weil, M.D.

Herbal remedies have been the mainstay of folk medicine in many cultures throughout history and are still in common use by most people in less developed countries, where pharmaceutical drugs are unavailable or unaffordable. In recent years popularity and use of medicinal herbs have increased greatly in the advanced nations. Why? The trend is part of a larger sociocultural change that is also responsible for growing interest in complementary and alternative medicine and integrative medicine.

In Europe and North America, more and more consumers question the safety and efficacy of synthetic drugs, prefer more "natural" therapies, and want to feel more empowered in managing their health. Because information about botanical medicine is no longer included in the education and training of physicians and pharmacists, those professionals are rarely able to advise patients about the risks, benefits, and proper uses of medicinal herbs or tell them how to find products of good quality. Another consequence of that educational deficiency is that physicians and medical scientists in the West tend to be biased against natural remedies, ranking them less predictable and efficacious than purified compounds, more likely to cause harm than promote healing.

I am trained as a botanist and physician and for many years have practiced and taught integrative medicine to physicians, nurse practitioners, and medical students. I have studied medicinal plants worldwide and recommend them to patients more frequently than I prescribe pharmaceutical drugs. In my experience, whole plant preparations are less toxic than their purified, concentrated derivatives and often both effective and cost-effective for treating common health conditions. Some medicinal herbs have uses not obtainable from chemical drugs. For example, milk thistle (*Silybum marianum*) increases metabolism of liver cells and protects them from toxic injury (from excessive alcohol intake, fumes of volatile solvents, and drugs like acetaminophen and some chemotherapy agents). No available pharmaceutical products have those actions.

As consumer demand for herbal products has grown, the marketing of those products has become very big business. It is the manufacturers and distributors of medicinal herbs who provide most of the information on them that consumers read—in books, magazine articles, advertisements, and on the Internet. I'm afraid that much of that information is inaccurate, particularly with regard to therapeutic claims that purport to be backed by scientific studies and the latest research but all too often are based on nothing more than testimonials.

Because I have long worked to make accurate information on botanical remedies available to consumers as well as to doctors, pharmacists, and allied health professionals, I am delighted to see the appearance of the National Geographic Society's *Guide to Medicinal Herbs*. This excellent guide is the work of a team of highly qualified botanical and medical experts, including two of my colleagues from the Arizona Center for Integrative Medicine. The book offers reliable, up-to-date, practical information on 72 of the most important healing plants and medicinal herbs on the market today.

One way to help lower our staggering health care costs is to reduce dependence on costly, technology-based interventions, including prescription drugs. There is growing recognition that medicinal herbs can play a useful role in the maintenance of health and the management of common health problems. I want to see their potential realized and welcome this book as a significant contribution toward making that happen.

The World of Medicinal Herbs

✣

In our little sphere of modernity, the use of medicinal herbs may seem edgy and new, but the truth is that human beings have turned to the world of green for health and nurture from the beginning. The oldest known treatments for the ailments that still plague us today—from headaches to sore feet, from muscle cramps to melancholy—come from the world of plants. In becoming more knowledgeable about medicinal herbs, their powers, and their limitations, we join people throughout history who have harvested plant parts and prepared them according to their cultural traditions.

The advantage that we have, in these days of modern medical science, is that in many cases we have the ability to learn how and why these plants can do what they do for our minds and bodies. That is the purpose of this book: to draw together the ancient and modern, to recognize the remarkable healing properties of plants both familiar and rare, and to bring modern science to bear on understanding how the plant world interacts with the human.

Getting to Know Medicinal Plants

These days, healing herbs are never hard to find. Health food stores, organic food co-ops, and even mainstream groceries and drugstores offer prominent displays of capsules and tablets, tinctures and oils, labeled with the names of plants both familiar and exotic. Herbal teas sit side by side with familiar black teas and coffee. In the case of a few herbs—ginkgo, for example, as a memory aid—the claims have grown to the level of sensational, with promises far exceeding either traditional uses or scientific evidence. Herbal healing has become a commercial business, and in the process we risk forgetting what it is all about.

Indigenous healers had to identify, gather, and process the herbs that they found valuable. They knew the plants' growing cycles, and they knew which parts of the plants to harvest, and how. Those in the commercial herb business today are equally knowledgeable. Occasionally their products remind us of their earthy, botanical origins: Goldenseal powder gleams a mustard yellow; cayenne powder stings the tongue; aloe gel oozes as thick from the bottle as it does from the newly cut leaf. But herbal preparations today are often designed to deliver the remedy without any sensory overload: "Experience the miracle effects of garlic without any aftertaste!"

Knowledge of medicinal herbs and other healing plants can only make our use of them more valuable, effective, and long-lasting as part of our culture in the future. By recognizing that this substance, whether delivered in a pill or capsule, a tube or bottle, derives from a plant with distinct growing habits and a native range somewhere specific on the globe, one discovers new levels on which herbal medicine can enrich our lives and culture as well as heal our bodies. The more knowledge we have, the more precisely and appropriately we use these amazing plants—and the healthier we stay.

Growing Your Own Medicine Garden

There are many ways to make medicinal herbs part of your everyday life, but none is more satisfying than growing your own. If you are lucky enough to have a kitchen garden outdoors, designate one corner of it your herbal pharmacy.

A number of medicinal herbs, some already familiar as culinary herbs, are easy to start from

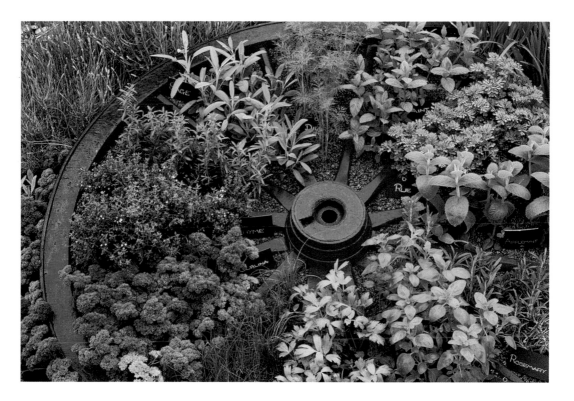

seed and grow year after year in temperate growing zones. Some are annuals or biennials, such as calendula and members of the carrot family—parsley or fennel, for example. Start these from seed and allow some seed to ripen and fall, and you may be able to nurture crops of these herbs year after year.

In establishing your own medicine garden, pay attention to the species and variety of plant you are growing. Always procure growing stock, whether roots, seeds, or whole plants, from reputable sources that clearly identify the plant variety. Some varieties developed for the garden differ from those with the most potential for healing. Compare the scientific species names, not just the common names, as you choose the ones to cultivate.

Just as the vigor of flowers and vegetables varies depending on soil, climate, weather, and other growing conditions, so the effectiveness of medicinal herbs will vary from plant to plant, garden to garden, year to year. While we celebrate the impulse to use simple homegrown herbs for remedies, we also recognize the value of controlled harvests and measured dosages.

The Business of Medicinal Herbs

The medicinal herb industry is today a five-billion-dollar business in the United States alone—even larger if you factor in research funds sponsoring ongoing searches for traditional medicinals with promise for modern pharmaceutical research. And in many developed countries beyond the United States, herbal remedies are even more accepted as a normal health regimen.

Debates continue as to how government regulators can interact with the medicinal herb trade, which accomplishes some measure of self-regulation through such organizations as the American Botanical Council and the American Herbal Products Association. Herbal remedies pose different regulatory challenges from pharmaceutical medicines. The World Health Organization is spearheading an effort to develop guidelines for good manufacturing practices (GMPs) of herbal products worldwide, and the U.S. Food and Drug Administration recently set rules for "dietary supplements"—a term that covers medicinal herbs as well as vitamins and minerals.

The Safe Use of Medicinal Herbs

Consumers of commercial herb preparations would do best to educate themselves about what they are buying and using medicinally. Herbs can be potent. Read labels, pay attention to recommended dosages, and avoid combining herbs on your own. Although in many cases this book identifies several herbs that may address the same health problem, in no way does it imply that a person should use all of them at one time. Many commercially available herbal teas contain blends of herbs to enhance flavor and benefit, but consumers should be cautious about mixing herbs on their own.

It is best to seek the advice of a health care professional before beginning the use of herbal therapies. Especially if you use prescription drugs, seek advice before turning to herbal remedies, because some combinations of herbs and pharmaceuticals can be dangerous or cause undesirable side effects. Pregnant and breast-feeding women should be especially careful about using herbal remedies, and parents should seek advice before giving herbal remedies to children.

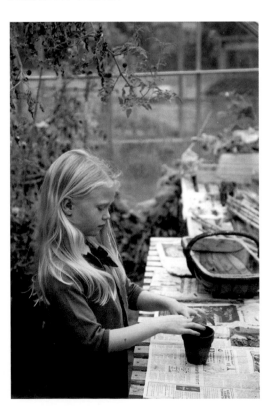

The Many Ways of Using Herbs

Herbal remedies come in many forms, and each has a strict definition:

INFUSION: A tea preparation: plant parts and hot water mix for a short time.

DECOCTION: A longer tea preparation: plant parts simmer in hot water for a longer time.

SYRUP: Plant parts added to sugar-water or honey-water mixture.

POWDER: Dried plant parts pulverized, traditionally by mortar and pestle.

TINCTURE: Essential plant components dissolved in water and alcohol solution.

ESSENCE: Essential plant fragrance added to alcohol.

OINTMENT: Powdered or essential plant parts added to an oily substance such as olive oil, petroleum jelly, lard, often mixed with beeswax.

POULTICE: Fresh or dried plant parts applied to skin with moist heat.

Today, with so many herbal preparations available commercially, it's important to read labels to confirm that the product contains a "standardized extract," which is the manufacturer's promise that from batch to batch a measure and control are placed on the level of active herbal ingredients in the tea, tincture, salve, or other product. Standardization assures proper, consistent, and effective levels. This measure is especially important in capsules and tablets, the method of delivery most often chosen by consumers of commercial herbal medicine today. Mention of specific products, companies, or organizations in this book does not imply that the publisher or the authors endorse them.

For the sake of simplicity, and to match current practices, this broad array of delivery methods has been narrowed down in this book to the five most common: tea, tincture, capsule or tablet, topical applications, and in or as food. For every plant in this book, you will see icons designating which of the five delivery methods is appropriate.

To those who wish to bring medicinal herbs into their daily lives, whether as part of a regular health regimen or as an alternative or supplement to modern medical treatments, we say: Read, learn, consider—and good health to you.

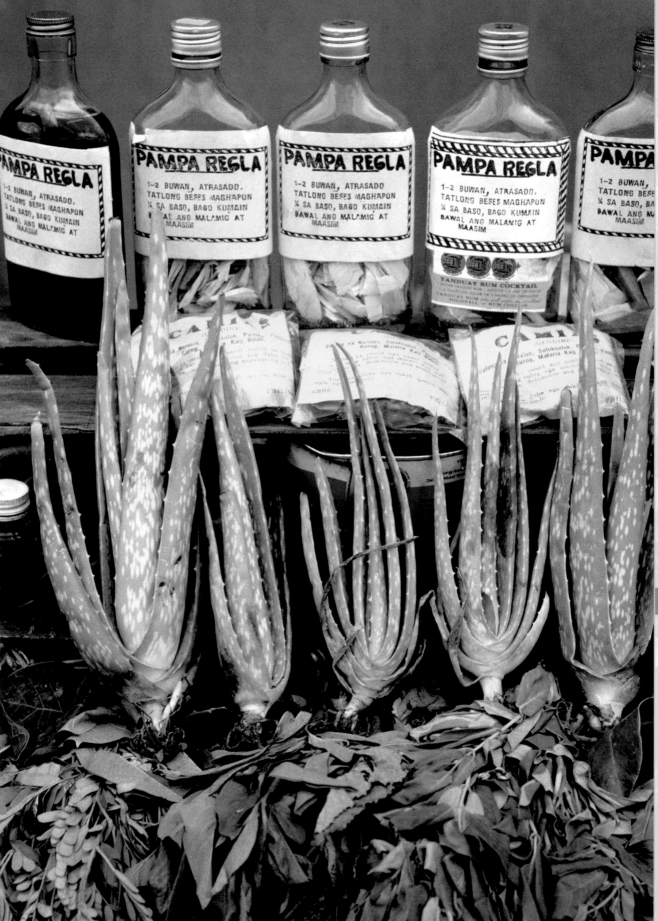

How *to* Use *this* Book

Each of the 72 plants featured in this book is represented by four pages. The first two pages introduce the plant's distinguishing characteristics, with an eye to geography, botany, history, culture, and medical science today. A time line puts the plant's recognition and use into the context of history. ⟨⟩ The next two pages in this "plant-ography" go into greater detail about the plant's botany and its medicinal effects. Botanical information includes detailed plant descriptions, the plant's native origins and present-day range worldwide, its growing habits, and the methods by which it is cultivated and harvested. Medical information includes the therapeutic uses of each plant, listed and explained with reference to the most current scientific literature and research; specific information on the most common preparations in use today; and important precautions regarding the use of this medicinal herb.

At the end of this book, an appendix offers several different ways of accessing information. First, an index of therapeutic uses (pages 352-60) allows readers to scan for health conditions of interest and to quickly locate them in the book. The righthand column of this chart refers readers to additional information on medicinal plants in another National Geographic book, *Desk Reference to Nature's Medicine,* also written by Rebecca L. Johnson and Steven Foster. A glossary (pages 362-66) defines all technical and scientific terms found in the book. Following that, an illustrated plant index (pages 367-73) allows readers to scan the book's contents by scientific name (rather than by common name) and botanical illustration. Finally a standard index (pages 374-83) lists all contents of this book alphabetically.

Since the influence of herbal medicine is holistic, affecting the entire body, many of these herbs can have broader and more complex effects than those highlighted by their placement in a particular chapter. It is impossible for a book to describe every individual's potential response to an herbal remedy, and so it is important to consult a reliable health care professional before using medicinal herbs and other plant remedies. The information here represents a starting point on the path to an understanding of the uses and functions of medicinal herbs and how our bodies respond to them. This guide is meant to be an important educational tool in every consumer's quest for health and longevity.

Delivery Methods

There are many ways in which the power of medicinal herbs can be added to your daily routine, and many delivery methods developed by those who prepare medicinal herbs commercially. On the third page of every plant feature, you will find a chart that highlights the most common delivery methods for that plant. Refer to page 10 for the traditional herbalists' definition of some of these preparations.

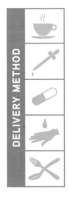

DELIVERY METHOD

TEA This symbol stands for infusions and decoctions, in which plant parts are prepared in hot water.

TINCTURE This symbol stands for tinctures, extracts, and essential oils.

PILL OR CAPSULE This symbol stands for tablets, pills, and capsules.

TOPICAL This symbol stands for ointments, lotions, salves, creams, and poultices.

FOOD This symbol indicates edible medicinal plants with healthful effects.

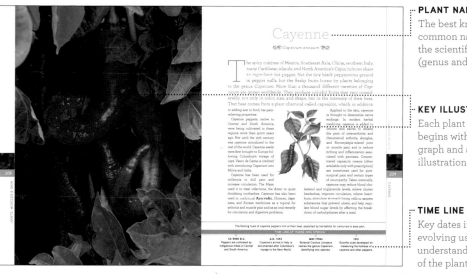

Cayenne
Capsicum annuum

The flaming hues of cayenne peppers hint at their heat, exploited by herbalists for centuries to ease pain.

TIME LINE OF USAGE AND SPREAD

CA 5000 B.C.	A.D. 1493	MID-1700s	1912
Peppers are cultivated by indigenous tribes in Central and South America.	Cayenne's arrival in Italy is documented after Columbus's voyage to the New World.	Botanist Carolus Linnaeus names the genus Capsicum, identifying two species.	Scoville scale developed for measuring the hotness of cayenne and other peppers.

PLANT NAMES
The best known common name and the scientific name (genus and species).

KEY ILLUSTRATIONS
Each plant profile begins with a photograph and a botanical illustration.

TIME LINE
Key dates in the evolving use and understanding of the plant.

PLANT BASICS
Basic information on names, botanical classification, medicinally effective parts, and growing range.

DELIVERY METHOD
Icons indicate delivery methods. For more information, see opposite page.

BOTANICAL INFORMATION
The most important features of a plant's physical characteristics and growing habits.

MEDICAL INFORMATION
The most important medicinal uses of this plant, including references to current research.

SPECIAL NOTE
Sometimes you will find a special note such as this on the page, with or without the red warning symbol. These may highlight an important precaution, add extra medical information, or feature an interesting detail about the plant.

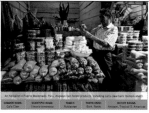

An herbalist in Puerto Maldonado, Peru, displays rain forest products, including cat's claw bark (bottom shelf).

COMMON NAME:	SCIENTIFIC NAME:	FAMILY:	PARTS USED:	NATIVE RANGE:
Cat's Claw	Uncaria tomentosa	Rubiaceae	Bark, Roots	Amazon, Tropical S. America

over the (kitchen) counter CAT'S CLAW TEA

SUGGESTIONS FOR USE
Best preparation methods for the various delivery methods of this plant.

PRECAUTIONS
General comments or warnings on the use of this plant.

GLOSSARY TERM
Words in bold are defined in the glossary of technical terms found on pages 362-66.

GROWING INFORMATION
Details on how this plant is grown and gathered, in gardens or commercially.

OVER THE (KITCHEN) COUNTER
Simple ideas and recipes for making use of this medicinal plant at home.

CHAPTER ONE

Mental Health
and the
Nervous System

Plants *and the* Brain

❧◉☙

ippocrates (460-370 B.C.) is often called the father of medicine and credited as being the first physician in ancient Greece, and thus the Western world, to reject the idea that illness is caused by supernatural or divine forces. He believed instead that any disease or ailment resulted from an imbalance in four principal bodily fluids, or "humors." These four substances—blood, phlegm, yellow bile, and black bile—were thought to be produced by various organs, to spread through the entire body like subtle vapors, and to affect not only physical health but the mind and emotions as well. When the humors were in balance, well-being naturally ensued. When they were out of balance, they exerted a negative influence on both physical and mental health. Hippocrates and his followers believed that the task of a physician was to restore the balance. Attempts to do so typically involved removing an "excess" of a particular humor by purging or bloodletting, or reestablishing its equilibrium through the use of medicinal herbs.

In fact, herbal medicine in the West evolved largely through attempts to use plants to help balance the body's four humors.

In our modern, high-tech world, the entire concept of humors and their effects on health might seem ridiculously archaic and far-fetched. Yet considerable scientific research has revealed that the proper functioning of many of our physiological systems does indeed depend on a balance—not of humors, but rather of various arrays of chemical substances. The human nervous system is a prime example. It is an incredibly vast and complex network that includes the brain and spinal cord, and threadlike nerves that reach deep into every part of the body. Each of these organs is made up of millions, even billions, of specialized cells called neurons that gather and transmit information using electrical impulses. Naturally occurring chemical compounds called neurotransmitters help relay these impulses from cell to cell at lightning speed—less than 1/5,000th of a second. Scientists have identified some 30 neurotransmitters, including serotonin, dopamine, and norepinephrine.

The nervous system is also intimately aligned with the endocrine system, the collection of organs and glands that release hormones such as insulin, cortisol, estrogen, and testosterone. These substances are also powerful chemical messengers that circulate through the bloodstream to specific target cells, where they generate a wide range of biological responses. Hormones help regulate many body functions and also influence mood, energy levels, and feelings of well-being.

Studies have shown that disruptions in the normal balance of neurotransmitters and hormones definitely affect health. For example, an imbalance in serotonin levels may influence mood in ways that can lead to depression, as well as anxiety, anger, and feelings of panic. In much the same way, hormonal irregularities can lead to problems such as a lack of appetite, insomnia, and mood swings.

One of the primary disruptors of the body's chemical messengers is thought to be stress. Stress manifests itself in many ways. Some of its symptoms are probably disturbingly familiar to most of us, because stress—especially the insidious, chronic form often generated by demanding jobs, hectic lifestyles, financial worries, and personal conflicts—seems to have become an integral part of everyday life. Signs of stress include irritability; high blood pressure; nervous tension; anxiety; headaches, including migraines; depression; insomnia. Prescription medications are available to treat these conditions, or at least their symptoms. Yet many of these drugs have side effects or can be habit forming. Medicinal herbs, on the other hand, are a time-tested, and in some cases scientifically supported, alternative.

Through the centuries, many herbs have been used to treat nervous conditions and help restore mental health. This chapter focuses on nine herbs that many herbalists consider particularly effective, and which are widely prescribed and commonly available. At least one has found its way into the conventional medical systems of European countries. Several have long and interesting histories, and a few have been used medicinally for thousands of years. Others are more recent additions to the herbalist's arsenal.

Preparations made from the roots and large, distinctive leaves of butterbur (*Petasites hybridus*) are used in modern herbal medicine to relieve stress-induced migraine headaches. Clinical trials have confirmed the herb's effects, and commercial preparations of butterbur have been available in the United States since 1997. Feverfew (*Tanacetum parthenium*) was introduced into the herbal pharmacopeia in ancient Greece primarily as a fever reducer, but it, too, is currently prized as an effective remedy for migraines.

Hops (*Humulus lupulus*) are often associated with beermaking. Medicinally, the herb is prescribed for those who struggle to fall asleep, as it can effectively help fight insomnia, induce sleep, and calm stress-jangled nerves. Kava (*Piper methysticum*), a relative newcomer to Western herbal medicine, is also used for treating sleep disorders and as an alternative to prescription drugs for anxiety and mild depression.

Lemon balm (*Melissa officinalis*) is often combined with hops, and another herb included in this chapter, valerian, in preparations used to promote sleep and ease tension; it may also help mental health in another way—by improving memory and enhancing learning. Both passionflower (*Passiflora incarnata*) and skullcap (*Scutellaria lateriflora*) are native to North America, used first for their healing properties by Native American tribes, and later adopted by European settlers. Modern herbal practitioners prescribe them both for problems associated with stress, including tension and anxiety.

No modern compendium of medicinal herbs would be complete without St. John's wort (*Hypericum perforatum*), the most widely used herb for treating mild to moderate depression. Many conventional European physicians regularly prescribe St. John's wort for elevating mood or relieving stress. In Germany, it is considered safe enough to give to teenagers and children. Some studies have shown preparations of St. John's wort are as effective as several common prescription antidepressants; both appear to work in a similar way, helping to balance levels of the neurotransmitter serotonin in the brain.

Last, valerian (*Valeriana officinalis*) has been included in the herbal repertoire of ancient Greek and Roman physicians, practitioners of Chinese and Ayurvedic traditional medicine, medieval healers—and now modern herbalists— as a gentle sleep aid with few side effects.

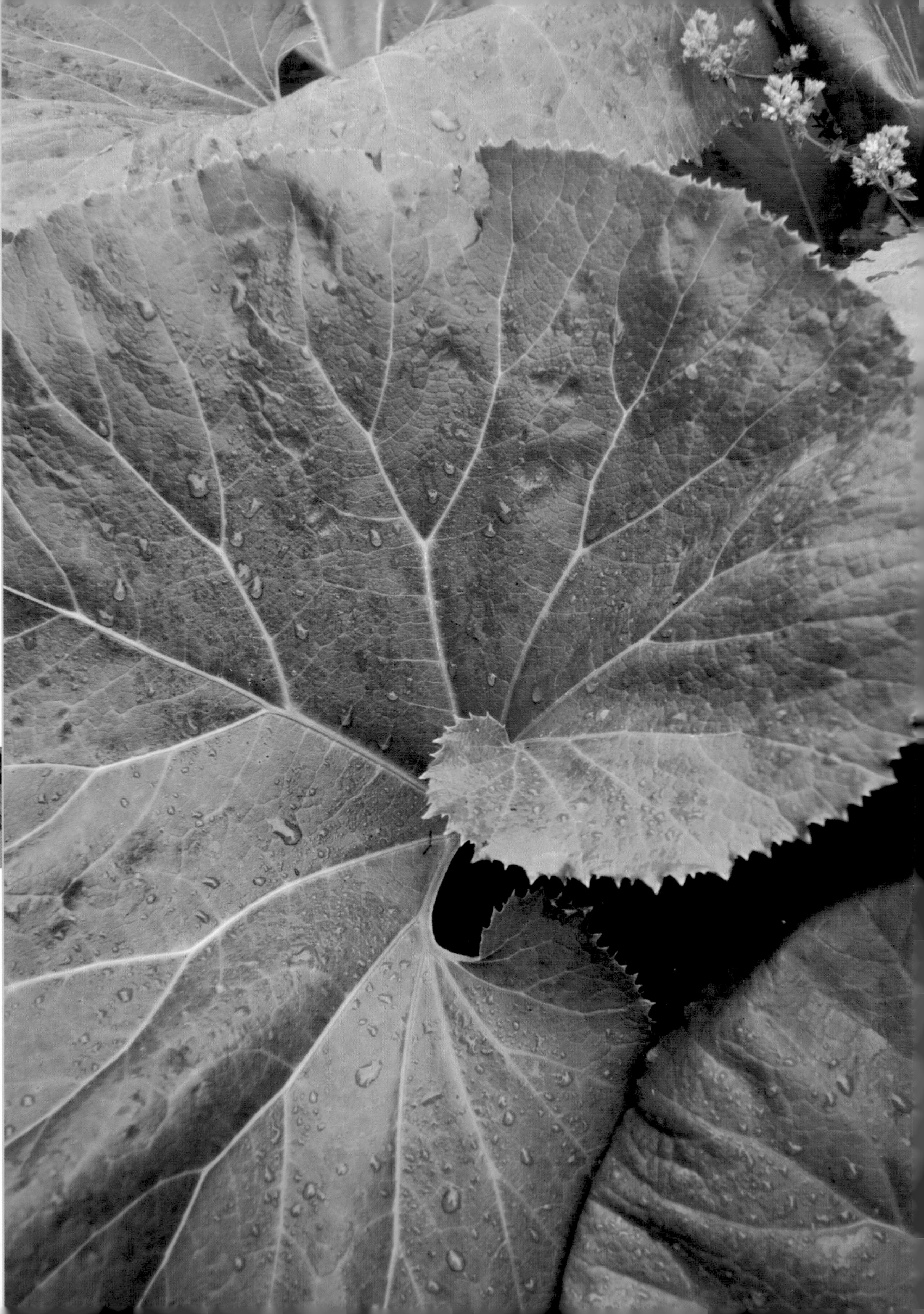

Butterbur

Petasites hybridus

I t's butterbur's foliage that first attracts attention. Green above and woolly gray below, the heart-shaped leaves may reach nearly 3 feet in diameter on plants growing under ideal conditions on marshy ground. Scientific names often capture the essence of a plant's appearance, and *Petasites* is no exception. The word is derived from the Greek *petasos*, which refers to a type of hat with a broad brim. In some parts of butterbur's range, its leaves are still used as impromptu umbrellas and sunshades. Butterbur leaves were once used to wrap fresh butter in summer as it was taken from

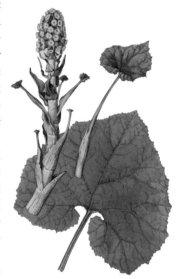

the churn, and this may account for its most familiar common name. Over the centuries, butterbur has been known by other names. Cough wort is one that is well deserved, as the plant has been used for millennia to relieve coughs and various other respiratory conditions.

Butterbur has been used medicinally for at least 2,000 years. The ancient Greeks used it to treat asthma. In medieval Europe, **infusions** of butterbur roots or leaves were a remedy for treating coughs, hoarseness, bronchial infections, and urinary tract complaints and to expel intestinal worms. It was given to lower fever and calm intestinal ailments. In the 1600s, fresh butterbur leaves went into **poultices** that were applied to swellings, painful joints, cramped muscles, rashes, wounds, and other irritations.

People even smoked dried butterbur roots or leaves to relieve nagging coughs.

The number of ailments for which butterbur is used in modern herbal medicine is considerable. One of its primary therapeutic applications is in treating migraine headaches. Butterbur **extract** may help reduce the frequency of migraines as well as their duration and intensity. It may also help prevent migraines from occurring. Herbal practitioners also recommend butterbur as a treatment for the symptoms of seasonal allergies (allergic rhinitis) without the drowsiness and other side effects associated with taking **antihistamines**. And today as in the past, butterbur is still taken to relieve joint pain, to soothe coughs and bronchitis, and to ease irritations of the small intestine.

The gargantuan leaves and creeping rhizomes of butterbur are sources of an extract for reducing migraine pain.

TIME LINE OF USAGE AND SPREAD

1633
English herbalist J. Gerard touts butterbur with wine as "a soveraigne medicine."

1951
Reports on butterbur lead to a resurgence of interest in its medicinal properties.

1954
In *The Lord of the Rings*, The Prancing Pony's innkeeper is named Barliman Butterbur.

1997
Commercial preparations derived from butterbur become available in the U.S.

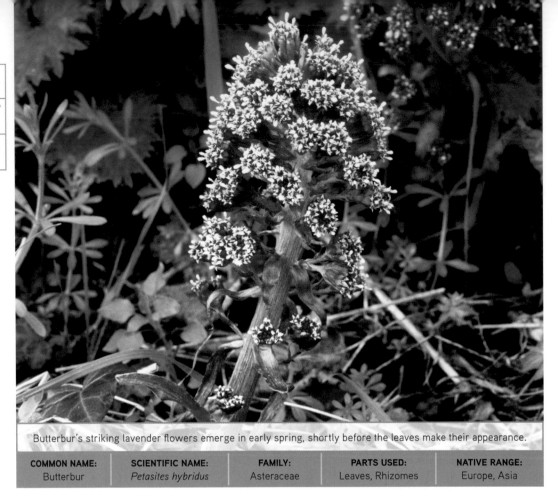

Butterbur's striking lavender flowers emerge in early spring, shortly before the leaves make their appearance.

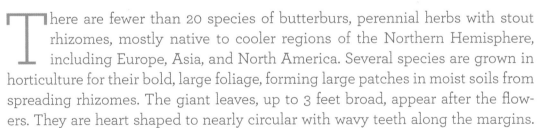

COMMON NAME:	SCIENTIFIC NAME:	FAMILY:	PARTS USED:	NATIVE RANGE:
Butterbur	*Petasites hybridus*	Asteraceae	Leaves, Rhizomes	Europe, Asia

There are fewer than 20 species of butterburs, perennial herbs with stout rhizomes, mostly native to cooler regions of the Northern Hemisphere, including Europe, Asia, and North America. Several species are grown in horticulture for their bold, large foliage, forming large patches in moist soils from spreading rhizomes. The giant leaves, up to 3 feet broad, appear after the flowers. They are heart shaped to nearly circular with wavy teeth along the margins.

As the leaves mature, they become nearly hairless and dark green above with grayish-downy hairs on the underside of the leaves. The rhubarblike leaf stalks are up to 18 inches long. Purple flowers, all without ray flowers, shoot up on a 3-foot stem in early spring before the leaves appear. Most plants in cultivation are male. More than 30 purple-tinged flowerheads appear on each male stalk, with up to 130 pink to lilac flowerheads on female plants. The flowers and flowering stalks of male and female plants have such different appearances that they were once classified as separate **species**. The resinous aromatic root has a bitter flavor.

Growing Habits

Butterburs usually grow in moist fields, stream banks, and riverbanks, where they produce large colonies. The large leaves make them easily recognizable in wild habitats. In fact, the leaves' size led 18th-century Swedish botanist Carolus Linnaeus to observe that chickens and other small farm animals would take shelter from rain beneath butterbur's large leaves.

In northern Europe, female plants are rare, and the dominant male plants are believed to have been introduced centuries earlier. Butterbur has escaped from cultivation in the northeastern United States, and is also established in Illinois and Washington.

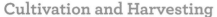

Common migraine triggers include ripe bananas, peanuts, MSG, red wine, champagne, aged cheeses, chocolate, anchovies, avocados, and sodium nitrate found in cured meats. If you suffer from migraines, in addition to trying butterbur, try keeping a diary for a few weeks to see if there are any foods that might act as triggers.

Cultivation and Harvesting

Butterbur needs plenty of room to spread. The soil should be moist and rich, and the planting situated in partial shade. It is easily propagated simply by dividing the roots and requires no special care. The vast majority of the world's supply is wild-harvested in Eastern Europe.

Therapeutic Uses

+ *Migraine headaches*
+ *Seasonal allergies*

Butterbur is gaining attention globally for its use in the prevention of migraines, a condition that affects roughly 28 million Americans, striking women three times more frequently than men. Standard treatments are designed to control symptoms by calming sensitive nerve pathways, reducing **inflammation**, preventing spasm of the cranial blood vessels, and preventing future attacks. Unfortunately, many conventional treatments also have side effects; a survey of migraine sufferers reveals only 21 percent as very satisfied with their current treatment options.

Thus, it is good news that the humble butterbur has been shown to reduce the duration, frequency, and pain of migraines by as much as 50 percent in human studies. One well-controlled clinical trial involving 245 people with migraines found that 150 mg per day of butterbur root extract cut the number of migraines experienced by the participants by almost half compared with the group taking a **placebo.** Butterbur has also been studied in children and adolescents. A study of 108 children (ages 6 to 17) reported that 77 percent of those receiving the butterbur extract (doses ranging from 50 to 150 mg per day) had fewer migraines, and 91 percent felt substantially or partially improved. Both of these studies reported that butterbur extract was very well tolerated.

Scientists do not completely understand how butterbur prevents migraines but believe it is due to a reduction of inflammation and spasm of the blood vessels, particularly in the brain.

Butterbur is also popular, particularly in Europe, for treating seasonal allergies. **Compounds** in the root reduce inflammation and appear to inhibit mast cells—a type of cell involved in nasal congestion and allergies. Well-controlled human studies in children and adults have shown that the extract works as well or better than pharmaceutical antihistamines, with fewer side effects.

How to Use

In Europe, where butterbur is used widely, regulatory authorities require manufacturers to guarantee extracts are free of pyrrolizidine **alkaloids**. Further, a consistent amount of the main active compounds is desirable. So users should look for products that guarantee a minimum of 7.5 mg of petasin and isopetasin. **EXTRACT:** According to the clinical trials, for migraine prevention, the dose is 150 mg butterbur extract per day for 30 days, and then 100 mg per day for adults and adolescents. For seasonal allergies the dose for adults is typically 50 to 75 mg of the extract taken twice a day. The dose used in the studies for children ages 10 to 12 was 25 mg twice daily.

 NOTE: Butterbur contains pyrrolizidine alkaloids (PA), a group of compounds that can be toxic to the liver. Only products labeled "PA free" should be used.

Precautions

Butterbur extracts that are PA free appear to be quite safe when used as directed. Use of butterbur in pregnancy and lactation is discouraged.

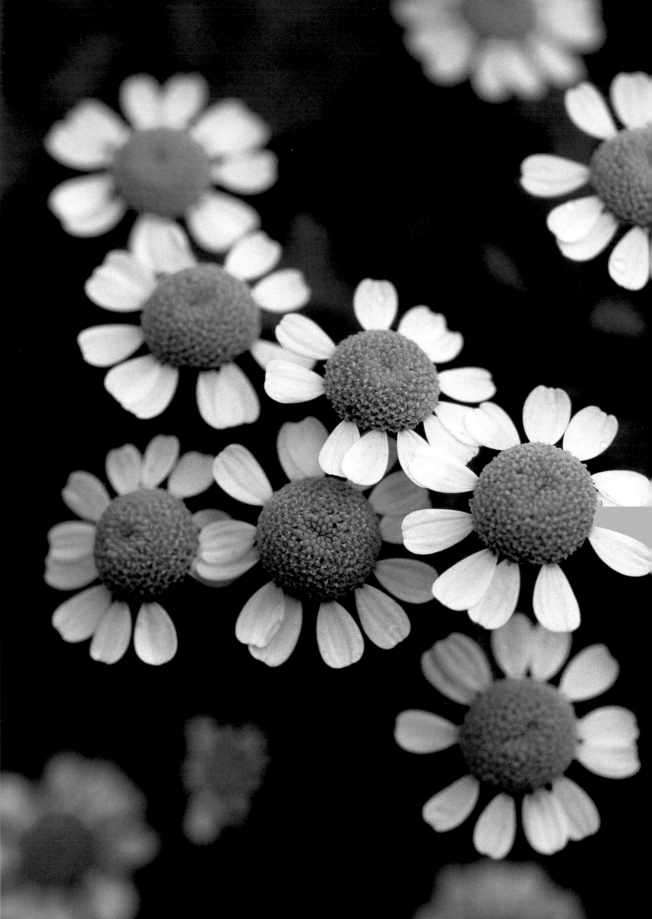

Feverfew

Tanacetum parthenium

A relative of dandelions and marigolds, feverfew is an unwavering perennial. It provides a profusion of tiny daisylike flowers year after year with only minimal attention. The entire plant exudes a strong, bitter scent, and people once believed that growing feverfew around a house was a sure way to purify the air and ward off infection. Feverfew found a place in herbal medicine some 2,000 years ago. Legend has it that the ancient Greeks called feverfew *parthenium* because the herb had been used to save the life of someone who fell from the Parthenon in Athens. Whatever the treatment, the herb's more recent common name may provide a clue. Feverfew comes from the Latin *febris*, for fever, and *fugure*, meaning "to chase away." For many centuries, feverfew has indeed been used to chase away fevers, along with a variety of other ailments, including migraine headaches.

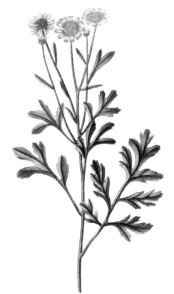

The Greeks used *parthenium* for more than just fever. Dioscorides, renowned Greek physician of the first century A.D., recommended the herb for many complaints, including headache, arthritis, and melancholy. It was also something of a woman's herb, used to help expel the placenta after childbirth and ease menstrual irregularities. By the 16th century in Europe, it had become well established as a remedy for headaches, stomach disorders, toothaches, and nerve pain. Europeans introduced feverfew to the Americas, and it was a part of herbal medicine until the early 20th century, when it fell into disuse.

Interest in feverfew abruptly revived in the 1970s, however, when the wife of a Welsh doctor who suffered from chronic migraines began experimenting with feverfew. After less than a year of eating just a few fresh feverfew leaves each day, her migraine attacks diminished, and ultimately ceased. This incident and others sparked intense interest and research in feverfew and its effects. Today, herbal practitioners regularly suggest feverfew as an alternative to conventional medications for migraine headaches, as well as the nausea and vomiting that frequently accompany them.

The dainty feverfew's flowers and leaves are a powerhouse for preventing and relieving headache pain.

TIME LINE OF USAGE AND SPREAD

1525
Banckes's Herbal advocates feverfew for stomach disorders, toothaches, bites

1787
Culpeper's *Herbal* recommends feverfew for "pains in the head."

1791
The *Edinburgh Dispensatory* suggests feverfew for hysteria and flatulence.

1973
Welsh woman experiments with feverfew to relieve migraines and finds relief.

The genus *Tanacetum* includes about 160 species of herbaceous plants found in northern temperate climates. Relatives of feverfew include aromatic herbs such as common tansy *(Tanacetum vulgare)* and costmary *(Tanacetum balsamita)*, among others. Feverfew is a strongly aromatic perennial herb growing from 1 to 2 feet with stiff, erect, round, smooth, striated stems. The greenish yellow alternate leaves are divided into 2 or more segments, giving a superficial resemblance to fern leaves. The lower leaves, up to 6 inches long, are oval in outline with 3 to 7 irregular oblong segments, further divided into smaller lobes with small rounded teeth or without teeth. Upper leaves are smaller. Numerous flowers crowded atop the plant in flat-topped, branching clusters look like small daisies. Flowering plants often droop under the weight of the flowering tops. The ray flowers are white, about ⅜ of an inch long (though variable in length), and have 3 small teeth at the end. Feverfew blooms from June through the first frost of the autumn.

Growing Habits

Feverfew is at home in the mountain scrub and rocky soils of the Balkan Peninsula. Cultivated for centuries as an ornamental and medicinal plant, it is now naturalized in fields, waste places, and garden edges throughout Europe. Brought to North America by early settlers by the mid-19th century, it has become naturalized throughout the eastern United States, south to South Carolina, and westward from Colorado to the Pacific Coast states. It is also found in eastern and western Canada.

Cultivation and Harvesting

Feverfew is an easy-to-grow perennial at home both in the flower and herb garden. It is not particular about soil type, as long as the soil is well-drained. Plants can be propagated either by dividing established clumps in spring or fall or by planting seeds. The tiny seeds should be lightly tamped into the soil surface, as germination is enhanced by light. Feverfew prefers full sun but will grow in light shade.

Commercially, feverfew is grown as a row crop, with leaves harvested before the plant comes into bloom. It is produced in Eastern Europe, the United Kingdom, China, and the United States. The chemistry is highly variable, so commercial growers often select chemotypes, varieties of a known chemistry, for commercial production to help ensure a product of consistent quality.

Therapeutic Uses

✤ *Migraine headaches*

Modern research confirms anecdotal evidence of earlier decades that feverfew can reduce the frequency and severity of migraines. Recent research on its **anti-inflammatory** properties also supports its historical use in easing menstrual cramps, arthritis, and fevers. But it is the traditional use of feverfew in preventing headaches for which the herb is best known today. During the 1980s, feverfew became very popular as an alternative treatment for migraine headaches, and a survey conducted in the United Kingdom found that 70 percent of migraine sufferers reported feeling better after chewing two fresh feverfew

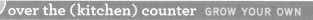

over the (kitchen) counter GROW YOUR OWN

Many migraine sufferers in Britain prefer to grow their own feverfew and chew ½ to 1 small leaf each day to ward off headaches. Make sure you purchase organic *Tanacetum parthenium* seeds. The seeds sprout readily in flowerpots or in your garden. Discontinue use of any feverfew leaf or product if mouth ulcers occur.

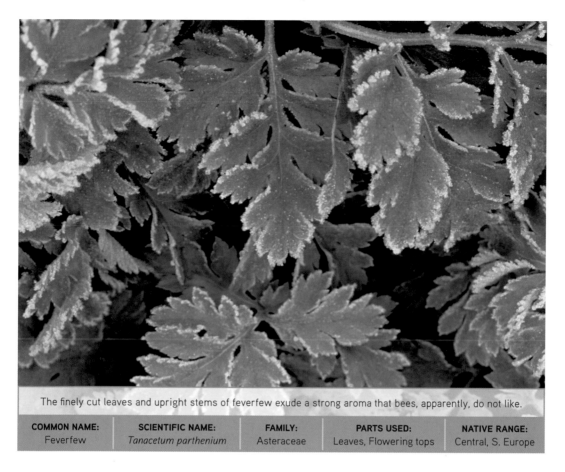

The finely cut leaves and upright stems of feverfew exude a strong aroma that bees, apparently, do not like.

COMMON NAME:	SCIENTIFIC NAME:	FAMILY:	PARTS USED:	NATIVE RANGE:
Feverfew	*Tanacetum parthenium*	Asteraceae	Leaves, Flowering tops	Central, S. Europe

leaves every day. This spurred a number of human studies on dried feverfew leaf. A review of all the published clinical trials found that the majority favored feverfew over **placebo** for the prevention of migraine.

How feverfew prevents migraine is not completely understood. One of the more than 40 **compounds** in the leaf is parthenolide, shown to ease smooth muscle spasms and prevent the constriction of blood vessels in the brain, one of the leading causes of migraine headaches. While there is little question that this compound is important, it appears that parthenolide is only one of a number of compounds that contribute to the overall effect.

How to Use

FRESH LEAF: Two leaves chewed daily to ward off migraines is the traditional treatment. But the fresh leaf can cause mouth ulcers.

CAPSULES: Studies showing benefits from feverfew used a freeze-dried formulation of 50 to 100

mg daily, typically standardized as 0.2 to 0.35 percent parthenolide content. In some countries such as Canada, parthenolide consistency is required for feverfew products. Sometimes feverfew is blended with riboflavin (vitamin B_2) and magnesium, as these have also been shown to reduce migraine frequency.

TINCTURE: Feverfew is available in **tincture** form; however, one clinical trial failed to note any benefit from this type of preparation.

Precautions

Clinical trials have shown feverfew to be safe and well tolerated. A few people experience mouth ulcers, primarily associated with chewing the fresh leaf; use should be discontinued if that occurs with any product. Withdrawal headaches have been reported by roughly 10 percent of long-term feverfew users when they abruptly stopped taking feverfew. Tapering off feverfew minimizes this adverse effect. Pregnant women should not use feverfew.

Hops

Humulus lupulus

Hops are the pale green, conelike fruits of a hardy, twining vine native to Europe, western Asia, and North America. They are probably best known by brewers—and beer drinkers—for giving aroma and flavor to beer. Interestingly enough, hops were originally added to beer for their natural preservative properties. Only later did they come to be valued for the bitter, but agreeable, taste they impart to the drink. The Romans ate the young shoots of the hops plant like asparagus, a practice that continued in rural parts of the British Isles well into the

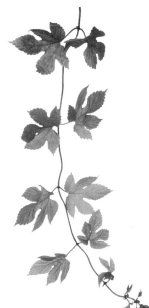

20th century. The Roman physician Pliny the Elder named hops *Lupus salictarius,* which means "willow wolf" and refers to the vine's habit of twining around other plants and strangling them, like a wolf does to sheep. The plant's **species** name, *lupulus,* is Latin for "small wolf," a similar reference. Hops were used medicinally in Europe and by Native Americans in North America. Today, their greatest value in herbal medicine is as a calming, natural sedative.

Hops have been put to numerous healing purposes over the centuries. Many Native American tribes used the herb to treat pain and insomnia. The Delaware applied small bags of heated hops leaves to aching teeth or ears. They also drank hops tea, as did the Cherokee, Mohegan, and Fox, to hasten sleep. In Europe,

hops were used to ease pain in rheumatic joints; cure fevers; and treat heart conditions, diarrhea, and hysteria. Hops was renowned as a sedative. King George III of England (aka the king who lost America) is said to have slept on a pillow stuffed with hops to ease his porphyria, a condition that can cause anxiety and mental illness.

In modern herbal medicine, hops are valued for their soothing, sedative effect. Under a pillow, a sachet of dried hops is considered an effective tool for fighting insomnia and inducing sleep. Tea made from hops is good for calming nervous tension. The bitter flavor of hops is thought to help strengthen and stimulate digestion, and may ease muscles spasms in the digestive tract associated with irritable bowel syndrome.

The female flower clusters on a hops vine—called strobiles—are the source of hops' healing properties.

TIME LINE OF USAGE AND SPREAD

1067
The oldest surviving written record of the use of hops in brewing dates from this year.

1428
Hops are planted in English soil.

1516
Wilhelm IV decrees all German beer must have malt, hops, and water.

1629
The Massachusetts Bay Company orders hop seeds shipped from England.

The fruiting bodies of common hops, known as strobiles, are famous for the bitter flavor they impart to beer. There are only three species in the small genus *Humulus,* all native to the Northern Hemisphere. Along with *Humulus lupulus,* there is an Asian species, *Humulus japonicus,* that is sometimes grown as an ornamental and is naturalized in some parts of North America. A third species was discovered recently in central China, deemed *Humulus yunnanensis.*

Common hops is a climbing perennial **herbaceous** vine. The leaves are stalked, opposite, and heart shaped at the base, with 3 to 7 lobes, typically with 3 major lobes. Ovate and circular, the leaves are about as wide as long, ranging 2 to 4 inches broad and long. Male and female flowers grow on the same plant on separate branches. When female flowers mature into fruiting heads (hops), they are harvested and used for brewing beer and in herbal medicine.

Growing Habits

Humulus lupulus and its varieties are found throughout the temperate Northern Hemisphere. Early European settlers to the American continent brought hops for planting, and this plant material (*H. lupulus* var. *lupulus*) has naturalized in the Northeast and adjacent Canada, along roadsides, in waste places, and in moist thickets. This **variety** is also widely cultivated as a flavoring for alcoholic beverages. However, once Europeans arrived, they found hops already growing in America. Three native varieties include *H. lupulus* var. *neomexicanus,* most of the wild hops found in the western prairies, south to Arizona and north to Saskatchewan; *H. lupulus* var. *pubescens,* which grows in woods and wet thickets of the Midwest; and *H. lupulus* var. *lupuloides,* the main native strain in thickets and riverbanks of the Northeast.

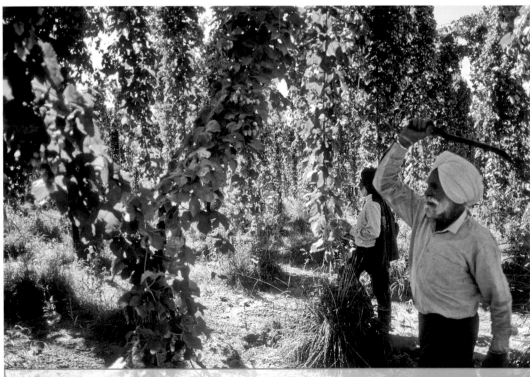

Prior to harvesting of hops vines, workers in British Columbia sever the strings holding vines to their supports.

COMMON NAME:	SCIENTIFIC NAME:	FAMILY:	PARTS USED:	NATIVE RANGE:
Hops	*Humulus lupulus*	Cannabaceae	Female flowers (strobiles)	Northern Hemisphere

While brewing a cup of skullcap bedtime tea (see page 47), assemble a hops pillow to ensure a good night's sleep. Pour 1 cup of fresh dried hops into a cotton or satin drawstring sachet bag (available at most craft stores). Cinch the drawstring and tie tightly. At bedtime, tuck beneath the pillowcase and snuggle in for a restful night.

Cultivation and Harvesting

Hops are a hardy perennial, propagated by seeds, or more frequently by dividing the rooting suckers. Hops likes a rich, well-drained garden soil with high humus to encourage vigorous growth. The **genus** name *Humulus* comes from the Latin *humus* meaning "soil," referring to the fact that if the plant is not supported on trellises it sprawls over the ground. Typically, hops are supported with strings, fencing, or other structures to allow them to climb for easier harvest of the female fruits. Hops are widely grown in northern Europe and the United States. Large-scale commercial cultivation occurs in the Pacific Northwest and in adjacent British Columbia.

Therapeutic Uses

+ *Digestion*
+ *Nervousness*
+ *Insomnia*
+ *Menopause*

Though most famous as an ingredient vital to brewing beer, hops has been used to improve appetite and digestion, relieve toothache and nerve pain, and treat insomnia around the world. It is said that Abraham Lincoln relied upon hops pillows to relax and improve sleep.

Today, Germany's health authorities continue to approve the use of hops for "discomfort due to restlessness or anxiety and sleep disturbances." Most of the scientific research evaluating the effectiveness of hops for anxiety and sleep has been conducted on a combination of hops and valerian, another popular sedative herb. Three controlled studies have shown that this combination is more effective than **placebo** and similar in effectiveness to **benzodiazepines** (sleep medication) for shortening the time it takes to fall asleep and for improving sleep quality. None of the studies reported any rebound insomnia when the participants stopped taking the herbs, nor excessive morning sleepiness.

One area that is garnering attention is the potential use of hops for the relief of menopausal symptoms. Researchers have identified at least one key **compound** in hops, 8-prenylnaringenin, linked to significant hormonal activity. A six-week study in menopausal women found that a standardized hops **extract** decreased the number of hot flashes, night sweats, and insomnia. Another study found that a topically applied gel containing hyaluronic acid, vitamin E, and hops extract significantly improved vaginal dryness in postmenopausal women. Hops might prove to be an attractive option to conventional hormone therapy, but more research is needed to determine long-term safety.

How to Use

TEA: Steep 1 teaspoon hops strobiles (female flowers) in 1 cup water for 5 to 7 minutes. Add honey to taste. Drink 30 minutes before bed.
CAPSULES: 500 mg, 1 to 3 times daily; often taken in combination with valerian root.
TINCTURE: 2 ml **tincture**, 1 to 3 times daily.

Precautions

Given the potential for increased hormonal activity stimulated by hops, women who had breast cancer or who are at risk for it should avoid hops until more is known. Safety in pregnancy is not known. Hops may have sedative effects, so driving or operating heavy machinery should not be attempted while using hops.

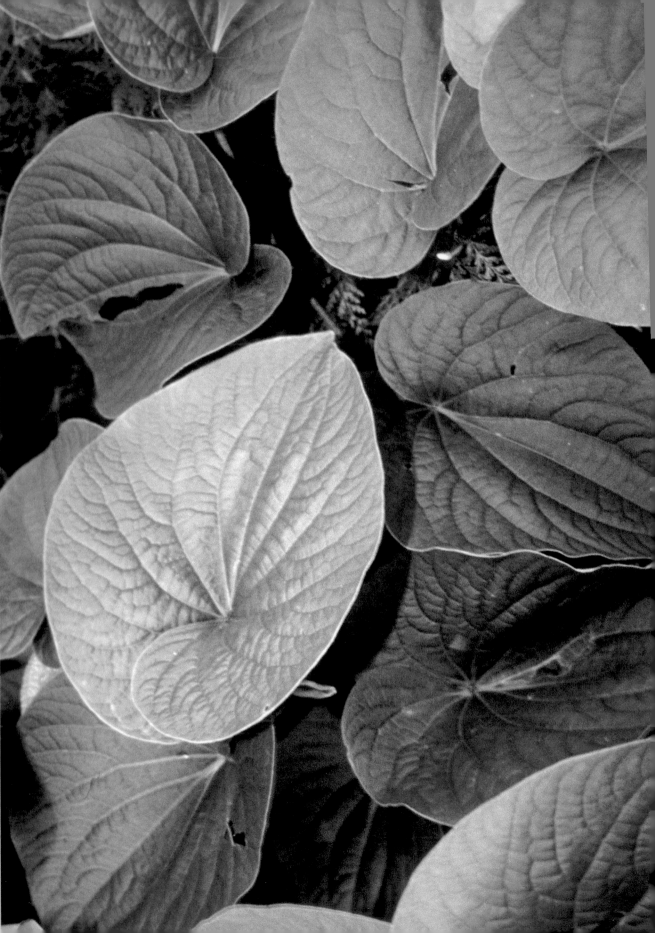

MENTAL HEALTH & THE NERVOUS SYSTEM

Kava

❧ Piper methysticum ❧

During his second voyage across the Pacific Ocean in the 1770s, Capt. James Cook encountered the inhabitants of several Pacific islands drinking a thick, bitter brew made from the pounded rhizome of a robust tropical plant. The native islanders called it kava, a word that may be derived from the Hawaiian name for the plant, *'awa*, which means "bitter." Kava's preparation was unique. The rhizomes were chewed by a child or young woman, spat out into a container, and then mixed with water or coconut milk until the proper consistency was achieved.

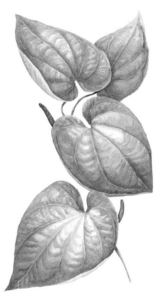

A few sips of kava left a person's mouth slightly numb and entire body infused with a feeling of calm contentment. Drunk in large quantities, it produced a state of euphoria. Kava is believed to have originated in Melanesia, and spread from there to other Pacific islands. It was originally a drink reserved for royalty or served to honored guests, as it was to Cook and members of his crew. Kava also had great religious significance. By drinking it, the islanders believed they could gain access to the spirit realm of both ancestors and gods. The ritual use of kava continues on a number of Pacific islands today.

On almost every island where kava grew, islanders also employed it medicinally. Its primary use was in relieving nervous tension and elevating mood. Taken in larger quantities, kava induces sleep and so was taken as a cure for insomnia. People also drank kava as a health-promoting tonic and to combat fatigue, alleviate weakness, and treat chills and colds. Islanders chewed the **rhizomes** to relieve headache pain.

Captain Cook went on to introduce kava to Europe. However, it wasn't until the 1990s that the herb became popular in the West. Today it is used in herbal medicine as an alternative to prescription medications in treating symptoms associated with anxiety, nervous tension, and depression without disrupting mental clarity. It may help reduce symptoms of anxiety associated with menopause and premenstrual syndrome. Herbal practitioners also recommend kava for insomnia and certain types of sleep disorders.

Kava's heart-shaped leaves grow from gnarled, aromatic roots used medicinally and ceremonially for centuries.

TIME LINE OF USAGE AND SPREAD

1777
A naturalist on Cook's second Pacific voyage describes kava preparation in detail.

1992
Hillary Clinton participates in kava ceremony conducted by Samoans in Hawaii.

2002
European, British, and Canadian authorities ban kava sales.

2008
The ban on kava in European countries is lifted.

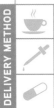

The genus *Piper* includes more than a thousand species of tropical herbs, shrubs, lianas, and small trees, the most familiar of which is *Piper nigrum*—source of the black pepper of commerce. *Piper* is the classical Latin name for pepper. Kava (*P. methysticum*) is a shrub found on a number of islands in the South Pacific, where the root is used ceremonially to prepare a somewhat intoxicating and medicinal beverage.

Kava is typically harvested when it is 6 to 8 feet in height, but left to grow, it can reach up to 20 feet. It is a much branched robust plant, the stems somewhat succulent, hairless, and with distinct swollen nodes. The alternate leaves range from broadly heart shaped to nearly circular in outline, with prominent veins beneath. The deep green leaves are mostly smooth above, with lighter coloration and fine hairs beneath. They are typically 4 to 10 inches wide and 4 to 8 inches long. The leaf stalk is up to 2 inches long, and is winged for about half its length. The flowers are often terminal, either solitary or in small groups. It is not known to produce viable seed. The most important part of the plant is the strongly aromatic root, which has many rootlets.

Growing Habits

Botanists deem kava a cultigen, a plant that has evolved over a long period of time under cultivation by humans. One theory is that it originally derived from *Piper wichmannii* native to the island of Vanuatu, which is where the greatest diversity of kava varieties is currently found. Kava has been cultivated by Pacific islanders for at least 3,000 years. Many local varieties are found throughout tropical Pacific islands.

Cultivation and Harvesting

Kava cannot be grown in temperate climates except in a greenhouse. On Pacific islands it is grown in traditional multicrop agricultural systems, usually partially shaded beneath taller plants such as bananas. The plant requires adequate shade, wind protection, and fairly high temperatures and high humidity. It likes a deep, friable soil that is rich in humus, and well drained. Free movement of air and moisture is essential. Kava is propagated by stem cuttings. The root, weighing 10 to 100 pounds fresh, is harvested after three or four years' growth.

Therapeutic Uses

+ *Anxiety*
+ *Menopause*

Kava, native to the South Pacific islands, has been used medicinally and ceremonially for centuries. In 1877, the Parke-Davis pharmaceutical company introduced kava to the Western world. Today, it is predominantly used to relieve tension and anxiety. Anxiety affects approximately 40 million Americans in a given year and can be very disruptive to an individual's life. There are many strategies for relieving anxiety, such as meditation and breathing exercises, as well as medications such as **benzodiazepines**. Kava has been subjected to rigorous human clinical trials and shown to be as powerful as prescription antianxiety drugs. There have been at least 11 published studies confirming its effectiveness. Two smaller studies showed that kava reduced anxiety and irritability, while improving sleep in women going through menopause.

over the (kitchen) counter KAVA COCO SHAKE

In a small bowl, pour 1 cup hot lowfat milk or soy milk over 1 teaspoon dried kava root. Let steep for at least 10 minutes. Strain the liquid through some cheesecloth or a piece of muslin into a blender. Add 1 teaspoon lowfat coconut milk, 4 teaspoons chocolate syrup, and 1 cup ice. Blend on high for 30 to 60 seconds. Pour into a glass and enjoy a stress-relieving chocolate shake!

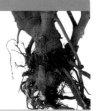

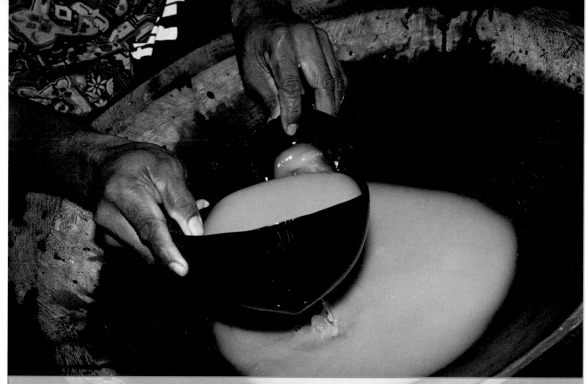

In kava-consuming countries, the fresh beverage is traditionally served in drinking vessels made from coconut shells.

COMMON NAME:	SCIENTIFIC NAME:	FAMILY:	PARTS USED:	NATIVE RANGE:
Kava	*Piper methysticum*	Piperaceae	Rhizomes, Roots	South Pacific islands

While there is little question about kava's effectiveness, there are questions regarding its safety. Kava was banned in the United Kingdom and in several European countries after concerns that it might cause liver damage. In a number of cases people taking kava **extracts** had laboratory abnormalities in liver function tests and some went into liver failure. While the numbers were very small given the widespread use of kava in both Europe and the United States, a number of regulatory agencies decided that any risk was too much. Kava is still available for sale in the United States, though the Food and Drug Administration has asked doctors to report possible cases immediately.

Traditionally, kava was made into tea by adding water to the roots. Almost all cases of liver damage reported were from kava products extracted with alcohol and/or acetone. Some scientists believe that these solvents allowed toxic **compounds** into the final product. Further, manufacturers may inadvertently have used leaves and stems—known to contain potentially toxic compounds—instead of or in addition to the root, as they are cheaper to use.

How to Use

Purchase kava from a reputable manufacturer and use only dried powdered root (not an extraction), or until the evidence is clearer, look for products sold as "aqueous" extracts (meaning water, instead of acetone or alcohol, was used as a solvent). The better companies often include a statement that they do not use any stem or leaf in their kava products.

TEA: Simmer 1 to 2 teaspoons root in 1 cup water for 10 minutes. Strain. Drink 1 cup daily.

EXTRACT: The dose used in clinical trials is 100 to 200 mg of root extract taken 3 times per day.

 NOTE: Consult a health care professional before using kava if you have liver problems, use alcohol, or take **acetaminophen** or prescription medications.

Precautions

See a doctor if symptoms develop that may signal liver problems, such as fatigue, abdominal pain, vomiting, dark urine, pale stools, or yellow eyes or skin. Use during pregnancy or lactation or by those under 18 is not recommended.

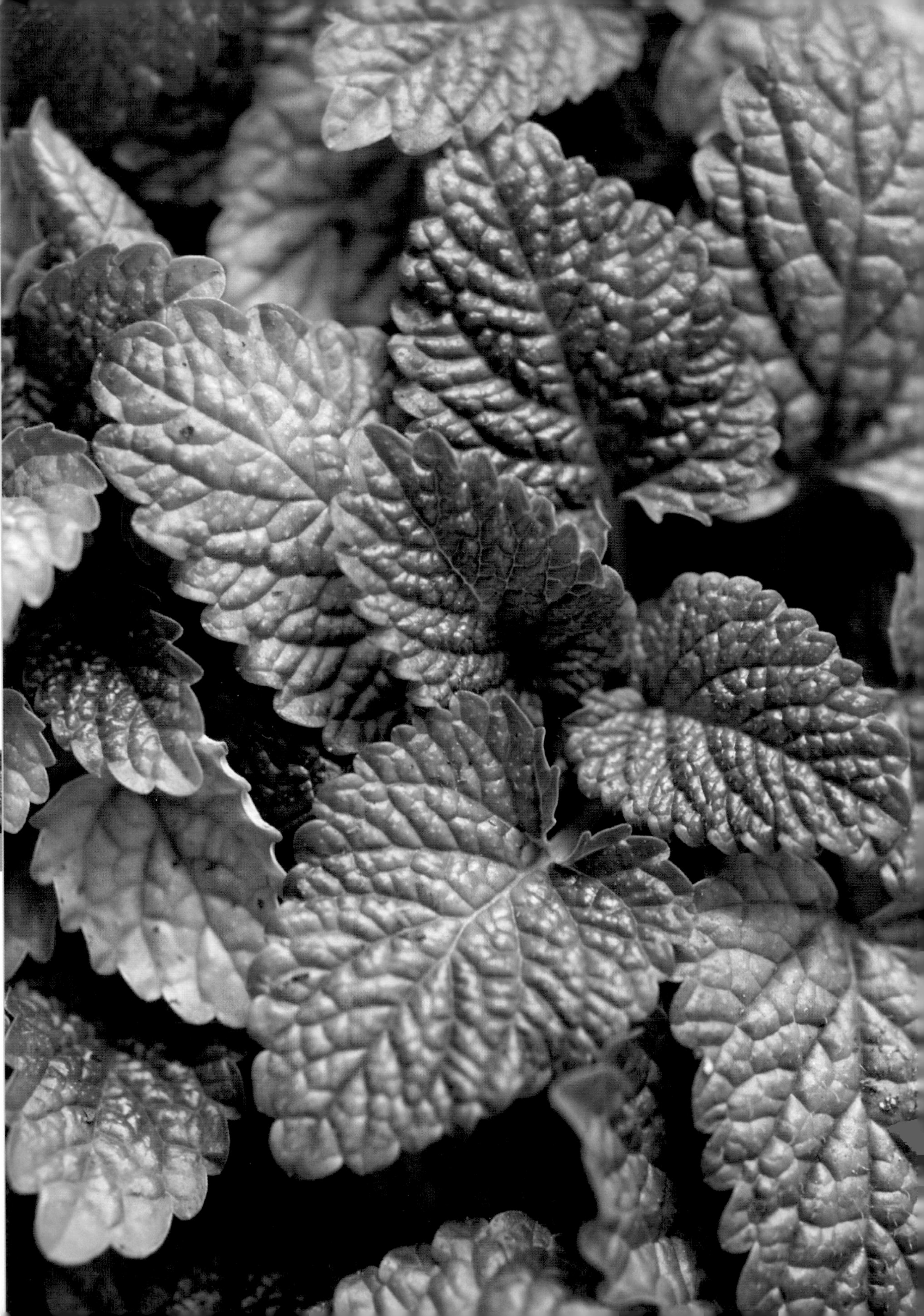

Lemon Balm

~ Melissa officinalis ~

Brushing the leaves of lemon balm fills the air with a minty, lemony scent. The fragrance is almost irresistible, especially to bees. That fact is reflected in the herb's genus name, *Melissa*, which comes from the Greek word for honeybee. Lemon balm has been cultivated as a bee plant for over 2,000 years. According to Dioscorides and Pliny the Elder, both renowned physicians in their day, the Greeks and Romans valued lemon balm as a flavoring for food as well as a medicinal plant. They drank wine infused with lemon balm for fevers and used the

crushed leaves to treat wounds and bites. The Greeks may have introduced the Arabs to lemon balm, who praised it as a remedy for heart conditions and depression and for strengthening the memory and the mind.

In the ninth century, the emperor Charlemagne was so impressed by the herb's healing properties that he ordered it planted in all monastery apothecary gardens. During the Middle Ages and Renaissance, lemon balm was used for treating wounds and digestive upsets and easing anxiety and sleeplessness. A number of religious orders used lemon balm in special aromatic waters. The most famous, Eau de Melisse de Carmes, or Carmelite water, was first produced by French Carmelite nuns in the early 17th century. A mixture of lemon balm, angelica,

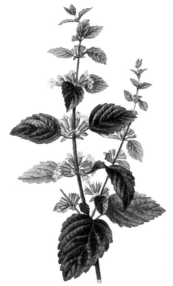

and various spices—infused in alcohol—was valued as a headache cure. European colonists brought lemon balm to the United States, but its use as a medicinal herb faded during the 19th century. However, it still is very popular in Europe.

In modern herbal medicine, lemon balm is combined with other calming herbs, such as valerian and hops, to reduce anxiety and promote sleep. Recent studies indicate that it may also improve secondary memory and the ability to learn, store, and retrieve information. Hence, herbal practitioners recommend lemon balm for Alzheimer's disease, dementia, and attention deficit/hyperactivity disorder (ADHD). Lemon balm is also used for digestive problems and hyperthyroidism, and externally as a treatment for cold sores.

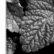

Lemon balm's leaves harbor profusions of tiny glands that, when touched, release a minty—and calming—fragrance.

TIME LINE OF USAGE AND SPREAD

1440
Lemon balm first mentioned in medieval manuscript as "Herbe Melisse."

1611
French Carmelite nuns create Carmelite water, which was sold up to 1840.

1696
The London Dispensary says lemon balm will "strengthen the brain."

2007
Lemon balm is chosen as International Herb Association herb of the year.

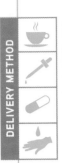

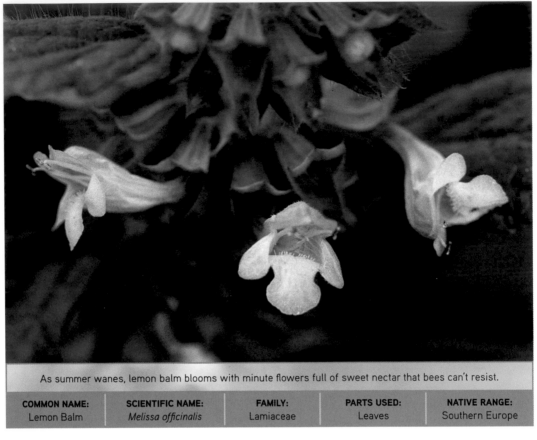

As summer wanes, lemon balm blooms with minute flowers full of sweet nectar that bees can't resist.

COMMON NAME:	SCIENTIFIC NAME:	FAMILY:	PARTS USED:	NATIVE RANGE:
Lemon Balm	*Melissa officinalis*	Lamiaceae	Leaves	Southern Europe

There are 3 or 4 species in the genus *Melissa* native to the Mediterranean region and Asia. Lemon balm is an erect herbaceous perennial that grows from 1 to 3 feet in height. The stems are either sparsely hairy or generally covered with small hairs. The opposite, toothed, broadly oval to diamond-shaped leaves are wrinkled and scalloped along the edges. When crushed, the fresh leaves have a distinctive, oily lemon scent, though it loses much of its fragrance upon drying. Depending upon the growing conditions, the leaves may be up to 4 inches broad, and 1 to 3 inches long. The flowers—barely ¼ inch long—are in whorls around the top of the stem, with 4 to 12 flowers in each whorl. The pale yellowish, pink, or white flowers appear in late summer.

Growing Habits

Historically, fresh crushed lemon balm leaves were rubbed in an empty bee skep to attract a swarm of bees to the hive. Worker honeybees have a **pheromone**-releasing gland at the tip of the abdomen called the Nasonov gland, which releases a scent used to mark good sources of food. Lemon balm contains some of the same chemical constituents as those released by the honeybee's scent-producing Nasonov gland.

Originating from southern Europe, lemon balm is now found throughout much of the European continent as far north as England, Sweden, and east to central Russia. It is widely naturalized in North America, found in most eastern states and Canadian provinces. In California, it is commonly naturalized in coastal redwood forests, where in search of sunlight the plant stretches and becomes leggy with large leaves, giving it a different appearance than if grown in the sun. However, simply stroking the lemon-scented leaves makes it easy to identify.

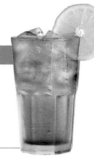

Pour 4 cups boiling water over an herb combination of 1 teaspoon dried lemon balm leaves, 1 teaspoon dried peppermint, and 1 teaspoon chamomile flowers. Mix in large pitcher or bowl. Let steep for 10 minutes. Strain. Pour into clean pitcher. Add 1 tablespoon honey and 1 to 2 cups ice cubes. Drink on a hot day!

Cultivation and Harvesting

Lemon balm is an easy-to-grow perennial. Fragrant and flavorful when fresh, it is a good plant to have in the herb garden or on a porch, where leaves can be plucked to make a pleasant hot or iced tea. It is propagated by seeds, stem cuttings, or divided clumps. Once established, it self-sows freely. Seedlings can be replanted or potted as gifts for family and friends. It prefers a relatively rich, moist, well-drained garden soil, though it is adaptable. In full sun it has a compact, bushy growth; in partial shade it becomes more sprawling.

The leaves can be harvested throughout the growing season; or, just before flowering, cut the plant 6 inches aboveground, then tie in a bundle and dry. It dries quickly and easily. Most commercial production is on a relatively small scale for local consumption. It is grown in Eastern Europe for export.

Therapeutic Uses

+ *Anxiety and stress*
+ *Colic*
+ *Digestion*
+ *Fever blisters*

Once referred to as the gladdening herb, this gentle member of the mint **family** has been used to relieve stress and anxiety for millennia. European and German authorities approve the use of lemon balm for tension, anxiety, and poor sleep. Studies in children and adults confirm that the combination of lemon balm and valerian, also prized as a calming agent, reduces restlessness and improves sleep. A study in people with Alzheimer's disease found that lemon balm **extract** decreased agitation and improved cognition when taken internally. Even the topical application of lemon balm **essential oil** produced a calm affect in elders with dementia.

Lemon balm is also a digestive aid suitable for all ages. Lemon balm gently relaxes the muscles of the gastrointestinal tract. The European and German health authorities approve lemon balm for minor gastrointestinal spasms and for easing bloating and gas. A study of 93 breast-fed babies with colic found a combination of lemon balm, fennel, and chamomile decreased crying time by more than double compared with the babies receiving a **placebo** over a period of one week! Studies in adults of lemon balm in combination with other herbs have shown that it eases indigestion.

Another area of exciting research is the use of lemon balm extract for the treatment of oral herpes, or fever blisters. Scientists have identified several **compounds** in the herb that block the herpes simplex virus. Two clinical trials in volunteers found that lemon balm extract shortens duration and severity of a herpes outbreak when applied topically 3 to 4 times daily.

 NOTE: Do not give honey to children less than 18 months of age and substitute chamomile or spearmint for peppermint in children under three.

How to Use

TEA: Pour 1 cup boiling water over 5 to 6 fresh leaves or 1 teaspoon dried leaf and steep for 5 to 7 minutes. Strain. Add honey or stevia if desired. Delicious with mint. Drink several times a day.

TINCTURES AND EXTRACTS: Widely available. Use as directed.

LIP OINTMENT: Lemon balm ointments can be found at many health food stores and pharmacies. Apply as directed.

Precautions

Lemon balm is safe and tolerated by all ages.

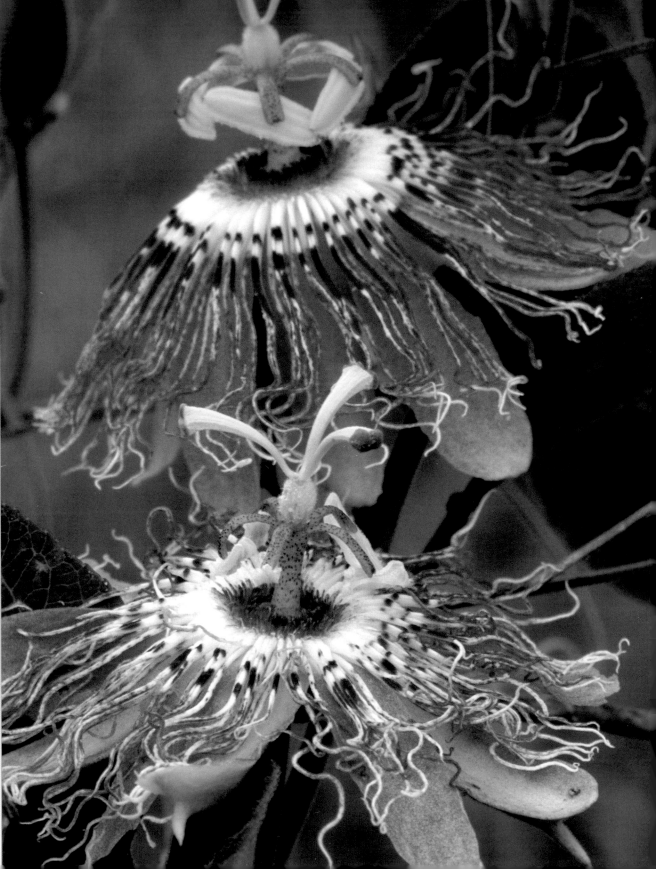

Passionflower

⟨⟨ Passiflora incarnata ⟩⟩

There is nothing understated about passionflower. This twining vine produces a large violet-and-white flower of astounding complexity that can be several inches across. The flowers are succeeded by yellow-orange egg-shaped fruits that are filled with small seeds embedded in an edible, sweet yellow pulp. In the early 1600s, Spanish Jesuit missionaries gave passionflower its name when they encountered one or more species in South America and claimed to see symbols of Christ's Crucifixion, or Passion, in the plants' showy blossoms.

Passiflora incarnata is the **species** native to the southern and eastern United States, where the fruits are called maypops. Archaeological evidence suggests that Native Americans ate passionflower fruits a thousand years before Europeans arrived. The Cherokee, Houma, and other tribes used preparations of passionflower roots to draw inflammation from wounds and help correct liver problems and as a tonic. Babies were given passionflower tea during weaning and ear drops made of a root **infusion**. Passionflower was also given as a sedative for nervous conditions. The Spanish conquistadores learned of passionflower's healing properties from the Aztec in Central America, who used parts of the vine to treat insomnia. The Spanish introduced passionflower to Europe. It found its way into conventional North

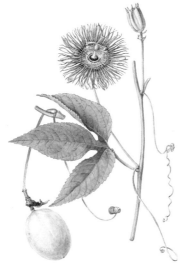

American medicine in the mid-1800s, and in the following decades was prescribed for anxiety and insomnia. It was an ingredient in many over-the-counter sleep aids and sedatives for much of the last century. But in 1978, the U.S. Food and Drug Administration withdrew approval for use of the herb in these products. Passionflower remained popular in Europe.

Modern herbal practitioners use passionflower as a sleep aid and gentle sedative to relieve nervous tension. Passionflower may exert these effects by stimulating a chemical that lowers activity in some brain cells, thereby promoting relaxation. In Europe, passionflower, combined with hawthorn and valerian, is used for digestive upsets and irritations and in a sedative tea for children.

All the aboveground parts of passionflower vine, including its extravagant blossoms, are used in herbal preparations.

TIME LINE OF USAGE AND SPREAD

1787	**1800s**	**1916–1936**	**1978**
Materia Medica Americana mentions passionflower as treatment for epilepsy.	Passionflower becomes fashionable conservatory plant in Victorian England.	Passionflower is listed in the *National Formulary* of the United States.	FDA withdraws support for passionflower in over-the-counter sedatives.

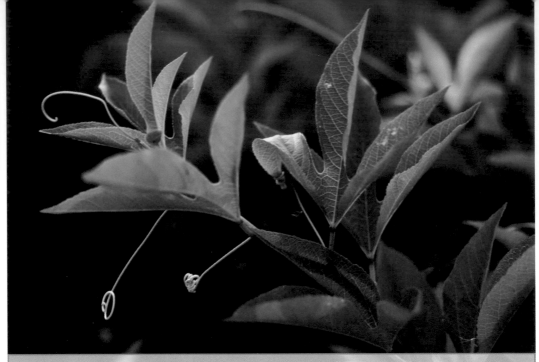

Passionflower vines are vigorous climbers that anchor themselves to supports with slender, twining tendrils.

COMMON NAME:	SCIENTIFIC NAME:	FAMILY:	PARTS USED:	NATIVE RANGE:
Passionflower	*Passiflora incarnata*	Passifloraceae	Flowers, Leaves, Stems	E., S. North America

Passionflower is one of only a handful of the more than 450 species of *Passiflora* that grow in temperate North America. The vast majority of passionflower plants are found in the American tropics. Some 20 species are native to tropical Asia. Passionflower is a perennial herbaceous vine with stems stretching to 30 feet or more once they become established. The dull green, deeply lobed leaves are 4 to 6 inches long, with serrated margins.

The fantastic floral assemblage—up to 3 inches across—is one of the most intricate of the plant world. Above the 10-part receptacle is a corona with white-purple threadlike filaments. Five stamens with hammerlike anthers surround a 3-part style, topped with reddish stigmas protruding from the flower's center. The edible fruits, the size and shape of a hen's egg, are filled with black seeds in sweet flesh. About 20 species of *Passiflora* are grown in the tropics for edible fruits, most notably *P. edulis*.

Growing Habits

This fast-growing vine is found in fields and along fences, ditches, and the edges of woods from Virginia to Florida, west to Texas, and north to Ohio. Outside of its native range in the Southeast, it can be grown as far north as Boston if given a protected southern exposure.

What natural or evolutionary event could create a flower of such unusual beauty? Early European explorers to the Americas described the flower in terms of religious symbolism. Passionflower's floral structure was seen to represent the Passion of the Christ—the period of suffering following the Last Supper and Crucifixion. The three styles atop the stigma represent the three nails by which Christ was attached to the cross. The five anthers atop the stamens exemplify hammers used to drive the nails. Beneath these parts is a fringe of colored filaments, known as the corona, seen as a halo or perhaps a crown of thorns. Beneath the corona sits the corolla with 10 petals, representing the 10 apostles at the Crucifixion—except for Peter and Judas. The common name and the scientific name, *Passiflora*, reflect the religious symbolism.

Combine 1 cup dried chamomile, ¼ cup lavender buds, ¼ cup dried passionflower, ¼ cup dried lemon verbena, ¼ cup rose hips. (Dried herbs are available in bulk.) Add 1 tablespoon of mix per cup of tea in teapot, plus 1 tablespoon for the pot. Pour boiling water in pot and steep for 5 minutes. Strain, sweeten, and enjoy!

Cultivation and Harvesting

Passionflower is most easily propagated by stem cuttings or layering (placing a 6-inch section of the growing stem beneath the soil so it will root). After about 6 weeks, the rooted stem can be cut from the mother plant and replanted. The plant likes full sun and well-drained soil. Once established, it is a vigorous grower. Leaves and stems are harvested in late summer and dried in the shade. Most passionflower herb is wild-harvested in the southeastern U.S., along with limited commercial production in Guatemala and Italy.

Therapeutic Uses

+ *Anxiety*
+ *Insomnia*

Passionflower is one of the calming herbs, providing a soothing effect on the nervous system. **Extracts** of its flowers, leaves, stems, and fruits are used to combat anxiety and sleep problems. The exact way passionflower exerts its psychological effects is unknown but may involve inhibiting **enzymes** in the brain with known psychological effects. Also, **compounds** in passionflower bind to the same areas of the brain affected by a calming **neurotransmitter** called GABA. These effects would explain why passionflower is able to tone down the nervous system, leading to relaxation and sleep.

In animal studies, preliminary research supports the assumption that passionflower extracts have antianxiety and sedative effects. But more definitive research is needed on humans. In one study, 32 people suffering with anxiety were given either 45 drops daily of a passionflower liquid extract plus a **placebo** tablet or placebo drops plus 30 mg daily of oxazepam, a medicine similar to diazepam (Valium). Over the course of a month, both groups had less anxiety, though similar rates of dizziness and drowsiness; the group taking passionflower seemed to have less impairment of job performance.

Passionflower contains various **flavonoids**, compounds that are well-known **antioxidants** and may also contribute to antianxiety effects; flavonoids may be more concentrated in the leaves than other plant parts. Passionflower also contains **alkaloid** compounds, bitter-tasting chemicals found in many plants that have a range of medicinal activities.

How to Use

INFUSION: Boil 1 to 2 teaspoons dried passionflower herb (excluding roots) in 2 cups of water for 5 to 10 minutes. Strain and take 3 times daily and before bed for its calming and antianxiety effects.

CAPSULES/TABLETS: 1 to 2 350-mg capsules, 1 to 2 times daily; often combined with other herbs.

TINCTURE: 1 to 2 ml, 1 to 3 times daily; often combined with hops or with lemon balm.

Precautions

Some people experience drowsiness and dizziness with use of passionflower. It may increase effects of other sedative herbs or medications. Alkaloids in passionflower may possibly stimulate the uterus, so it is generally not recommended during pregnancy. Passionflower also may increase the activity or otherwise interact with anticoagulant, or blood-thinning, medications.

Passiflora incarnata

41

PASSIONFLOWER

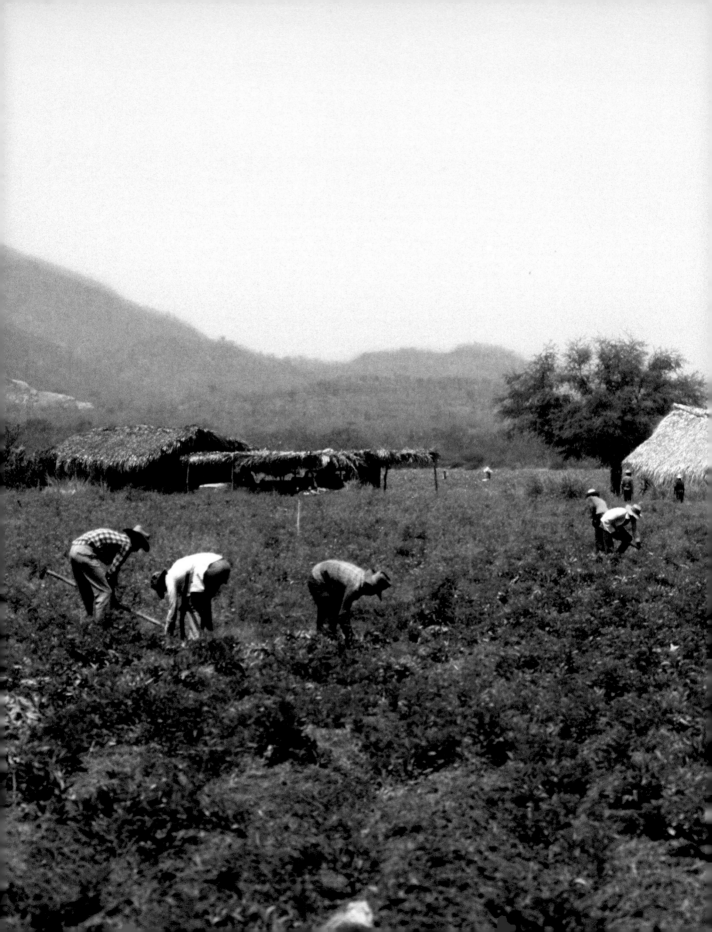

Passionflower Harvest

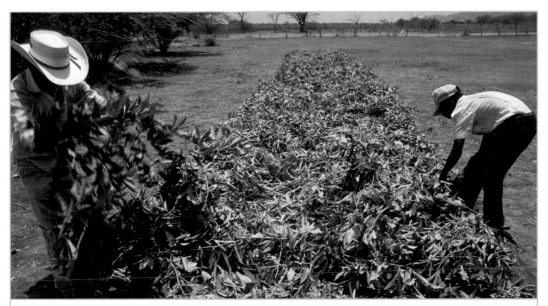

Under a china blue summer sky, workers cultivate a field of passionflower plants in Guatemala (opposite). Supports for the vines are unnecessary, as they sprawl across the soil as they grow. Harvesting of the aboveground parts begins when the plants are in full flower. A tangle of freshly cut passionflower vines (above) forms a fluffy green carpet across hard-packed ground as workers ready plants for loading onto trucks bound for industrial herb dryers. When the vines are sufficiently dry (below), they are baled and hand-stitched into white cotton bags. The bags are stored in dry, well-ventilated warehouses to be shipped to extraction and processing facilities in Europe.

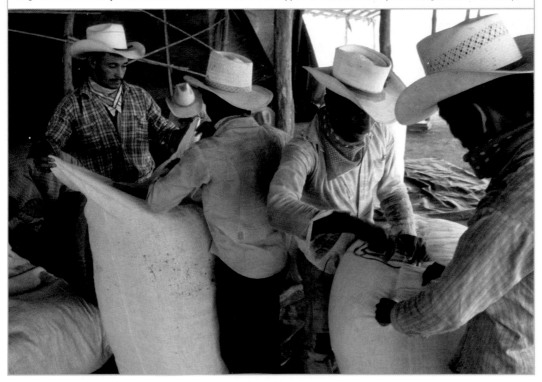

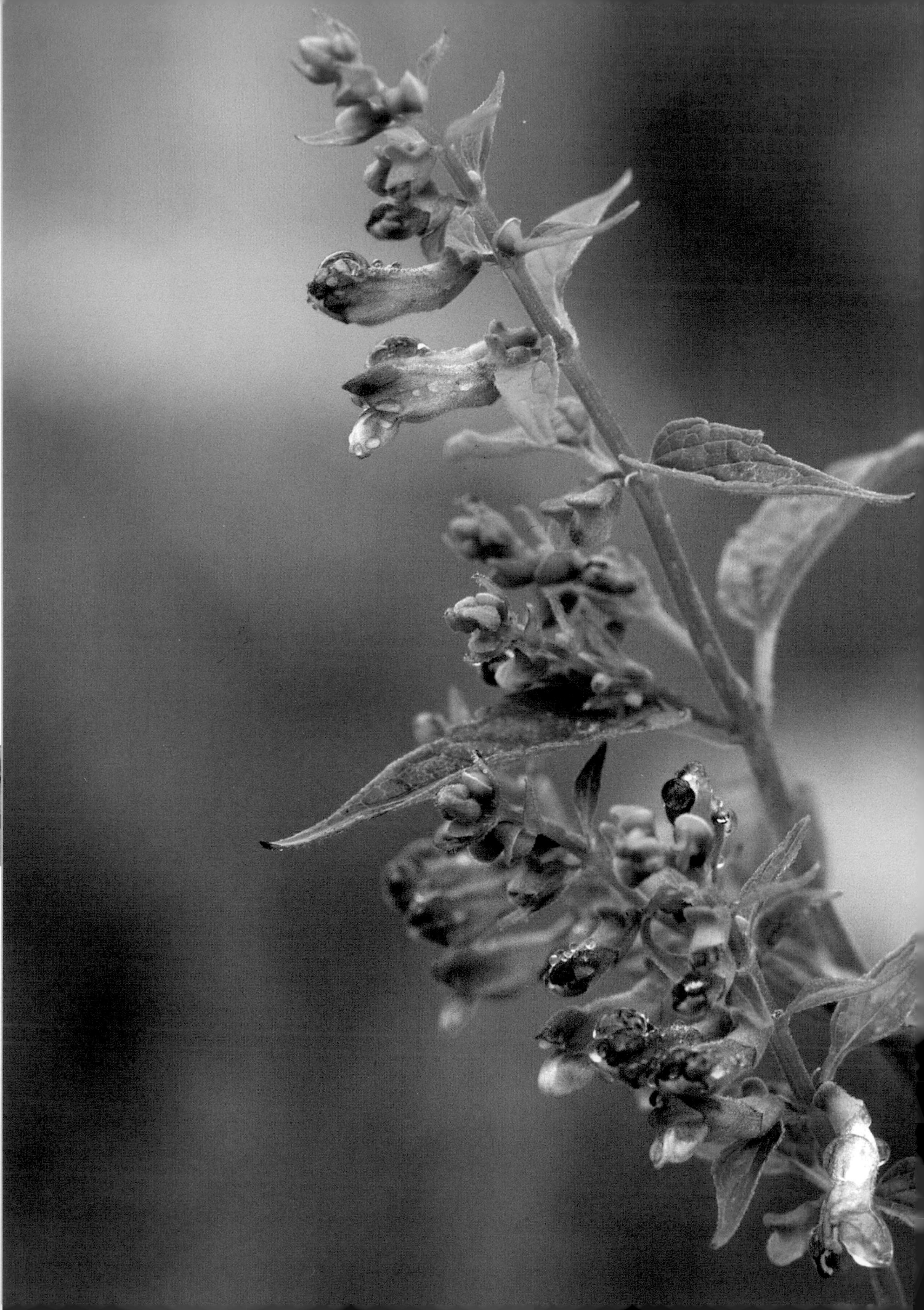

Skullcap

Scutellaria lateriflora

American skullcap (also scullcap) is a member of the mint family and native to eastern North America. The common and scientific names help paint a picture of skullcap's appearance. The common English name refers to the hooded, violet-pink-to-white blossoms that resemble the sort of close-fitting helmets that soldiers wore in medieval times. *Scutellaria* is derived from the Latin *scutella,* meaning "little dish." Sepals form this dish at the base of the flowers. *Lateriflora,* meaning "flowering on the side," reveals that skullcap's blooms grow along just one side of its short flower stalks.

The story of this unassuming plant's place in herbal medicine begins with the Native Americans. Several tribes steeped skullcap leaves to produce a tea drunk to promote menstruation. Preparations of the roots were a remedy for diarrhea, kidney problems, and breast pain and were used to expel afterbirth.

When American settlers adopted herbs from Native Americans, they typically used them for the same purposes. Not so with skullcap. In American folk medicine, skullcap was valued as a sedative and nerve tonic—a nervine, in the vernacular of the day. Steaming cups of skullcap tea were downed to cure fevers, calm nerves, and ease anxiety. In the 1770s, Lawrence Van Derveer of New Jersey began promoting

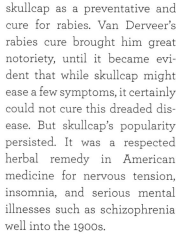

skullcap as a preventative and cure for rabies. Van Derveer's rabies cure brought him great notoriety, until it became evident that while skullcap might ease a few symptoms, it certainly could not cure this dreaded disease. But skullcap's popularity persisted. It was a respected herbal remedy in American medicine for nervous tension, insomnia, and serious mental illnesses such as schizophrenia well into the 1900s.

Modern herbalists and naturopaths suggest skullcap as a mild relaxant for treating nervous tension, anxiety, insomnia, and muscular tension. It is also used for tension headaches, fibromyalgia, and anorexia nervosa. Skullcap may also be used as a calming therapy for people withdrawing from excessive use of alcohol and certain prescription drugs.

Scutellaria lateriflora is a native North American herb valued for its ability to calm anxiety.

TIME LINE OF USAGE AND SPREAD

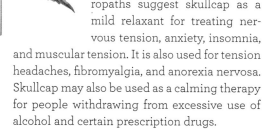

1773
Lawrence Van Derveer introduces skullcap as a cure for rabies.

1806
Lewis and Clark expedition collects first American samples of skullcap.

1863
Skullcap is added to the *United States Pharmacopeia* but removed in 1916.

1991
Two cases of liver damage reported in Norway by users of skullcap supplements.

More than 350 species of *Scutellaria* are found worldwide. Over 100 species occur in the Americas stretching from the Arctic Circle to the southern tip of South America. Most species are found in Europe and northern Asia. In North America, *S. lateriflora* is used in herbal medicine. The root of the Chinese skullcap *(S. baicalensis)* is the traditional medicine *huang-qi*. American skullcap is a wiry perennial 1 to 3 feet tall, with opposite, oval to lance-shaped toothed leaves. Chinese skullcap is a perennial growing 1 to 2 feet tall with opposite, lance-shaped to linear leaves, with black glandular dots beneath. The blue or violet attractive two-lipped flowers are in pairs on one side of the stem. The **species** name *baicalensis* signifies that botanists described it from plants collected in the vicinity of Lake Baikal in Siberia. Both species flower from July through August.

Growing Habits

S. lateriflora is found in rich woods and moist thickets in much of North America (absent from Colorado, Utah, Nevada, and Alberta), often occurring in small populations of just a few plants. *Scutellaria baicalensis* grows in northeastern China and adjacent Russia, and in mountains of southern China. It is found in dry, sandy soils, in fields and along roadsides.

The **genus** name *Scutellaria* refers to the helmetlike or skullcaplike form of a small hump atop the flowers. That characteristic also gives rise to its common name, skullcap.

Cultivation and Harvesting

North American skullcap is not commonly grown in herb gardens. It likes a relatively rich, moist but acidic soil and is propagated by seeds or cuttings. The leaves and stems, harvested

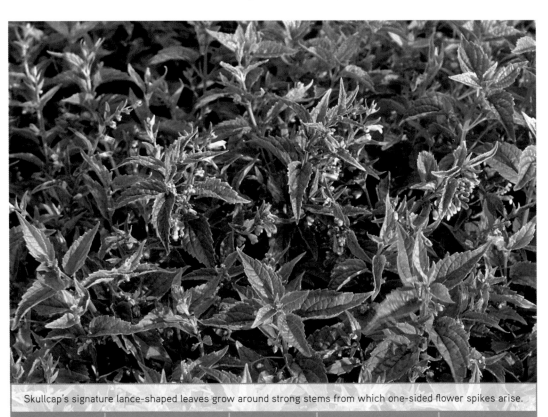

Skullcap's signature lance-shaped leaves grow around strong stems from which one-sided flower spikes arise.

COMMON NAME:	SCIENTIFIC NAME:	FAMILY:	PARTS USED:	NATIVE RANGE:
Skullcap	*Scutellaria lateriflora*	Lamiaceae	Aboveground parts	E. North America

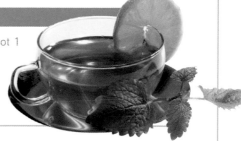

over the (kitchen) counter BEDTIME TEA

To make sleep-inducing, anxiety-reducing tea, combine in a teapot 1 tablespoon of dried lemon balm leaves, 1 teaspoon each of dried passionflower and dried skullcap leaves, and ½ teaspoon chopped valerian root. Fill the pot with 2 cups boiling water. Steep the mixture for 10 minutes and strain tea into a cup. Sweeten with honey or stevia leaf.

in flower, are the skullcap of commerce. Most of the commercial supply is wild-harvested, though there is limited cultivation in the Pacific Northwest.

Chinese skullcap is a drought-tolerant perennial that enjoys full sun in cooler climates and partial shade in warmer regions and likes a well-drained gravelly or sandy soil. It is propagated by seeds. It has showier flowers than *S. lateriflora* and is more suitable and desirable for the herb garden. In Western horticulture, it has been grown as a specimen plant among rock gardening enthusiasts.

Shanxi and Hebei provinces in China produce the bulk of the commercial supply of the root, the part that has been used in traditional Chinese medicine for more than 2,000 years. The root is harvested in spring after 3 or 4 years' growth, then dried until 50 percent dry. The bark is then scraped off, and the root fully dried.

Therapeutic Uses

+ *Anxiety*
+ *Insomnia*

Skullcap was traditionally used as a calming plant effective for headaches. Today, herbalists use its calming actions not only for soothing anxiety but also for sleep difficulties. **Compounds** in skullcap may bind to the receptor of a **neurotransmitter** in the brain responsible for modulating anxiety. This neurotransmitter, GABA, and its receptor, GABA-A, may be affected by **flavonoid** compounds in skullcap. This group of strong compounds, often **antioxidant** and **anti-inflammatory**, in this case also exhibit effects on the nervous system. Skullcap also contains the **amino acid** glutamine, which provides both sedative and anxiety-fighting effects.

Some animal research demonstrates decreased anxiety when **extracts** of skullcap are ingested, but few clinical research studies back up the traditional use of skullcap for any of its uses, including anxiety and insomnia. One small preliminary study lends credence to the traditional lore. Nineteen healthy volunteers were given either a **placebo** capsule or 100-, 200-, or 350-mg capsules of a freeze-dried extract of skullcap and asked to rate their anxiety an hour later. The volunteers taking the 2 higher doses of skullcap showed a reduction in anxiety levels. Further testing will be necessary before adequate conclusions can be drawn from this trial. Also, it is unknown if skullcap will be helpful for people with sleep problems if they take it every day for several months.

How to Use

CAPSULE: Generally, 850-mg capsules (containing leaves, stems, and fruits) twice a day, or 850- to 1,275-mg capsules (just leaves) 3 times daily, or follow manufacturer's directions.

TINCTURE: Some herbal experts recommend alcohol **tinctures** of the fresh plant to capture more of the healing compounds lost in drying the plant. Dosages range from 1 to 4 ml, taken 1 to 3 times throughout the day.

TEA: Steep 1 tablespoon of dried leaves (with or without stems, flowers, fruits) in a cup of hot water. Strain, cool, and drink 1 to 3 times a day.

Precautions

Though cases of severe liver toxicity have been reported, experts agree that they were caused by adulteration of skullcap products with a similar-appearing but dangerous plant, germander. Drowsiness may result from a sedative herb like skullcap; caution is advised for those taking pharmaceuticals for sleep or anxiety.

MENTAL HEALTH & THE NERVOUS SYSTEM

St. John's Wort

⤷ Hypericum perforatum ↩

The sunny yellow flowers of St. John's wort (SJW) harbor a strange secret. Bruise the delicate petals and they seem to bleed. The blood-red liquid is an oil released from tiny, dark-colored glands scattered along the petal margins. In ancient times, a plant that "bled" was assumed to possess great powers. During the rise of Christianity, the herb came to be associated with John the Baptist (*wort* is the Old English word for plant). It was said to bloom on the saint's birthday, June 24, and to bleed on August 29, the anniversary of his beheading. The earliest use of the name may date to the sixth century, when the Irish missionary St. Columba carried the herb with him into northern Scotland. The **genus** name, *Hypericum*, is from the Greek, meaning "over a picture or icon"—a reference to the custom of draping the herb over religious images to strengthen their powers in banishing demons. For many centuries, St. John's wort was a symbol of protection against evil, but also a prized medicinal herb, with the power to heal the body and ease the troubled mind.

Ancient Greek and Roman physicians used St. John's wort to dress battle wounds, as well as treat burns, bruises, and inflammations. Hundreds of years later, as battles raged in the Holy Land, the crusaders treated their wounds with St. John's wort in much the same way. Throughout the Middle Ages, heart conditions, jaundice, dysentery,

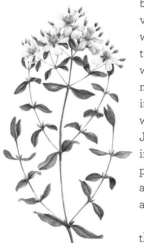

bleeding, urinary troubles, and nervous depression were all treated with the herb. Also popular at this time, and for centuries afterward, was hypericum oil, a preparation made from the flowers and rubbed into the skin to heal bruises and wounds. By the late 17th century, St. John's wort had been incorporated into American herbal medicine, prescribed externally for wounds and sores and internally for nervous anxiety and depression.

After falling into disuse early in the last century, St. John's wort has seen a remarkable revival in the past few decades. It is currently the most widely used herb in modern herbal medicine for treating mild to moderate depression. St. John's wort is also used to relieve anxiety, nervous exhaustion, seasonal affective disorder, premenstrual syndrome, and to help heal minor wounds and skin irritations.

The brilliant blooms of St. John's wort are the source of its gentle and well-documented antidepressant effects.

TIME LINE OF USAGE AND SPREAD

1650	**1696**	**1793**	**CA 1900**
English herbalist Nicholas Culpeper describes SJW as a "singular wound herb."	SJW is brought to Philadelphia by Rosicrucian pilgrims.	First recorded specimen of SJW is collected in Pennsylvania.	Hypericum oil, or red oil, available at pharmacies, though popularity has waned.

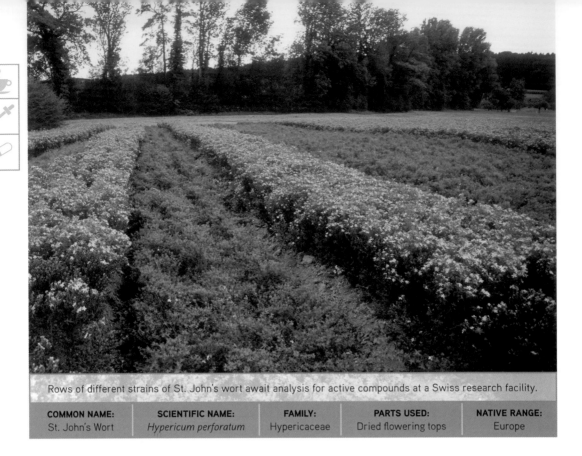

Rows of different strains of St. John's wort await analysis for active compounds at a Swiss research facility.

COMMON NAME:	SCIENTIFIC NAME:	FAMILY:	PARTS USED:	NATIVE RANGE:
St. John's Wort	*Hypericum perforatum*	Hypericaceae	Dried flowering tops	Europe

Among the 370 temperate and tropical species in the genus *Hypericum*, which includes trees, shrubs, and herbaceous plants, *Hypericum perforatum* is best known. An erect perennial growing up to 2 feet in height, it has smooth stems that typically display ridges, dotted with tiny black spots. The opposite inch-long leaves, oblong to linear, tightly hug the stems. They have netted veins and are without teeth or have wavy teeth. Holding the leaves up to the light reveals translucent dots; the leaves appear perforated, hence the **species** name *perforatum*. The showy yellow, 5-petaled flowers, about an inch across, bloom in flat-topped clusters from early June to mid-August. The petal edges are dotted with dark glands containing a red pigment, hypericin, an active constituent and a **compound** associated with photodermatitis in farm animals. When animals eat the flowers, hypericin reacts with light and oxygen to cause skin welts and lesions, a condition generally not associated with human use of plant products.

Growing Habits

To wildflower enthusiasts St. John's wort is a glorious wildflower dappling roadsides and old farm sites. To traditional herbalists it is a valued herb garden plant with many uses. To the modern practitioner it is a natural choice for treating depressive moods. To the rancher, however, it has long been a noxious weed.

Native to Europe, it migrated with settlers to temperate climates worldwide, becoming widespread in Asia, eastern and western North America, Argentina, North and South Africa, and Australia. First reported in North America in 1793, it quickly escaped from gardens to become naturalized. By the 1940s the wildflower transformed into a weed, choking out native vegetation. In the early 1960s a natural enemy, the Chrysolina beetle, imported from Europe successfully reduced the plant in western North America by 98 percent.

Little did ranchers know that 30 years later, St. John's wort would become a best-selling herbal product. Supply and demand created volatile prices rising to more than $20 per pound in the 1990s, then plunging to pennies per pound by 2003. Today, limited commercial supplies come from regions with cheap farm labor such as Eastern Europe or China.

Cultivation and Harvesting

An attractive perennial for the herb garden, St. John's wort thrives in well-drained soils; it is propagated from seed or by dividing root clumps. St. John's wort likes full sun. The flowers, leaves, and stems are harvested in full bloom in mid- to late July. The herb is dried under shade or by forced heat in dryers. Commercial standardized **extracts** are made from the fresh or dried tops, calibrated to a defined chemical profile, depending upon manufacturer's specifications to ensure consistency.

Therapeutic Uses

+ *Minor depression*
+ *Muscle aches*
+ *Fever blisters*

Modern science is confirming what the ancients knew. In 2009, researchers evaluated 29 clinical trials conducted on St. John's wort for mild to moderate depression and concluded that it is more effective than a **placebo** and as effective as standard prescription antidepressants with fewer adverse effects. St. John's wort has gained global recognition as an effective treatment for minor depression, with 2007 worldwide sales exceeding $100 million.

Antidepressant medications are also used to treat severe forms of premenstrual syndrome. A pilot trial using St. John's wort for PMS at University of Exeter in England reported a majority of women experienced a 50 percent reduction in symptoms, including anxiety and depression.

St. John's wort oil is highly regarded as a topical agent. When the flowering tops are infused in oil—olive oil is best—the oil turns ruby red after sitting in the sun for several weeks. It is massaged into the skin to relieve pain or made into an ointment for wounds, burns, and insect bites. Basic science and animal studies have confirmed that the oil eases inflammation of the skin and fights bacteria.

St. John's wort is being investigated for use in viral infections. Hypericin, one of its active constituents, has been shown to be highly active against the human immunodeficiency virus (HIV) and herpes simplex 1—the virus known to cause cold sores and fever blisters.

How to Use

TEA: Pour 1 cup boiling water over 1 teaspoon herb. Steep 5 to 10 minutes. Strain. Drink 1 to 3 times per day.

TINCTURE: Use 2 to 3 droppersful in 1 cup of hot water or lemon balm tea.

CAPSULES/TABLETS: Most research has been done on products guaranteed to contain specific levels of key ingredients. To find a supplement, look for one standardized to 0.3 percent hypericin or 3 to 5 percent hyperforin. The dose for these products is 900 to 1,500 mg per day.

NOTE: Individuals taking medication vital to their health should not use St. John's wort before consulting a doctor because of potential herb-drug interactions.

Precautions

St. John's wort appears to be safe. The main risk is the potential for interaction with prescription medications. Safety in pregnancy has not been established.

over the (kitchen) counter ST. JOHN'S WORT OIL

Gather the flowers of St. John's wort just as the plant is coming into bloom. Put them in a glass jar and completely cover the flowers with olive oil. Place in the sun for 2 to 3 weeks. Strain the oil and store in a dark, closed glass container for up to 1 year. You can use the oil to massage aching joints or for back pain.

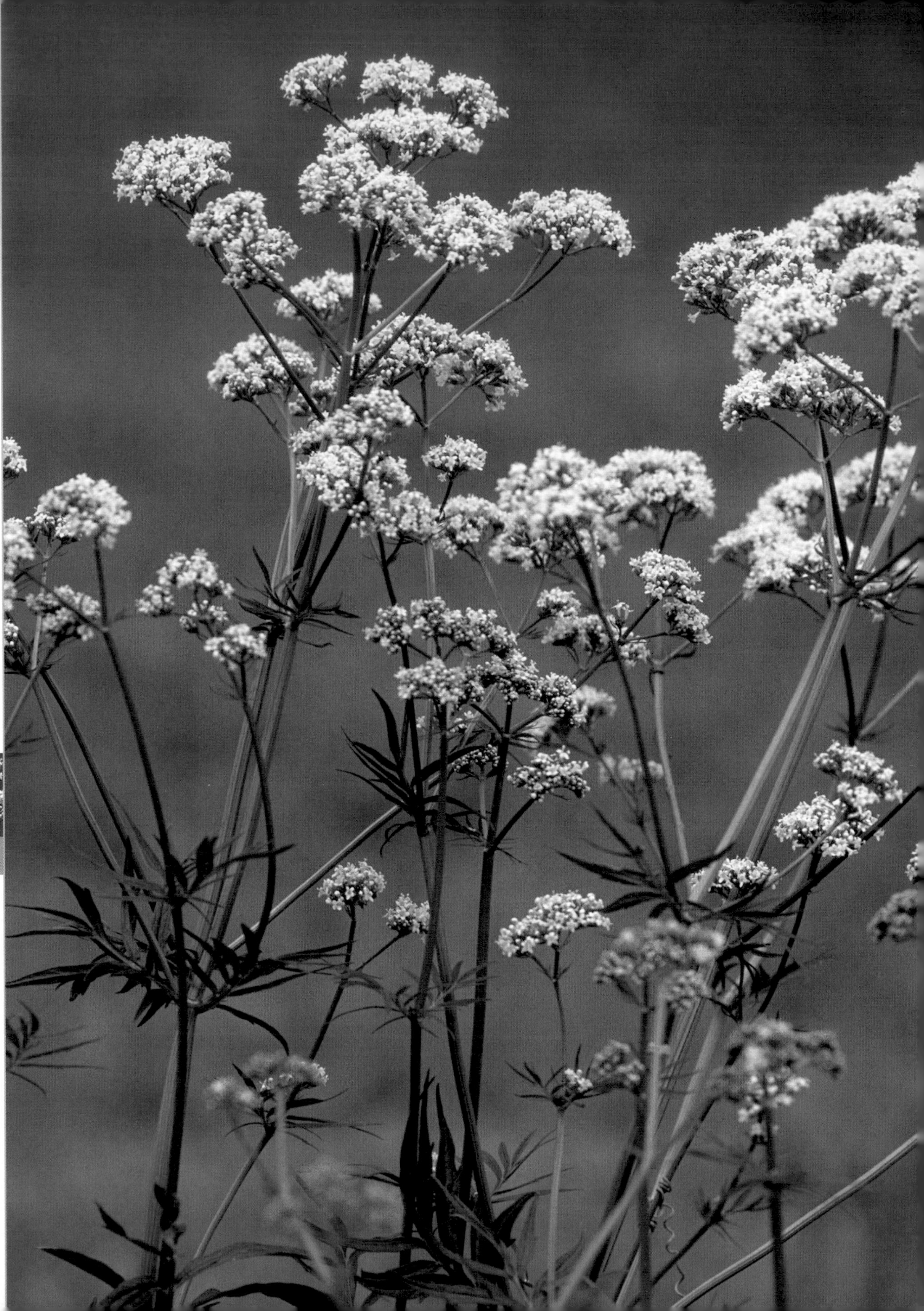

Valerian

Valeriana officinalis

It is common knowledge that cats are attracted to catnip. Some even go crazy over it. It's less well known that valerian has much the same effect. Something in the scent of valerian sends cats—and strangely enough, rats—into an intoxicated frenzy. Most people, however, find the musky odor of valerian offensive. The ancient Greeks certainly did. Their name for valerian was *phu*, a word that aptly communicates the typical reaction people have after smelling the plant's leaves or roots. Unpleasant smell aside, the Greeks valued valerian greatly as a medicinal herb. They used it to cure a variety of ills, notably insomnia. Some 2,000 years later, valerian is one of the best sleep-inducing sedatives in the modern herbal medicine chest.

It was Galen, a Greek physician practicing in the second century A.D., who first wrote of valerian's tranquilizing effects. The ancient Greeks also used the herb as a **diuretic**, and for digestive upsets, liver disorders, and urinary tract complaints. *Valeriana officinalis* and other **species** of the herb were used in both traditional Chinese and Indian **Ayurvedic medicine**. During the Middle Ages, valerian's popularity soared in Europe, and the herb became something of a cure-all. Over time, though, its calming effects came to be valued most. From the 1600s onward, valerian was widely used in Europe and later the United

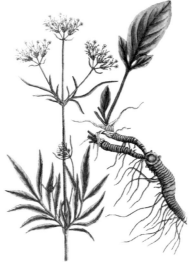

States as a sedative, to ease nervous tension and treat many nervous disorders, for insomnia and depression, even to lessen the severity of epileptic seizures. Valerian's popularity in conventional medicine lasted until the mid-20th century, when it was largely replaced by prescription sedative drugs such as Valium. Once valerian was omitted from the *National Formulary*, it was all but forgotten.

However, it remained a constant in herbal medicine. Today valerian is widely available in health food stores as a dietary supplement. Herbalists and naturopathic doctors suggest valerian as a safe and gentle alternative to commonly prescribed medications for insomnia and other sleep problems.

Airy blooms crown stately valerian, but it's the roots that have been used since antiquity to promote peaceful sleep.

TIME LINE OF USAGE AND SPREAD

2ND CENTURY A.D.	11TH CENTURY	1942	1950
Roman physician Galen recommends valerian for insomnia.	*Valeriana* is mentioned in an Anglo-Saxon leechbook, a book of medicinal recipes.	Writer Agatha Christie includes valerian as evidence in *Murder in Retrospect*.	Valerian is dropped from the *National Formulary* of the United States.

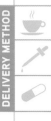

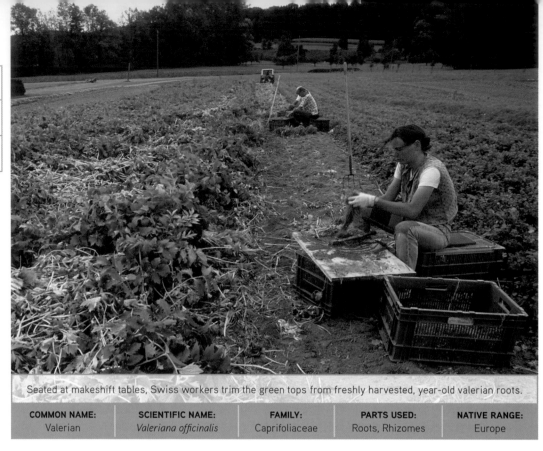

Seated at makeshift tables, Swiss workers trim the green tops from freshly harvested, year-old valerian roots.

COMMON NAME:	SCIENTIFIC NAME:	FAMILY:	PARTS USED:	NATIVE RANGE:
Valerian	*Valeriana officinalis*	Caprifoliaceae	Roots, Rhizomes	Europe

More than 200 species of *Valeriana* are found worldwide, most in northern temperate climates, as well as South Africa and the Andes. Most are herbs, though some are shrubs. Common valerian is a highly variable perennial usually growing from 1 to 4 feet in height, with a short, branched root, which in some variations produces lateral creeping underground stems known as rhizomes. The leaves at the base of the plant are divided into 3 to 25 leaflets, either linear or lance shaped. They are without teeth or coarsely toothed. The tiny white or pink flowers, crowded atop a flat-topped cluster on a robust stalk, have a sweet vanilla-like fragrance. They bloom from June through August.

Growing Habits

Valerian is native to most of Europe, though in extreme southern Europe it is rare, mostly limited to mountain habitats. Found in damp and dry meadows, along the edge of woods, or in small openings in forests, the plant exhibits great adaptability. Valerian has naturalized in eastern North America, from Newfoundland south to Maryland and West Virginia, west to Iowa, and north through Minnesota and adjacent Canada. In western North America, it is naturalized in Montana, Idaho, Oregon, Washington, and southern British Columbia. More northerly naturalized populations in North America tend to have pink flowers.

Cultivation and Harvesting

Valerian is an easy-to-grow perennial propagated by seeds or by dividing the rootstocks. Established root clumps will produce 6 to 8 strong plants from the division. Seeds must be planted soon after maturing. They germinate in about 20 days. Valerian grows well in full sun or partial shade in a rich, well-drained garden soil.

Some commercial operations mow back the flowering tops before they mature—a practice that seems to produce more vigorous, larger roots. The roots and **rhizomes**—the plant parts used in herbal medicine—are usually harvested in the fall of the second year. After harvest, the roots are washed, then dried under shade. Valerian is grown commercially in Belgium, Germany, France, the Netherlands, and Eastern Europe. It is also produced commercially in China as an export crop and in the U.S.

Therapeutic Uses

+ *Nervousness*
+ *Insomnia*
+ *Anxiety*

Valerian is the most widely used sedative in Europe, where more than a hundred preparations are sold in pharmacies across Germany, Belgium, France, Switzerland, and Italy. Now researchers are getting closer to understanding the **compounds** in valerian, as well as the mechanism responsible for its sedative effect. GABA is one of the major inhibitory **neurotransmitters** in the central nervous system and its receptor, GABA-A, is the target of many drugs used to reduce anxiety or aid sleep, such as **benzodiazepines**. Valerenic acid and valerenol are two compounds in valerian root that have been shown to strongly bind GABA-A receptors and are likely to be key players in its therapeutic effect.

There have been numerous clinical trials studying the effect of valerian on insomnia. Two studies administering valerian every night for 2 to 4 weeks found that those taking it had significant improvement in sleep and sleep quality compared with a **placebo**. Other studies yielded contradictory results, especially those that tested valerian for shorter periods for "acute" insomnia. It appears that if valerian does improve sleep, it must be taken for at least 2 weeks to achieve a benefit.

The majority of valerian preparations sold in Europe contain other sedative herbs such as hops, lemon balm, or passionflower. The combination of valerian and hops is popular in Europe and has been shown in several studies to shorten the time it takes to fall asleep and reduce waking up during the night. A clinical trial of valerian and lemon balm was shown to improve sleep in children 12 years of age and under. It appears that valerian is a safe herbal choice for treating mild insomnia. Valerian in combination with hops and/or lemon balm may be more effective than valerian alone.

How to Use

TEA: Steep 1 teaspoon dried valerian root in 1 cup water for 10 minutes. Strain. Drink 30 to 60 minutes before bed.

CAPSULE: Take 2 to 3 g of dried valerian root 30 to 60 minutes before bed.

EXTRACT: Doses of 300 to 900 mg of valerian **extract** standardized to valerenic acid were used in clinical trials.

TINCTURE: Generally, 5 to 10 ml, 30 to 60 minutes before bed.

Precautions

The American Herbal Products Association gives valerian a class 1 safety rating, indicating that it is a very safe herb with a wide dosage range. Valerian does not appear to be habit-forming, which is an important advantage over many other sleeping medications. A small number of people may experience adverse reactions to valerian such as restlessness after taking the herb. This is believed to be an idiosyncratic reaction, however, and limited to individual hypersensitivities.

over the (kitchen) counter VALERIAN HOPS TINCTURE

Chop 1 ounce dried valerian root and 1 ounce hops flowers. Grind herbs in a coffee grinder and put into a 1- or 2-quart jar. Add 12 ounces vodka. Make sure herbs are thoroughly moist. If they are not, add 2 more ounces of vodka. Screw on lid and shake daily for 14 days. Strain liquid tincture using a muslin cloth and then store in a dark bottle. Label and use according to directions above, generally 5 to 10 ml, 30 to 60 minutes before bed.

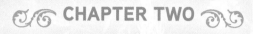

CHAPTER TWO

Respiratory System

Plants *and* Breathing

"It is in vain to describe an herb so commonly known," begins the entry for thyme *(Thymus vulgaris)* in *The Complete Herbal*, penned by the 17th-century English botanist, herbalist, and physician Nicholas Culpeper (1616-1654) and published in 1653. Culpeper's description of thyme continues, relating that the herb is "a noble strengthener of the lungs, as notable a one as grows; neither is there scarce a better remedy growing for that disease in children which they commonly call the Chin-cough [whooping cough], than it is. It purges the body of phlegm, and is an excellent remedy for shortness of breath." It is probably safe to say that nearly every English herb or kitchen garden during this period in history had its patch of thyme. Commonly known and commonly grown, thyme was a good herb to keep close at hand, because respiratory afflictions were common, too. Like many of the body's systems, the respiratory system goes about its job somewhat outside our conscious awareness, at least most

of the time. We hardly notice the regular inhalations and exhalations that are so fundamental to its functions and that form a rhythmic accompaniment to daily life, much like a beating heart. Remarkably, the average person breathes in and out about 22,000 times each day. With help from the diaphragm, the lungs form the core of the respiratory system, drawing in air, and in so doing, supplying the body with oxygen. From the lungs, oxygen enters the bloodstream and is rushed to organs, tissues, and cells. Oxygen is what drives cell respiration, the chemical transformation that provides cells with the energy they need. The process produces carbon dioxide as a toxic by-product, one that cells release into the bloodstream so it can be carried back to the lungs and exhaled.

The lungs, and the respiratory system to which they belong, are absolutely fundamental to health and life. The ancient Egyptians believed this to be true both in this world and the next. When mummifying the dead, they typically left the heart in the body so that it could be weighed against the feather of truth in

the afterlife. But four other organs—the spleen, stomach, intestines, and lungs—were considered so important that they were removed and preserved separately in special sacred containers. In traditional Chinese medicine, which has been practiced since at least 2000 B.C., the lungs are one of five organs believed to govern qi, the vital, animating force that flows through all living things.

Despite its strengths, however, the respiratory system possesses a vulnerability not shared by the body's other systems, a sort of physiological Achilles' heel. In drawing in air, the lungs and the passageways that lead to them are constantly exposed to the external environment and any airborne disease organisms it might contain. Thus, the respiratory system is susceptible to a host of bacterial and viral infections. In Nicholas Culpeper's day, one of the most devastating was tuberculosis, known in the 1600s as phthisis (from a Greek word meaning "to waste away"), white plague, or consumption. It was a disease with which the herbalist was intimately familiar, for he died

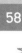

from it at age 38, just a year after *The Complete Herbal* was published. While tuberculosis is far less of a concern today in the Western world, many other respiratory infections still hound us, as they have for centuries.

Influenza, or flu, is a virus-caused illness that often starts with a sore throat followed by fever, chills, and cough. Bronchitis, characterized by cough and a feeling of tightness or congestion in the chest, is an inflammation of the lining of the bronchial tubes, the airways that connect the trachea, or windpipe, to the lungs. Inflamed sinuses and nasal passages are often termed sinusitis, which can be accompanied by headache or pressure around the eyes and nose, as well as cough, fever, and nasal congestion. Asthma is a long-term, inflammatory lung disease that causes airways to tighten and narrow when a person with the condition encounters irritants such as dust, pet dander, or cigarette smoke. Even the healthiest of us occasionally succumb to the most universal of all respiratory ailments—the common cold. More than 200 different viruses are responsible for this inflammation of the upper respiratory tract and its annoyingly familiar symptoms of sneezing, cough, sore throat, and runny nose.

Yet as long as there have been respiratory illnesses, people have used medicinal herbs to combat them, and with much success. This chapter highlights nine herbs selected from many that herbalists and naturopaths commonly recommend to treat respiratory system complaints. Astragalus or *huang qi (Astragalus membranaceus),* which has its origins in Chinese herbal medicine, is used both to help prevent colds and other frequently contracted respiratory infections and to ease their symptoms. To most people, however, it will probably be less familiar than echinacea *(Echinacea purpurea* and several closely related species), which is routinely prescribed by medical doctors in many European countries for colds and flu. Echinacea preparations are also widely used in the United States; their sales are believed to represent approximately 10 percent of the dietary supplement market.

Using elder *(Sambucus nigra)* to treat coughs and colds—and many other complaints—is a practice that dates to at least the Middle Ages, and the herb is still a popular remedy for these illnesses, as it is for sinusitis and allergy relief. Australia's Aborigines used eucalyptus *(Eucalyptus globulus)* for thousands of years before it was introduced to the West. Its head-clearing vapors are prized for relieving congestion, and sore throats, bronchitis, and sinusitis typically respond well to eucalyptus tea. Licorice *(Glycyrrhiza glabra)* has served as a remedy for respiratory ailments since the time of the ancient Greeks. Mullein *(Verbascum thapsus)* is another old respiratory medicinal herb, favored for its congestion-relieving properties. Pelargonium *(Pelargonium sidoides)* is a much more recent introduction into Western herbal medicine. Research has shown that pelargonium, native to southern Africa, has powerful bacteria-fighting properties, making it a viable alternative to antibiotics for treating bronchitis and some other conditions.

Chapter 2 concludes with two herbs, sage *(Salvia officinalis)* and thyme *(Thymus vulgaris),* familiar to many cooks as classic seasonings for savory dishes. Yet by the time they found their way into Nicholas Culpeper's herbal, they had been easing respiratory ailments for many hundreds of years.

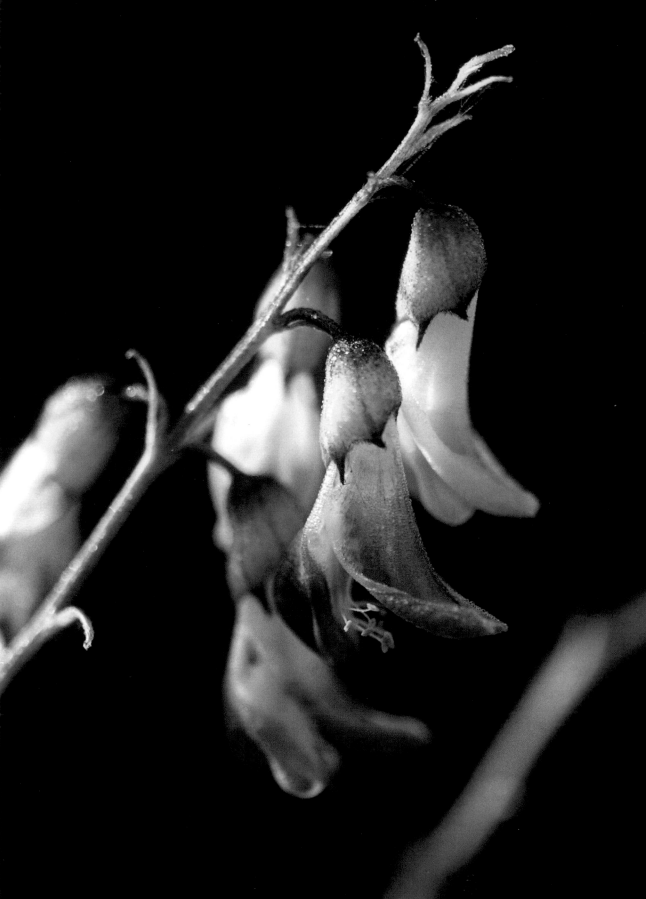

RESPIRATORY SYSTEM

Astragalus

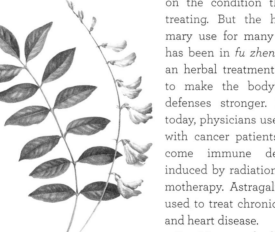

Astragalus membranaceus

Native to Mongolia and northern China, astragalus is a shrubby legume with pastel, pealike flowers that produce small pods. Many of the more than 2,500 species of plants in the genus *Astragalus* produce similar fruits. The name is derived from an ancient Greek word meaning "anklebone." The Greeks once used the anklebones of animals as dice, and the connection to these plants lies in the fact that when dry, the seed pods rattle with a sound that resembles rolling dice. *Astragalus membranaceus* also has thick, fibrous roots.

Peeling back the dark brown skin of the roots reveals a pale, yellowish core. The herb's Chinese name is *huang qi*, meaning "yellow leader," which refers to the color of the root's interior and its status as one of the most important tonic herbs in Chinese medicine. The first written reference to its use comes from the *Shen Nong Ben Cao Jing*, or *The Divine Husbandman's Classic of the Materia Medicia*, an herbal compendium from the first century A.D. that documents 365 medicinal plants. Many ancient Chinese herbals praise huang qi for its ability to stimulate the body's vital protective energy, known as qi, and in doing so help fight fatigue and strengthen resistance to disease.

In traditional Chinese medicine, astragalus root is often mixed with other herbs, depending on the condition that needs treating. But the herb's primary use for many centuries has been in *fu zheng* therapy, an herbal treatment designed to make the body's natural defenses stronger. In China today, physicians use fu zheng with cancer patients to overcome immune deficiencies induced by radiation and chemotherapy. Astragalus is also used to treat chronic hepatitis and heart disease.

In Western herbal medicine, practitioners recommend astragalus as an **adaptogen**, an herb that helps protect the body against physical, mental, and emotional stress by strengthening the immune system. Astragalus is also suggested for preventing and treating colds, upper respiratory infections, influenza, asthma, allergies, and digestive disturbances.

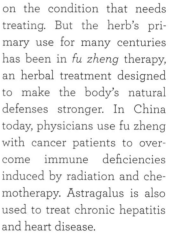

Astragalus's roots hold its medicinally important compounds; its pealike flowers reveal its link to the legume family.

TIME LINE OF USAGE AND SPREAD

1531
Shi Shan Yi An, a medical casebook, notes astragalus and ginseng used for fatigue.

1860s
Russian physician Alexander von Bunge describes use of astragalus for Western world.

1925
Astragalus membranaceus is introduced to U.S. through Department of Agriculture.

1980s
Astragalus gains popularity in the United States as an herbal medicine.

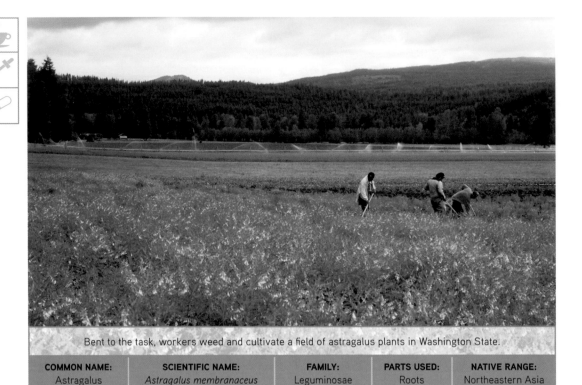

Bent to the task, workers weed and cultivate a field of astragalus plants in Washington State.

COMMON NAME:	SCIENTIFIC NAME:	FAMILY:	PARTS USED:	NATIVE RANGE:
Astragalus	*Astragalus membranaceus*	Leguminosae	Roots	Northeastern Asia

A*stragalus* is the largest genus of flowering plants, with some 2,500 species, most of which are indigenous to northern temperate regions. Europe is home to more than 130 species; another 250 *Astragalus* species range across the Middle East from Turkey to Iran; nearly 300 species grow in China. In North America, there are close to 400 species of *Astragalus,* most from desert regions of the western United States.

The Chinese traditional medicine huang qi is the root of *Astragalus membranaceus*, a perennial herb growing to about 2 feet. The alternate leaves are divided into 12 to 24 oval or elliptical leaflets, each about 1 inch in length. The tiny, pale to cream yellow flowers are borne on stalks arising from the leaf **axils**.

Growing Habits

This famous medicinal plant of Chinese traditions ranges from the mountains of Sichuan to the plains of Xinjiang province, the most northwesterly province in China. Its range extends eastward and south to the Shandong Peninsula. Astragalus also occurs in adjacent areas in Russia. It typically grows along the edges of forests; thin, open woods; grasslands; and shrub thickets.

Cultivation and Harvesting

Astragalus is propagated by seeds, which grow in two-valved, papery pods. Like many other members of the pea **family**, astragalus has a seed with a hard, impermeable coat. To facilitate germination, the seed coat can be nicked with a file, or rubbed between sandpaper, then soaked in water overnight before planting. Astragalus prefers a well-drained, deep, slightly alkaline sandy soil and full sun.

The roots—which look somewhat like tongue depressors on display in Chinese herb shops— are harvested in the fall of the fourth or fifth year of growth by hand or machine. Roots are carefully dried in the shade, and then thinly sliced along their lateral length. Astragalus is a rare plant in American horticulture, and nearly all commercial production of its root

over the (kitchen) counter ASTRAGALUS BUTTER

In a double boiler, gently warm 1 cup tahini and 7 tablespoons of pumpkin seed butter (available at health food stores). Stir in 3 tablespoons powdered astragalus root. Add 3 tablespoons sesame oil and stir to smooth consistency. (If too stiff, add up to 1 tablespoon of sesame oil.) This peanut butter substitute will keep 2 weeks in the fridge.

comes from herb farms in China. For medicinal purposes, the herb is marketed as dried roots, ground roots in capsule and tablet, as a liquid **extract**, or as an ingredient in herbal teas.

Therapeutic Uses

+ *Immune support*
+ *Viral infection*
+ *Tonic*

If an ounce of prevention is worth a pound of cure, astragalus is the medicinal herb that proves it. With the common cold, some plants, such as echinacea, are best used as soon as an upper respiratory infecton develops. Astragalus root works better as a preventive, helping to fend off viruses and bacteria before they make you sick. Laboratory studies support this: Extracts of astragalus root improve the function of white blood cells, even increasing **antibody** levels in healthy people. The success of astragalus in preventing infections and treating bacterial or viral infections once they get started may come from increases in **interferon** levels. Interferons are immune-activating proteins that fight viral infections and tumors. The benefits astragalus confers on the immune system help prevent upper respiratory infections, especially in those prone to colds and flus, during the peak winter season for such viruses.

Astragalus roots contain several **compounds** most likely responsible for its medicinal effects; these include **flavonoids**, **saponins**, and **polysaccharides**. The flavonoids belong to a family of compounds that occur in many medicinal plants and have been shown to exhibit **anti-inflammatory** and **antioxidant** activity. The polysaccharides boost several aspects of the immune system, while the saponins protect the liver, inhibit viruses, and help with **insulin** and glucose metabolism.

Much of the research on astragalus's medicinal properties has been conducted in China. One study of 1,000 patients showed that astragalus exhibits a **prophylactic** effect against colds and upper respiratory infections. Other research has focused on the immune-boosting effects in cancer patients after chemotherapy. For example, when white blood cell levels drop after chemotherapy, over the course of eight weeks, astragalus can increase those levels.

How to Use

In traditional Chinese medicine, astragalus is usually combined with several other plants in a tea, capsule, or **tincture**.

TEA: The daily dose of astragalus varies greatly; a typical dose is 3 to 6 tablespoons of dried chopped root, simmered in 2 to 4 cups water for 10 to 15 minutes. Under guidance of an herbal expert, significantly higher doses of astragalus are occasionally used.

CAPSULE: Generally, dosage is 1 to 3 g of dried, powdered root daily, depending on manufacturer's processing methods and medical condition being treated.

TINCTURE: 2 to 4 ml, 3 times a day.

Precautions

Astragalus is generally safe and very well tolerated. In fact, many think of astragalus as a food, adding pieces of the dried root to soups to get a daily tonic effect. However, anyone suffering an acute infection should not use asatragalus, particularly in large amounts. Those with autoimmune diseases should consult with a health care provider before using any herbal medicine that could have immune-boosting effects.

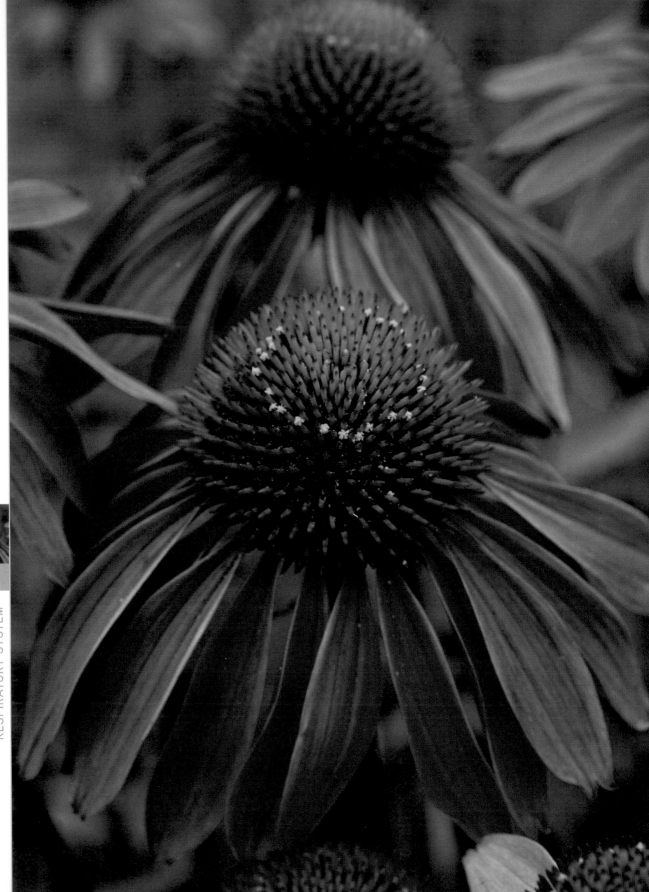

Echinacea

No sunny perennial border or herb garden is complete without echinacea, a robust and distinctive wildflower native exclusively to North America. Echinacea's flowers consist of prickly, domed centers encircled by a single layer of lavender-hued petals, the source of the herb's most common name, purple coneflower. The "cone" is the characteristic perfectly captured by the genus name, as *Echinacea* comes from the Greek *echinos*, meaning "hedgehog." Centuries before European settlers arrived in North America, native tribes were using

at least three **species** of echinacea medicinally. The herb was something of a universal remedy to Indians of the Great Plains and neighboring regions. It was used for more therapeutic purposes than almost any other herb.

The Omaha-Ponca chewed fresh echinacea root to dull toothache pain. Bathing the skin with the juice of echinacea roots helped heal burns and wounds, and made the fiery heat of a sweat lodge more tolerable. The Cheyenne used a tea brewed from powdered echinacea leaves and roots, or chewed the roots to soothe sore gums, mouths, and throats. Other tribes used various echinacea preparations to treat colds, coughs, colic, even snakebite. In the late 1800s, many

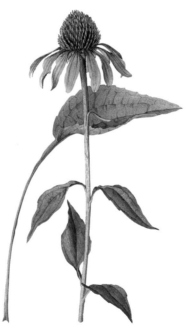

American **Eclectic** physicians, who relied on the use of American medicinal plants in their practices, began prescribing echinacea primarily for respiratory infections and skin conditions. In the 1930s, however, echinacea fell from favor in the U.S. while gaining popularity in Europe, particularly in Germany.

Today, echinacea remains popular in Europe and has made a dramatic comeback in American herbal medicine. Herbal practitioners prescribe echinacea to shorten the duration of the common cold and flu, and to reduce symptoms, including cough, fever, and sore throat. People also take echinacea to help strengthen the immune system and enhance the body's ability to resist infection.

In herbal medicine, echinacea is used in its entirety, from roots to stems and leaves to dazzling coneflowers.

TIME LINE OF USAGE AND SPREAD

1870
Physician H. Meyer creates echinacea preparation, Meyer's Blood Purifier.

1895
Ohio drug firm manufactures first preparations of echinacea in U.S.

1939
German physician G. Madaus launches *E. purpurea* into European herbal medicine.

1994
German physicians prescribe echinacea over 2.5 million times.

In the herb trade, echinacea is the root or aboveground parts (harvested in flower) of three species of large, robust plants with purple daisylike flowers. There are nine species in the genus *Echinacea*, three of which are used in herbal preparations. The most commonly used is *E. purpurea*, widely grown as a flower garden perennial and available at most nurseries. It grows 2 to 4 feet in height, and unlike other echinaceas has oval, coarsely toothed leaves with a heart-shaped base; its root is fibrous. All other echinaceas have **taproots**. The showy flowerheads have purple ray flowers surrounding a conelike disk, with numerous orange-tipped blunt spines at the top. Pale purple coneflower, *E. pallida*, is a perennial with long, slender, toothless leaves, much longer than broad. The purple, pink, or white ray flowers, up to 3½ inches, are long and drooping. *Echinacea angustifolia* is smaller than other *Echinacea* species, growing 6 to 20 inches high.

Growing Habits

Echinacea purpurea is the most wide-ranging species, usually growing in small populations in open woods, glades, and edges of fields and roadsides from Georgia west to Oklahoma, north to Michigan, and east to Ohio. Numerous cultivars, or cultivated varieties, are available in the nursery trade. *Echinacea pallida* grows in prairies, glades, and open woods and ranges from Michigan to Nebraska, south to Arkansas, and west to Texas. *Echinacea angustifolia* grows farther west than other echinaceas, along roadsides, prairies, and outcrops from Texas north through the Dakotas and southern Saskatchewan, west to eastern Montana and Colorado.

Cultivation and Harvesting

Echinacea purpurea is by far the easiest of the three commonly used species to grow. It can be propagated by seeds, which usually germinate in about 30 days, or by dividing root clumps and replanting in spring or autumn. It thrives in well-drained garden soil. It prefers full sun but will do well in dappled shade. *Echinacea pallida* is available from nurseries specializing in native midwestern plants. *Echinacea angustifolia* can be grown from seed; however, the seed requires a pregermination treatment to break dormancy, usually accomplished by putting it in moist sand in a refrigerator for three months before planting. It likes a drier, more alkaline soil than other species.

The entire world's supply of *Echinacea purpurea* is cultivated. It is grown commercially throughout Europe, as well as in North America. Additional supplies come from plantations in China and elsewhere. The whole flowering plant is harvested about 6 inches aboveground, or the root is dug in autumn of the second or third year. Most of the supply of *E. pallida* and *E. angustifolia* is wild-harvested from their native ranges.

Therapeutic Uses

+ *Colds and flus*
+ *Wounds*

Echinacea is one of the most well-studied herbs in herbal medicine today. It has gained a reputation for decreasing the severity and length of the common cold. It has been shown to have numerous effects on the immune system—from

over the (kitchen) counter COLD CARE TEA

Mix together 2 parts echinacea root, 1 part hyssop, 1 part peppermint leaf, and 1 part thyme. Steep 2 tablespoons of this mixture in 2 cups of boiling water for 15 minutes, strain, and drink. Take three cups a day whenever you are experiencing cold or flu symptoms. (If you are allergic to ragweed, you should avoid echinacea; if you're pregnant, you should avoid hyssop.)

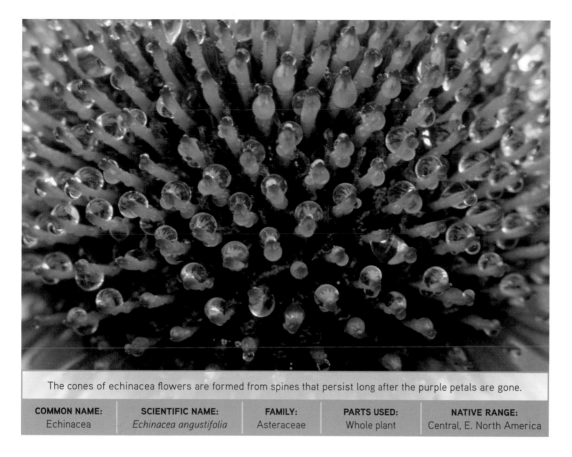

The cones of echinacea flowers are formed from spines that persist long after the purple petals are gone.

COMMON NAME:	SCIENTIFIC NAME:	FAMILY:	PARTS USED:	NATIVE RANGE:
Echinacea	*Echinacea angustifolia*	Asteraceae	Whole plant	Central, E. North America

increased **antibody** responses to elevated **interferon** levels for fighting viruses to stimulation of white blood cells to work harder to fight infection. There are several chemical **compounds** in echinacea that vary among the three species of the plant, plant parts, and extraction techniques: **Polysaccharides**, **glycoproteins**, and **alkylamides** all have medicinal effects that boost the immune system and inhibit viruses and bacteria. How echinacea works continues to be investigated.

Daily use of echinacea does not seem to protect against getting a cold; however, some studies point to an effect of shortening a cold's length by 1 to 2 days. In order to see benefits, take adequate doses of good product at the first sign of illness.

How to Use

TEA: Steep 1 to 2 teaspoons of echinacea leaf/flower in 1 cup of boiling water, or boil 1 teaspoon of root in 1 to 2 cups water for 10 minutes. **TINCTURE:** When coming down with a cold, take either a **tincture** of echinacea root or the expressed juice from fresh *E. purpurea* aboveground parts stabilized in alcohol. Every 2 hours, take 1 to 2 ml directly or diluted in water. **CAPSULE:** The dose varies with each echinacea product, depending on the plant part used and the species.

Precautions

Anyone with an autoimmune condition must exercise caution in taking an immune-boosting herb like echinacea. Echinacea may inhibit certain liver **enzymes**, theoretically increasing blood levels of medications such as itraconazole (for fungal infections), lovastatin (for lowering cholestrol), and fexofenadine (for allergies); so it is important to be careful when taking echinacea with these and other medications, including birth control pills. A rare allergic reaction can occur in people who are allergic to other plants in the Asteraceae (daisy) **family**. Some people experience very mild stomach upset or dizziness. High doses of echinacea can cause nausea.

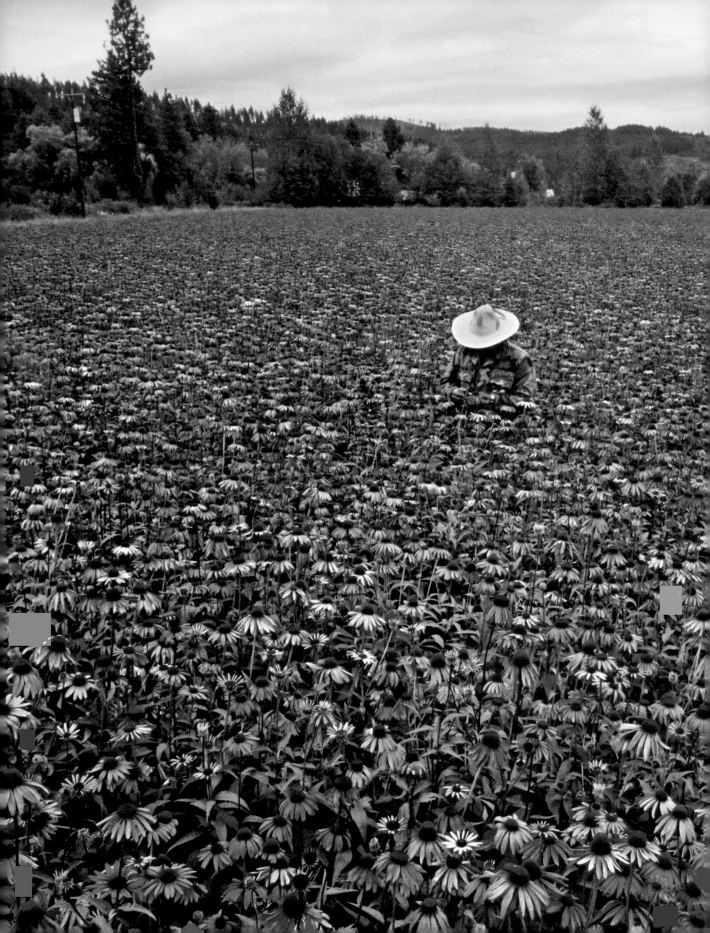

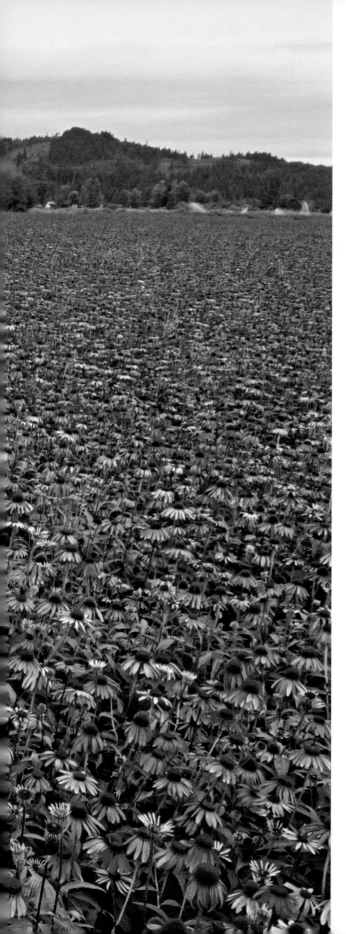

Echinacea Harvest

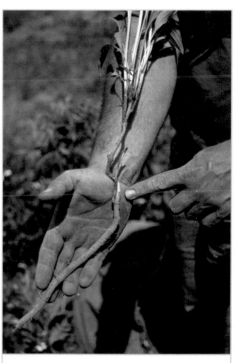

Nearly 30 acres of blooming *Echinacea purpurea* (left) lift their blossoms at an herb farm near Washington's Cascade Mountains. *E. purpurea* flowers, depending on where they are grown, appear from July to October. Flower harvesting for the herbal market, typically done by machine, occurs when flowers on cultivated plants are fully open, ensuring that key chemical constituents are at their peak. Harvesting of echinacea roots is in late fall during the third or fourth year of a plant's life. The roots are dried before any processing or extraction of the herb's active compounds takes place. A wildcrafter—who harvests herbs from their wild habitat—displays (above) a freshly collected *Echinacea pallida*. To address fears that wildharvested plants do not regrow, the wildcrafter points to the place where the upper plant part grew from rootstock left in the ground after a previous harvest. Scientific research coupled with firsthand reports from wildcrafters confirms that after careful harvesting roughly half of all wild echinacea plants regrow from pieces of roots left in the ground.

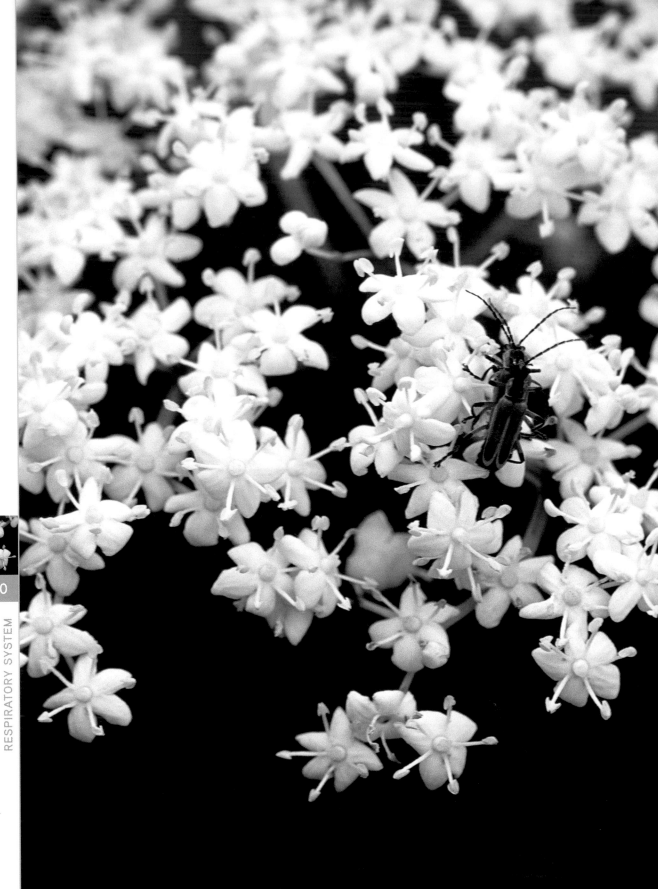

Elder

Sambucus nigra

Many centuries ago, conflicting superstitions surrounded elder. In some places, people thought that cutting or otherwise harming elder trees could anger supernatural beings who dwelled within them. Particularly frightening was the Elder Tree Mother, who sought revenge by haunting houses where elder wood was used and harming infants she found lying in elder wood cradles. Elsewhere, elder was a symbol of protection. Planting elder near a house or nailing elder branches above the windows and doors kept witches at bay.

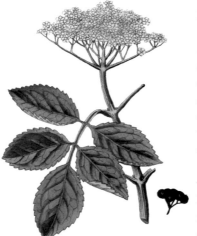

At burials, elder branches were interred alongside coffins to protect the dead from malevolent spirits. In medieval Europe, not only was the Cross on which Christ was crucified said to be made of elder wood, but his betrayer, Judas, supposedly hanged himself on an elder tree.

Superstitions aside, dark purple elderberries have been stewed into preserves, baked into pastries, and made into wine for millennia. The cosmetic and medicinal uses of elder date to at least the first century A.D. Medicinally, the Romans used elder primarily as a **purgative** and an emetic. During the Middle Ages, however, elder's reputation as a medicinal herb blossomed, and for centuries it was viewed as a plant that could cure almost anything. Elder roots were turned into remedies for reducing swelling. Elder leaves went into ointments applied to sprains, wounds, and bruises. Teas and **infusions** made from elder flowers were drunk for rheumatic aches, and to treat coughs and colds. Externally, they were used to treat wounds and heal skin conditions.

Elderberries are rich in vitamin C and **antioxidants**. Herbal practitioners recommend elderberry syrup and **extracts** to fight infection and shorten colds' duration. They suggest teas and infusions made from elder flowers for easing symptoms of colds, flu, and bronchitis. These preparations are also used in modern herbal medicine to reduce swelling in mucous membranes—and so relieve nasal and sinus congestion—and to lessen sneezing, itchiness, and other symptoms of allergies.

Elder's creamy white flowers and the purple berries that follow have a history of medicinal use in many cultures.

TIME LINE OF USAGE AND SPREAD

4TH CENTURY B.C.
Greek physician Hippocrates recommends elderberry for a wide variety of complaints.

1597
English herbalist J. Gerard writes of elder's medicinal and magical uses.

1751
Thomas Short writes in *Medicina Britannica* that elder is "useful and despised."

1820-1831
Elder is included in the *United States Pharmacopeia*.

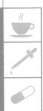
*S*ambucus is a small genus of 9 species of temperate and subtropical shrubs and small trees, all of which have pithy stems. Some species are toxic, while others, including *S. canadensis (S. nigra* var. *canadensis)*, have edible fruits, if properly prepared by cooking or drying. European elder is a shrub or small tree growing 4 to 25 feet in height, with stout rootstocks, often spreading from suckering sprouts from the roots. The trunk is light yellowish brown, with warty bumps. Inside the center of the weak, woody stalks is white pith. Leaves are opposite, with a smooth stalk (though hairy along the central groove), 1 to 2 inches long. The leaves are divided into 5 to 9 leaflets, and are about 2 to 4 inches long. The leaflets are generally lance shaped to oblong, smooth above, minutely hairy beneath, and irregularly toothed along the margins. The whitish to cream yellow, star-shaped flowers are borne on crowded clusters, making elder easily recognizable in summer. It blooms from June to August. The small bluish black to purplish black fruits have a pleasant flavor. European and common elder are very similar in appearance; European elder leaves almost always have 5 leaflets, while common elder leaves usually have 7 leaflets.

Growing Habits

European elder is found throughout most of Europe except in the extreme north, growing in habitats similar to its North American counterpart. *Sambucus,* the classical and botanical name for elder, refers to a type of harp made from elder wood. *Nigra,* meaning "black," refers to the color of the wood, and "canadensis" means "of Canada."

Common elder is exactly that—common. It is found in rich forest bottoms, drier upland forests, banks of rivers and streams, and the edges of ponds and lakes, as well as pastures, fields, and gardens and along roadsides. It ranges throughout eastern North America, from Nova Scotia and Quebec south to Florida and west to California, Wyoming, and Montana. It is absent from the Pacific Northwest.

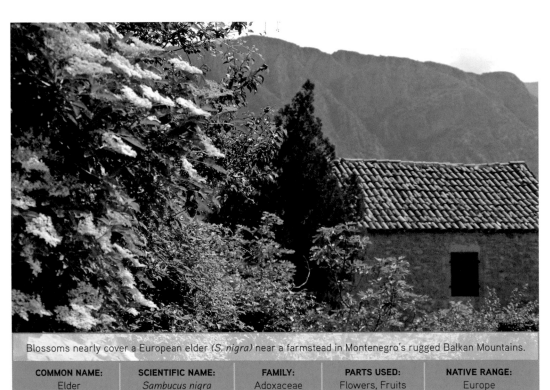

Blossoms nearly cover a European elder *(S. nigra)* near a farmstead in Montenegro's rugged Balkan Mountains.

COMMON NAME:	SCIENTIFIC NAME:	FAMILY:	PARTS USED:	NATIVE RANGE:
Elder	*Sambucus nigra*	Adoxaceae	Flowers, Fruits	Europe

Combine 2 pounds of rinsed, stemmed, edible elderberries with 4 cups of water in a large saucepan. Bring to a boil. Reduce heat and simmer for 20 minutes. Place cooled berry mixture in a large, fine-mesh strainer over the saucepan. Press out juice. Discard the seeds. Stir in 2½ cups sugar and cook over medium heat, until juice thickens into syrup. Refrigerate in a covered container. Yummy on pancakes!

Cultivation and Harvesting

Elders are easy to grow and make an attractive addition to landscape plantings. They prefer moist, fertile, well-drained soils, with a slightly acid pH between 5.5 and 6.5. Although they can be propagated from seed, buying plants from a nursery and planting in the spring is the easiest way to establish them. They can also be propagated from cuttings when the plant is dormant, or suckers severed from a mother plant can be replanted. Elders should be kept well watered during the first growing season, as the roots are relatively shallow.

The shallow root system can hamper commercial cultivation, as it is difficult for effective mechanical weed control, which may damage the roots. Both the flowers and the fruits are used. Elder flowers are harvested when in full bloom, simply by shaking the flower heads into a bag or basket. Once ripe in August or early September, the fruits are easily harvested by snipping off the entire **inflorescence**, usually with a basket or bucket beneath to catch the falling fruits.

Therapeutic Uses

+ *Colds and flus*

Ripe elderberries—once known as the Englishman's grape—have famously been used for making elderberry wine for centuries. Today, however, the elder plant's notoriety comes from preparations for treating colds and flu. The berries contain **flavonoid compounds** that are known antioxidants, exhibit **anti-inflammatory** properties, and are beneficial to the immune system. Laboratory studies have also shown that elder extracts act as antivirals, inhibiting replication of flu and other viruses.

Human studies have found that the syrup from the juice of an elderberry can help decrease the duration of flu symptoms. For example, in one study elder led to a faster resolution of flu symptoms in 15 people taking 4 tablespoons daily of syrup of elder, raspberry, glucose, honey, and citric acid (brand name Sambucol), when compared with 12 people taking a **placebo** syrup. In another study, the same dose of this syrup was tested in 60 adults with influenza, helping to decrease symptoms by 3 to 4 days when compared to the placebo group. It is possible that these results translate to people suffering from other viruses, such as those that cause the common cold, though more research is need to clarify that.

How to Use

SYRUP: Sambucol is an elderberry syrup on the market that has been the subject of several research trials. The syrup contains 38 percent of an extract made from elder fruits. Recommended dosage is 2 teaspoons 4 times daily, although clinical trials have used up to 1 tablespoon 4 times daily for flu treatment.

LOZENGE: Elder is combined with zinc, and often with other herbs, in a lozenge form. The lozenges may be used numerous times daily at the onset of a cold.

Precautions

Ripe elderberries and products made from them appear safe when used for a few days to ease symptoms of colds and flu. Do not eat unripe berries or consume products made from other plant parts. All contain dangerous compounds that may cause nausea, vomiting, diarrhea, dizziness, or confusion. As with any substance that may stimulate the immune system, caution is advised in people with autoimmune conditions.

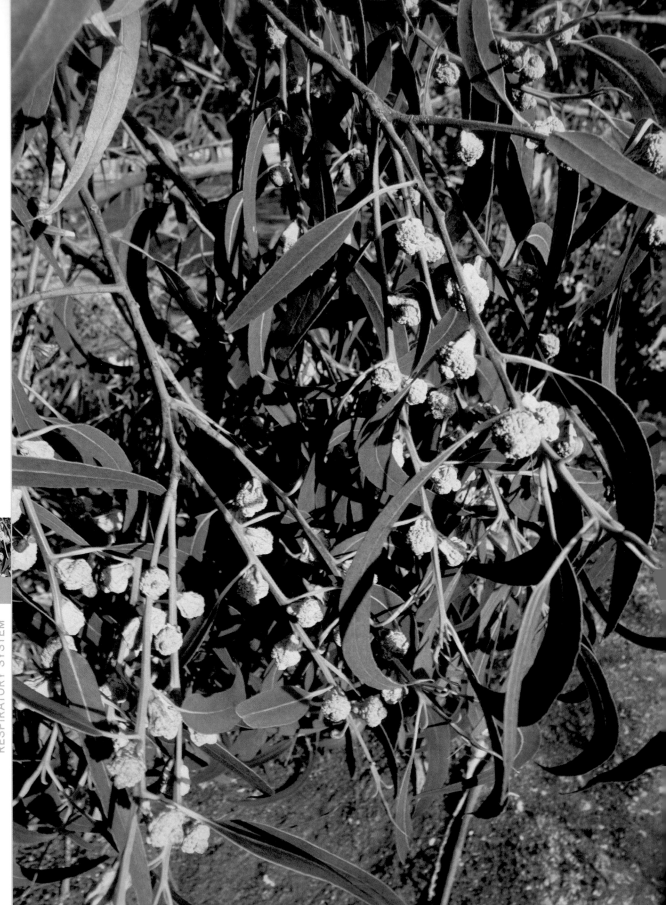

Eucalyptus

Eucalyptus globulus

On a hot summer day, the scent of eucalyptus fills the air in many parts of Australia. Most of the more than 680 species belonging to the genus *Eucalyptus* are indigenous to that continent. From scraggly shrubs to towering trees, they make up more than three-quarters of Australia's vegetation. Eucalyptus has played a significant role in Australian Aboriginal culture for many thousands of years. Some smaller species of eucalyptus have edible roots that indigenous tribes once used for food. They also ate the seeds of numerous species. Larger trees store considerable quantities of water in their roots, and during droughts were a handy source of drinking water. But the Aborigines valued eucalyptus primarily for its bark and leaves. The leaves, in particular, are a rich source of a volatile oil that has a pungent, heady fragrance and remarkable healing properties.

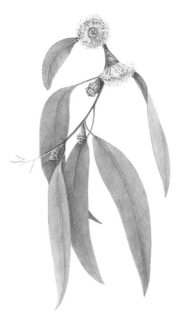

Aborigines made ointments and rubs containing eucalyptus oil taken from crushed leaves. These were applied to the skin to heal minor wounds and cure fungal infections. Leaves were bound over deeper wounds. The vapors released from fresh, macerated leaves were inhaled to clear the sinuses and nasal passages. To help ease rheumatism, patients lay on heated leaves and breathed in the volatile oils. Once commercial distillation of eucalyptus oil began in the mid-1800s, the oil was exported and quickly incorporated into both Western conventional and herbal medicine.

Today, eucalyptus is an ingredient in many over-the-counter cough and cold remedies, including cough drops, chest rubs, and vapor baths. Laboratory studies have shown that eucalyptus oil has strong anti-bacterial and **anti-inflammatory** properties. Herbalists recommend using fresh leaves in gargles to soothe sore throats, and in teas for bronchitis and sinusitis. Bronchitis, coughs, and the flu may also be helped by inhalation of eucalyptus vapors. Applied to nose and chest, ointments containing eucalyptus help relieve congestion. Rubbing the oil into the skin can relieve arthritis pain and ease tension headaches.

The medicinal properties of eucalyptus reside in oils contained in its surprisingly tough, gray-green leaves.

TIME LINE OF USAGE AND SPREAD

1852
Pharmacist J. Bosisto starts commercial eucalyptus oil industry in Australia.

1870
Chemist F. S. Cloez identifies major constituent of eucalyptus oil, eucalyptol.

1880s
Surgeons begin using eucalyptus oil as an antiseptic.

1930s
British firm Halls invents Mentho-Lyptus cough drops, with menthol and eucalyptus.

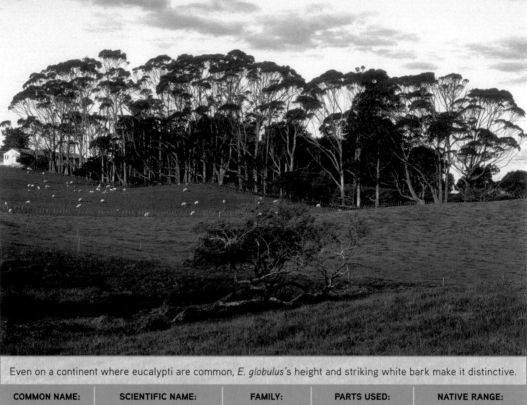

Even on a continent where eucalypti are common, *E. globulus*'s height and striking white bark make it distinctive.

COMMON NAME:	SCIENTIFIC NAME:	FAMILY:	PARTS USED:	NATIVE RANGE:
Eucalyptus	*Eucalyptus globulus*	Myrtaceae	Leaves, Oil	Southeastern Australia

RESPIRATORY SYSTEM

The genus *Eucalyptus* almost defines the woody vegetation of Australia, with more than 680 species, most native to Australia and others extending northward to Malaysia and the Philippines. Some eucalyptus species top 450 feet in height, making them among the tallest trees in the world. *Eucalyptus globulus* is the best known and most widespread species, planted and naturalized in warm temperate, subtropical, and tropical climates throughout the world. It can reach more than 300 feet and has distinctive smooth bark in a mottled pattern. The chief feature of the white, puffy flowers is their numerous stamens. The fruit is a single buttonlike sphere about an inch wide.

The leaves morph in shape and arrangement on the stalk from the juvenile to mature stage. Young leaves are stalkless, clasping the stem, and circular. The leaves are blue-green with a white film that rubs off when touched. Once mature, the leaves alternate on the stalk, becoming lance shaped to sickle shaped and up to a foot long. The changing leaf shape originating in the tree's native range is an adaptation—camouflage to prevent Australian adult tortoise beetles from attacking young leaves. Loaded with **essential oil**, which is also an insect deterrent, the leaves are strongly aromatic.

Growing Habits

Eucalyptus is native to southwestern Australia, generally found in damp gorges of Tasmania, Victoria, and New South Wales. Introduced to Europe by 1854, it was first planted in California in 1856. Today it is common in California, where it has become naturalized and spread throughout the warmer regions of the state. It is also common in warmer regions of southern Europe and North Africa. It was introduced to the Peruvian Andes in the late 19th century for erosion control and has become the dominant tree in the region. It is also commonly naturalized in South Africa and elsewhere.

To relieve chest and sinus congestion during a cold, try this trio of aromatic oils. Bring a large saucepan of water to a boil. Carefully pour water into a heatproof bowl and add 2 drops eucalyptus oil, 2 drops lavender oil, and 2 drops tea tree oil. Cover bowl and head with towel and, *keeping eyes closed*, inhale vapors for at least 3 minutes.

The name *Eucalyptus* is from the Greek *eu* and *kalypto*, meaning "to cover as a lid," in reference to the way the calyx encases the buds, which open like a small lidded box. The **species** name *globulus,* or globe shaped, refers to the juvenile leaves or alternatively the shape of the fruit.

Cultivation and Harvesting

Eucalyptus is one of the fastest growing trees on Earth. It prefers a soil wet a few feet beneath the surface; in California it thrives where the moist ocean air meets the coast. It requires a fertile garden soil with excellent drainage. It can also be grown from seed that germinates readily. The leaves, the part of the plant used, are harvested before flowering. Plantations where branches of leaves on pruned trees can be harvested en masse are used for the production of essential oils.

Therapeutic Uses

+ *Colds*
+ *Cough*
+ *Asthma*
+ *Emphysema*

Eucalyptus leaves and flowers yield a fragrant essential oil that offers relief for upper respiratory infections, colds, coughs, and asthma. The volatile oils, especially the cineole (also called eucalyptol), in eucalyptus leaf help to relieve coughs; oils in the leaf act primarily as an **expectorant,** stimulating removal of mucus from the lungs. Like thyme oil and other volatile oils, eucalyptus oil causes changes in lung secretions, allowing the mucus and phlegm to be removed more easily by coughing. A great deal of research focuses on the antiviral and antibacterial effects of eucalyptus oil, especially to combat the bacteria and viruses that normally cause upper respiratory infections. In addition, eucalyptus oil fights inflammation, making it a useful component in skin creams and other topical products for skin health and arthritis.

Eucalyptol is also being used to treat asthma and emphysema, due to its success in dilating airways and fighting airway inflammation. In a study of people with emphysema, eucalyptol capsules led to improvement in symptoms when compared with a **placebo** group. A clinical trial on asthmatics taking **steroids** daily found that a dose of eucalyptol 3 times a day facilitated the lowering of steroid doses.

How to Use

TEA: Steep approximately ½ teaspoon dried or fresh eucalyptus leaf in 1 to 2 cups of water for 5 minutes. Drink 3 times daily for a cough.

CAPSULE: Eucalyptol capsules—taken in 200-mg doses 3 times daily—help relieve both emphysema and the breathing problems that come with asthma.

Precautions

Ingested eucalyptus oil can cause nausea, vomiting, muscle weakness, breathing problems, increased heartbeat, and low blood pressure. These symptoms have been reported with ingestion of very small amounts—less than 1 teaspoon. Eucalyptus also may cause low blood sugar, so caution is urged for diabetics. Eucalyptus oil may interact with several medications. Those taking prescription medications should check with a health care provider before beginning any eucalyptus treatment.

Eucalyptus globulus

77

EUCALYPTUS

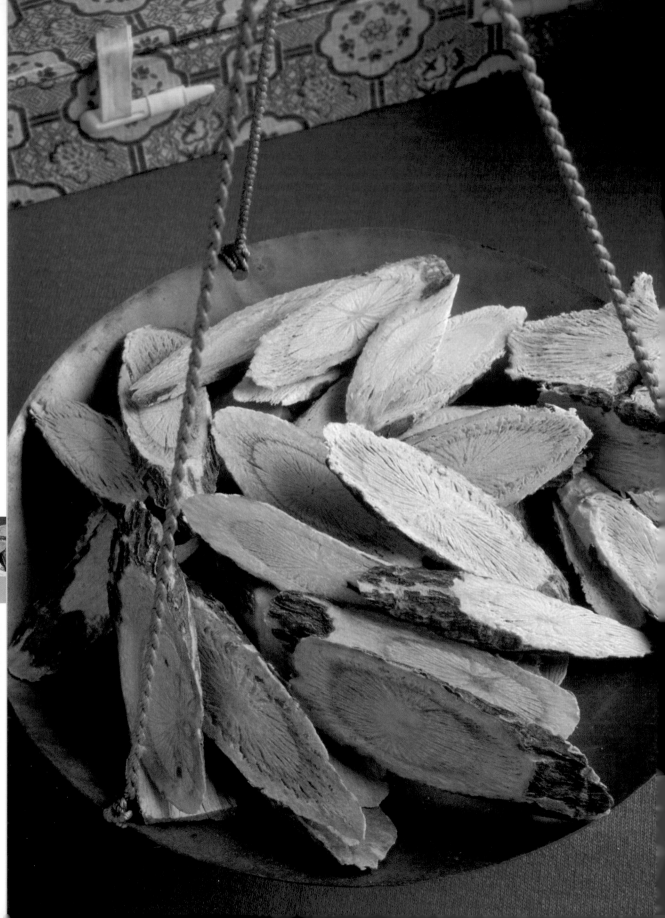

Licorice

Glycyrrhiza glabra

No one knows who first discovered that the tangled, fleshy roots (technically rhizomes) of licorice possess an intense sweetness. But evidence of licorice's use is widespread in ancient cultures. Archaeologists found bundles of licorice root sealed inside the 3,000-year-old tomb of Tutankhamun, presumably so the Egyptian king could brew *mai sus* in the afterlife, a sweet drink still enjoyed in Egypt today. The species known to both the ancient Egyptians and ancient Greeks was *Glycyrrhiza glabra*, commonly called European licorice. The genus name comes

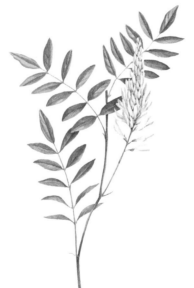

from Greek words meaning "sweet root." But there was more to licorice's appeal than its sweetness. Licorice root was also prized medicinally, primarily as a remedy for digestive and respiratory ailments.

In the third century B.C., Greek physician Theophrastus wrote that licorice was good for asthma, coughs, and diseases of the lungs. In both ancient Chinese medicine and Indian **Ayurvedic medicine,** licorice was given to soothe sore throats. Around A.D. 80, Roman physician Pliny the Elder recommended chewing licorice root to clear and strengthen the voice and to alleviate hunger. Greek and Roman soldiers were issued sticks of licorice root, chewed on long marches to quench thirst and improve stamina. Centuries later, Napoleon

Bonaparte habitually chewed licorice (purportedly it turned his teeth black). Dominican monks are said to have introduced licorice to England when they established a priory near Pontefract Castle in Yorkshire. The monks used licorice **extract** to ease coughs and settle upset stomachs. Eventually, the extracts were formed into lozenges that came to be known as Pontefract cakes.

Licorice root is used in modern herbal medicine for its **anti-inflammatory** properties and for reinforcing the actions of herbs combined with it. Herbal practitioners prescribe licorice root for mouth ulcers, sore throat, laryngitis, coughs, and bronchial infections. In both Europe and Japan, a synthetic form of licorice is prescribed for stomach ulcers.

Herbalists have valued aromatic licorice root—the creeping rhizomes under the soil's surface—since ancient times.

TIME LINE OF USAGE AND SPREAD

1305
Edward I of England taxes licorice imports to finance repairs of London Bridge.

1760
English apothecary adds sugar and flour to an extract to make licorice candy.

1914
American Licorice Company in Chicago produces Black Licorice Vines.

2008
Tom's of Maine discovers how licorice root extract can create foam in toothpaste.

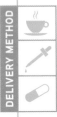

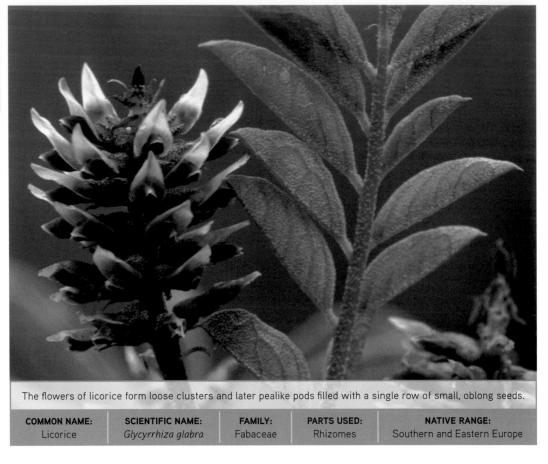

The flowers of licorice form loose clusters and later pealike pods filled with a single row of small, oblong seeds.

COMMON NAME:	SCIENTIFIC NAME:	FAMILY:	PARTS USED:	NATIVE RANGE:
Licorice	*Glycyrrhiza glabra*	Fabaceae	Rhizomes	Southern and Eastern Europe

The genus *Glycyrrhiza* includes 18 species native to drier regions of northwest China and Europe, and one North American species, *Glycyrrhiza lepidota*, not used in the herbal trade. Five species are native to Europe. European licorice (*G. glabra*) has escaped from cultivation and become naturalized in parts of North America. At least 6 species grow in China, 3 of which are source plants for Chinese licorice, known as *gan cao*.

European licorice is a perennial growing 3 to 7 feet tall. The leaves are divided into oval, inch-long leaflets, arranged opposite along a mid-rib. The small, yellow, blue, or purple pealike flowers are borne on short spikes. Chinese licorice (*G. uralensis*) and European licorice are used interchangeably.

Chinese licorice has 13 to 17 opposite leaflets; the stems and flower clusters are covered with glandular dots. The mauve flower blooms from June through August. The main rootstock is a deep, penetrating **taproot**, burrowing to 6 feet below the soil's surface. Creeping horizontal **rhizomes** (runners, or roots just below the surface) radiate from the rootstock. Rhizomes are the licorice root of commerce.

Growing Habits

European licorice is found in dry, open habitats in southern and eastern Europe. It has been cultivated throughout the continent and is naturalized in almost all of Europe, except Scandinavia. Chinese licorice (*G. uralensis*) is found in dry grassy plains and sunny mountainsides and is produced on lime-rich soils in the Chinese provinces of Gansu and Xinjiang and in Nei Mongol. It also occurs in Mongolia and Russian Siberia, eastward to northwest

Steep 1 teaspoon of licorice root in 1 cup of boiling water. Strain and reserve the liquid. Moisten 2 tablespoons of dried hyssop with 2 tablespoons of the licorice liquid. In a saucepan, stir together 1 cup honey, ¼ cup licorice liquid, and moistened hyssop. Bring to a boil, reduce heat, and simmer, covered, for 30 minutes. Strain and refrigerate. A teaspoonful several times a day will not only soothe a sore throat or cough but cater to your sweet tooth as well.

Pakistan. The long, creeping rhizomes are harvested after the third or fourth year of growth.

Cultivation and Harvesting

Licorice can be grown from seed sown in spring in well-prepared seedbeds, but seedlings are slow to develop. Licorice is usually propagated by dividing the root crown or by rhizome cuttings. The cuttings, of about 8 to 20 inches with a bud or "eye," are planted vertically in spring about an inch below the surface, with the plantings spaced 18 inches or so apart. Cuttings should be well watered until plants are firmly established. A moist, fairly rich, well-drained sandy loam is best. Soil pH should be slightly alkaline (7 to 8). Licorice is a plant for warm regions; mild climates ensure vigorous growth. European licorice is produced in Spain, Russia, and the Middle East. Most licorice in international trade originates in China.

Therapeutic Uses

+ *Sore throat*
+ *Cough*
+ *Heartburn*
+ *Gastritis*

This plant, better known as a candy and candy flavoring, also has some medicinal properties. Thanks to its demulcent, or tissue-coating, properties, licorice root can coat sore throats and soothe coughs, heartburn, and gastritis. It is possible that the thick **mucilage** from licorice provides the coating, or alternatively the body may build up secretions in response to **compounds** in licorice. A few research trials have been done, looking at combination products in the treatment of indigestion and asthma and topical treatments for canker sores. A group of compounds in licorice, the **triterpene saponins**, are responsible for the herb's sweetness and possibly also for its antiviral effects and its success in healing stomach ulcers.

How to Use

LOZENGE: For sore throat, a licorice lozenge used every few hours for several days allows the coating properties of licorice to soothe inflamed tonsils and throats.

TEA: To soothe a nagging cough, especially one due to an upper respiratory infection causing nasal drip, try a **decoction** of licorice. Add 1 to 2 teaspoons of chopped licorice root to 2 cups of boiling water. Boil for 10 minutes. Strain, cool, and drink a half cup 3 to 4 times a day for up to 1 week.

TABLET: Heartburn, gastritis, or related conditions requiring licorice treatment for more than a week respond well to deglycrrhizinated licorice, or DGL, tablets, generally, 1 to 2 380-mg tablets before meals and at bedtime.

Precautions

If taken for extended periods, a licorice compound called glycrrhizin can deplete the body's potassium and raise blood pressure. Generally, licorice is safe if taken for less than a week at the doses listed above. For those with gastritis or heartburn needing extended treatment, concerns about potassium and blood pressure can be avoided by taking a DGL product. Those with high blood pressure, kidney or heart troubles, or taking blood thinners or blood pressure medicines should be cautious with any amount of licorice. Not recommended during pregnancy or lactation.

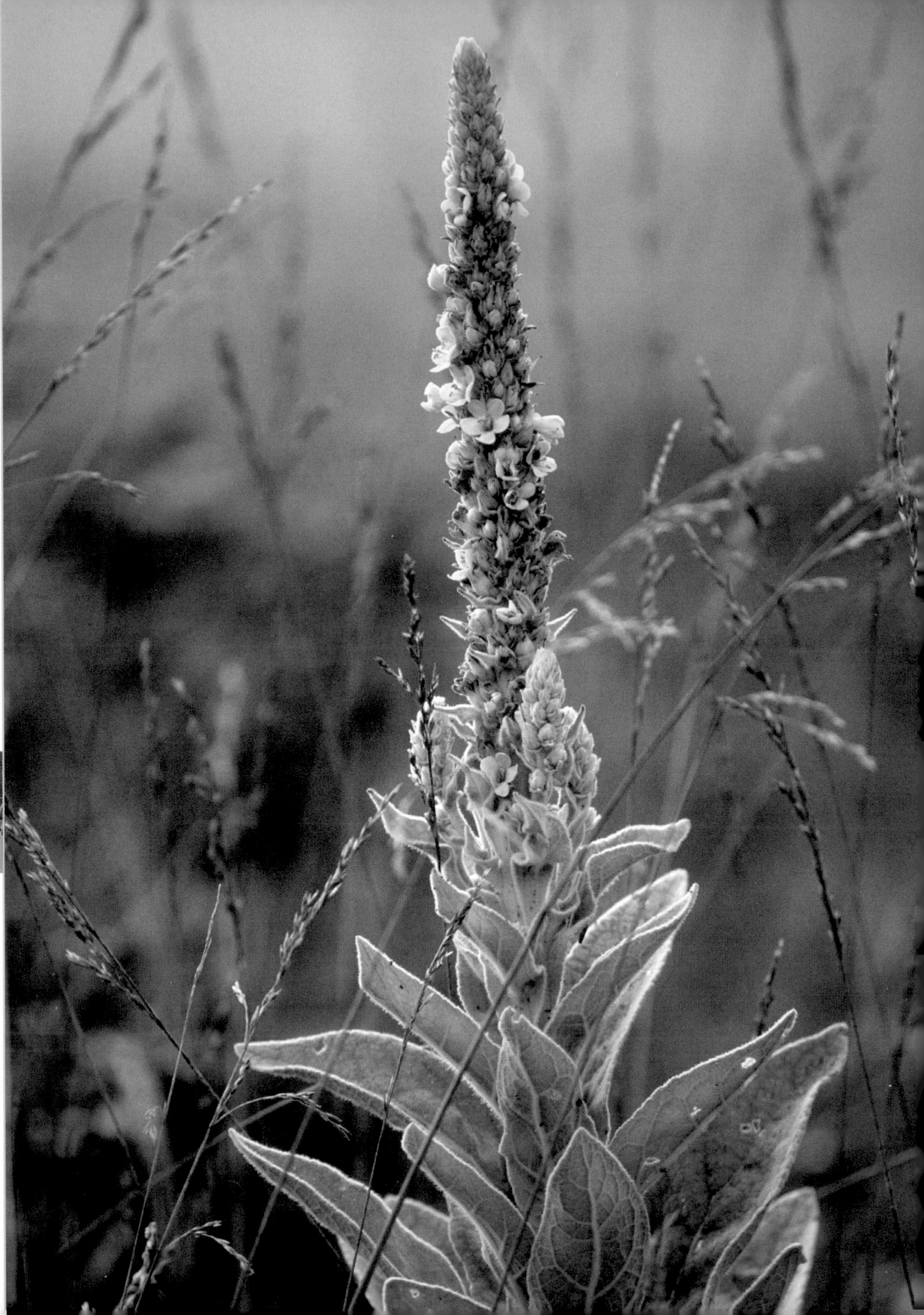

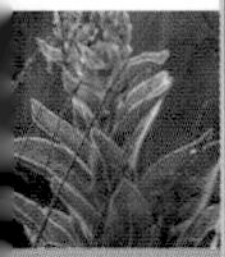

Mullein

⚶ *Verbascum thapsus* ⚶

Homely but charming, mullein has gray-green leaves and stems covered in a velvet cloak of soft, fuzzy hairs. The name mullein may come from the Latin word *mollis,* which means "soft"—an obvious reference to the plant's texture. Several other common names for *Verbascum thapsus* relate to this characteristic as well, including feltwort, flannel-flower, blanket leaf, bunny's ears, and velvet dock. Other common names, including Jupiter's staff and Aaron's rod, refer to mullein's tall flower spikes, which rise up in the second year of its biennial life and are covered in a profusion of small, sunny yellow flowers. The nickname candlewick originated during the Middle Ages, when people collected the downy hairs on mullein leaves and stems, dried them, and wound them into lamp and candle wicks. Dipping the flower stalks in melted fat and using them for torches is a custom that dates to ancient Rome. Over time, these herbal torches moved from the practical to the magical. Called hag tapers, they were supposedly either used by witches or employed by common folk to drive witches away.

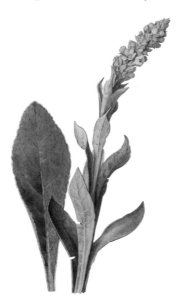

Mullein tea is a very old remedy for respiratory problems. It was brewed from the leaves or flowers, and then carefully strained through cloth to remove any fine plant hairs. During the Middle Ages, mullein tea was prized for its ability to soothe irritated membranes, relieve congestion, and break up phlegm. It was a common folk remedy for coughs, colds, bronchitis, and asthma. **Poultices** of fresh mullein leaves were bound over slow-healing wounds, and **infusions** of the flowers were dabbed on the skin to heal sores, burns, and fungal infections.

European settlers introduced mullein into North America. In the late 1800s, physicians in Europe, the United Kingdom, and the U.S. routinely prescribed mullein for the hacking cough and congestion associated with tuberculosis and other respiratory infections.

Mullein remains a respected remedy in herbal medicine today. Herbalists recommend it for coughs, colds, sore throat, laryngitis, tonsillitis, whooping cough, influenza, and asthma.

Mullein's velvety leaves and diminutive flowers are the sources of the respiratory remedies that come from the herb.

TIME LINE OF USAGE AND SPREAD

1753
Carolus Linnaeus describes *Verbascum thapsus* in his *Species Plantarum.*

1849
During the California gold rush, miners use mullein torches to light mine shafts.

1916
Mullein is listed in U.S. *National Formulary* (and removed in 1936).

2002
Clemson University researchers report mullein kills disease-causing bacteria.

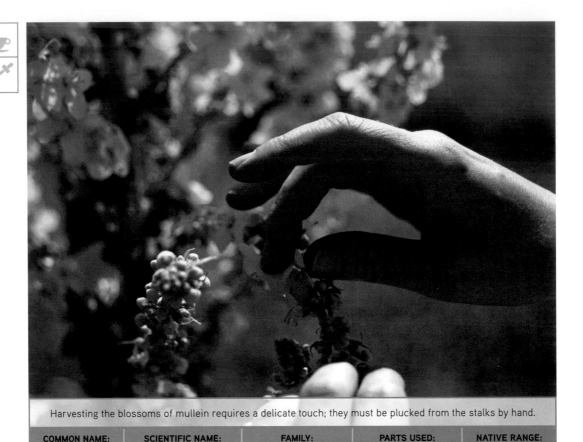

Harvesting the blossoms of mullein requires a delicate touch; they must be plucked from the stalks by hand.

COMMON NAME:	SCIENTIFIC NAME:	FAMILY:	PARTS USED:	NATIVE RANGE:
Mullein	*Verbascum thapsus*	Scrophulariaceae	Leaves, Flowers	Europe, Asia

The genus *Verbascum* contains more than 350 species of herbaceous plants, most native to Eurasia. Nearly 90 species occur in Europe, and in Turkey alone there are some 230 species. Usually biennial herbs (though sometimes annual) that are shrubby in habit, mulleins are often characterized by a distinct basal rosette of leaves. Common mullein is a biennial that in the first year produces a basal rosette of long, flannel-soft, fuzzy, lance-shaped leaves up to a foot long and 5 inches wide. The entire plant is covered with branching hairs. The edges have rounded teeth. In the second year, a flower stalk shoots up from the center, some 6 feet or more. This spike is crowded toward the top with yellow inch-long flowers, closely hugging the furry wand.

Verbascum is the Latin name for the plant, perhaps derived from *barbascum,* referring to the bearded filaments supporting the stamens. Olympic mullein (*Verbascum olympicum*) is grown for flower harvesting for herbal use. Its branching flower spikes produce far more flowers than does common mullein's towering stalk.

Growing Habits

Common mullein is native to Europe and Asia and undoubtedly arrived in North America with the first European settlers, its seeds likely stowaways in trouser cuffs. It quickly became naturalized over large areas. Officially deemed a noxious weed, it is found throughout the U.S. and Canada, in dry gravelly or sandy soils along roads, dry fields, and dry waste places.

Cultivation and Harvesting

Mullein is not generally grown as a garden plant, and is more likely to be found at the edge of a garden among the weeds, especially in sandy or rocky soil. However, it is easily grown from seed; in fact, part of its success as a **species** is that the seed remains viable for decades.

In a famous seed viability experiment in 1879, Professor William J. Beal of Michigan State University buried 1,000 seeds each of 20 plant species with instructions that the seeds be dug up and tested for viability every decade or so. One was moth mullein *(Verbascum blattaria)*, the seeds of which have remained viable for 120 years.

Mullein leaves are harvested at the end of the first year's growth. Mullein flowers are plucked from the stalks by hand when the plant is in full bloom.

Therapeutic Uses

+ *Ear infections*
+ *Respiratory infection (such as colds, bronchitis)*

The flannel-soft leaves and stems of the mullein plant have been used for millennia for a host of ailments. Mullein is known for its demulcent, or tissue-coating, properties as well as its **anti-inflammatory**, antiviral, and antibacterial effects. Several **compounds** in mullein combine to provide its medicinal benefits. The **polysaccharides** and **saponins** likely account for the demulcent activity; anti-inflammatory effects come from **glycosides**. The saponins also have an **expectorant** effect.

Despite its long history of use for medicinal purposes, mullein has not been researched extensively. Mullein is thought to ease symptoms of bronchitis, coughs, and other throat ailments. It does so by serving as both an expectorant and a coating and soothing herb for irritated respiratory tissues. Drinking

mullein leaf or mullein flower tea soothes the throat. The historical use of mullein for respiratory troubles such as bronchitis and asthma included smoking the dried leaves and inhaling the compounds. While this use has fallen out of favor due to the known dangers of smoke, it is thought that some respiratory benefits can be obtained by ingesting mullein as an infusion of the leaves or flowers. Various parts are used, including the leaves, flowers, and roots.

> **NOTE:** Mullein seeds are toxic and should not be a part of any mullein extract, capsule, or tea.

How to Use

INFUSED OIL: The classic mullein preparation involves putting mullein flowers in a small clear glass bottle of olive oil and leaving them in a sunny window for 2 to 3 weeks. The preparation can then be strained and placed in a dark brown bottle with a dropper dispenser and stored in a cool place for the long term. To ease the pain from ear infections, use 3 to 4 drops of the olive-oil-and-mullein extraction in the ear every few hours. (Plug the ear with cotton ball to prevent oil from running out. Don't instill if child has ear tubes or drainage from the ear.)

TEA: Pour 2 cups of boiling water over 1 tablespoon dried mullein leaf and flowers. Strain. Drink 1 cup, 2 to 4 times daily.

TINCTURE: Take 1 to 4 ml, 3 times daily, or follow manufacturer's directions.

Precautions

Aside from the seeds, mullein is considered to be safe and generally well tolerated.

---

over the (kitchen) counter TRIPLE GOOD TEA

Mix equal parts marshmallow root, mullein, and licorice root. Add 1 teaspoon of the mixture to a cup and add boiling water. Steep for 5 minutes, strain, and sweeten with honey, stevia, or rice syrup. A soothing tea for sore throats and laryngitis! Do not use for more than 7 days.

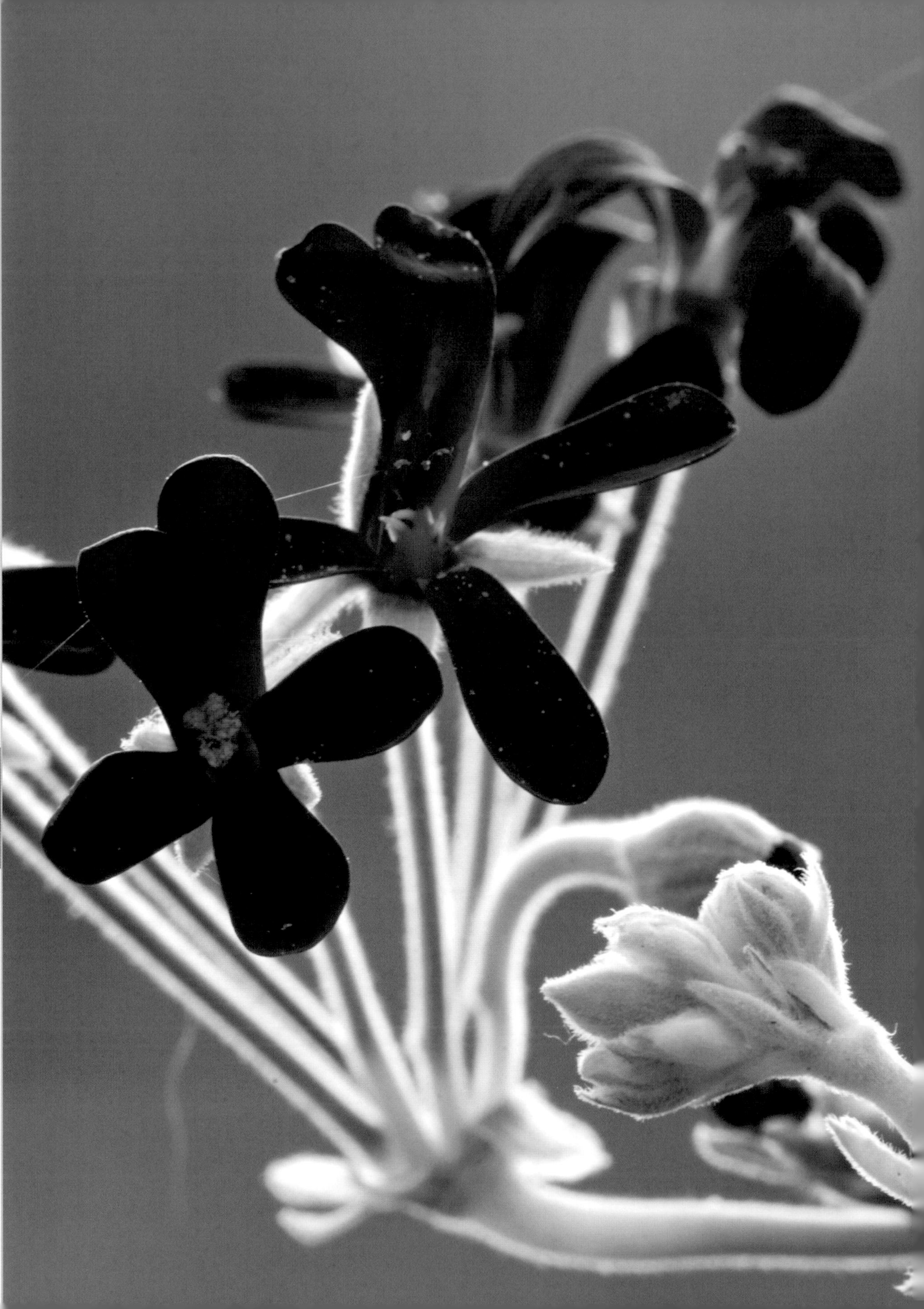

Pelargonium

Pelargonium sidoides

More than 280 species of flowering plants make up the genus *Pelargonium*. Most are native to southern Africa, and many of them are known as geraniums or, less commonly, storksbills because a part of the flower looks like a stork's beak. The resemblance was not lost on the ancient Greeks, as the name *Pelargonium* comes from *pelargós,* meaning "stork." The common name, geranium, came to be associated with pelargoniums as the result of an early botanical misclassification. True geraniums belong to the genus *Geranium* and are hardy perennials. Pelargoniums are grown for their flowers and pleasantly scented leaves. Other **species** have a long history of medicinal use in Africa. *Pelargonium sidoides*—known in modern herbal medicine simply as pelargonium—is one of these.

For centuries, traditional Zulu, Xhosa, Basuto, and Mfengu tribal healers used the plant's thick, brown roots to make herbal preparations to treat primarily respiratory ailments, but also diarrhea, intestinal problems, liver complaints, wounds, fevers, and fatigue. European settlers to South Africa may have known of these herbal remedies for some time, but pelargonium was not introduced to the West until 1897, when Englishman Maj. Charles Stevens was treated for tuberculosis with a pelargonium root preparation by a tribal healer. Pronounced

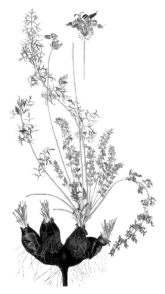

disease free on his return to England, Stevens marketed a patent medicine made from pelargonium called Stevens' Consumption Cure. It was used for a time to treat tuberculosis patients. Pelargonium was largely forgotten until the 1980s, when a European company began marketing an **extract** of pelargonium for colds and respiratory infections called Umckaloabo, a name derived from the Zulu. A similar product is now sold in the United States.

Herbal practitioners recommend pelargonium to help reduce the symptoms of respiratory infections such as coughs, colds, sore throats, pneumonia, tonsillitis, and acute sinusitis, and to prevent secondary infections such as chronic bronchitis. It is often used as an alternative to antibiotics in some of these conditions.

The deep purple blooms of pelargonium catch the eye, but it's the fleshy, tuberous roots that are used medicinally.

TIME LINE OF USAGE AND SPREAD

1920	1983	2002	2008
Swiss tuberculosis patients are successfully treated with Stevens' Consumption Cure.	German drug companies market *P. sidoides* root under the name Umckaloabo.	Sales of Umckaloabo top $55 million annually.	Zucol, a pelargonium-based cold remedy, is made available in the United States.

The genus *Pelargonium* is primarily a South African plant group with some 280 species. It is the source of many of the "geraniums" of greenhouses, as well as dozens of cultivated varieties and "flavors" of the common herb garden plants known as scented geraniums. Smaller than many Pelargoniums, *P. sidoides* is a perennial growing 8 to 20 inches tall, arising from a mound-like cluster of leaves. The evergreen, silvery gray, velvety, scented leaves are rounded to a heart shape and crinkled with scalloped leaf edges. The flower stalks hold loose groups of maroon, almost black flowers about an inch in diameter. *P. sidoides* generally flowers in late spring and early summer. The tuberous root is the part used. Other fleshy tuberous-rooted pelargoniums, including *P. antidysentericum, P. luridum, P. rapeceum,* and *P. reniforme,* are used interchangeably by **indigenous** groups and settlers of South Africa, most famously for the treatment of dysentery and diarrhea. Recently, the plant group has been useful for treating bronchitis and other lung conditions, particularly in children.

Growing Habits

Native to South Africa, *P. sidoides* is adapted to dry, bright, sunny grasslands, which are often subject to fires. The plant survives by retreating to the succulent tuberous root from which leaves spring forth as moisture reaches it. *P. sidoides* is often seen along rocky outcrops of the South African coast, and throughout the eastern Cape of South Africa, Lesotho, Free State, and southern and southwestern Gauteng.

Cultivation and Harvesting

Pelargonium sidoides is easy to grow as a potted houseplant. It is considered a tender perennial, but in its native habitat it experiences winter frost and snow cover. In warmer regions it can be planted outside in a rock garden in a gritty, well-drained, sandy, or rocky soil. The plant likes a hot, sunny situation and is drought tolerant. Propagation is by seeds

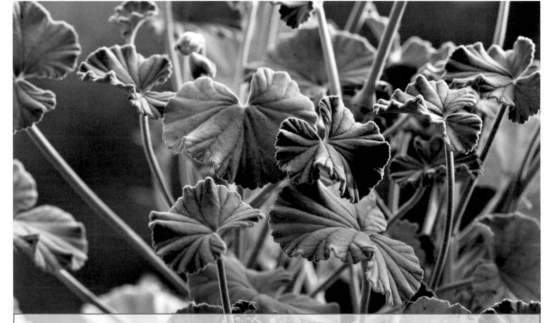

P. sidoides belongs to a group of plants often called scented geraniums for their remarkably aromatic leaves.

COMMON NAME:	SCIENTIFIC NAME:	FAMILY:	PARTS USED:	NATIVE RANGE:
Pelargonium	*Pelargonium sidoides*	Geraniaceae	Roots	Coastal South Africa

or cuttings taken from the base of the plant. Cuttings can be dipped in a rooting hormone and placed in coarse sand or pea gravel and watered until rooting occurs.

This species is grown on a small commercial scale in South Africa and exported to both Europe and the United States. Most locally used tubers in South Africa are supplied from wild-harvested plants.

Therapeutic Uses

+ *Bronchitis*
+ *Colds and flus*
+ *Sinusitis*

Pelargonium extracts and isolated **compounds** from pelargonium have been found to inhibit many of the bacteria commonly associated with sinus infections and bronchitis. Laboratory tests have also confirmed pelargonium's immune-boosting effects. Pelargonium's antibacterial and antiviral effects are thought to come from gallic acid and other **phenols**, compounds in plants that seem to play a protective role as **antioxidants**. Pelargonium's role in improving immune system function may stem from these same phenols, though compounds called **coumarins** are also thought to provide some of the immune-boosting effects.

In a study of 217 people with acute bronchitis, an improvement in symptoms, after just 3 days, was seen in the group taking 30 drops of an alcohol extract of pelargonium root (Umckaloabo) for 7 days, when compared with a group that was taking a **placebo**. Symptoms showing significant improvement included cough, phlegm production, fatigue, and hoarseness; people in the pelargonium group were able to go back to work sooner than those who were in the placebo group. Another analysis of 6 studies agreed with this result and reported the lack of serious adverse effects in people assigned to the pelargonium groups of clinical trials.

Fewer research results exist for the use of pelargonium for sinus infections or the common cold. One study of people with cold symptoms found that those who received 30 drops of Umckaloabo 3 times daily experinced greater improvement in cold symptoms than those in the placebo group. Subjects were surveyed at day 5 of treatment. In this study, pelargonium seemed to work better for stuffiness, sore throat, and hoarseness than for cough, muscle aches, and fever.

How to Use

EXTRACT: Umckaloabo is a clinically tested product that has been shown in clinical trials to be effective in the treatment of bronchitis and the common cold. The extract is available as an alcohol-based product and as an alcohol-free product as well. Follow dosing on the package.

LOZENGES: Zucol lozenges contain pelargonium and are recommended for treating cold viruses.

TINCTURE: Alcohol-based **tinctures** of pelargonium are becoming increasingly available in the marketplace; dosage is generally 1 teaspoon (5 ml) taken 3 to 4 times per day.

Precautions

Pelargonium root extracts are generally well tolerated, though some users report mild stomach upset, rashes, and nervous system disorders. Allergic reactions are occasionally reported. Umckaloabo may cause rash, itching, swelling, or more serious allergic reactions. Safety in pregnancy and lactation has not been established.

---

over the (kitchen) counter RESPIRATORY RELIEF

Add 2 tablespoons dried pelargonium root and 2 tablespoons dried mullein leaves to 2 to 3 cups boiling water. Reduce heat and simmer gently for 10 to 15 minutes. Strain and add 1 to 2 teaspoons honey. Drink 2 to 4 cups of the tea daily and as needed for congestion and cough.

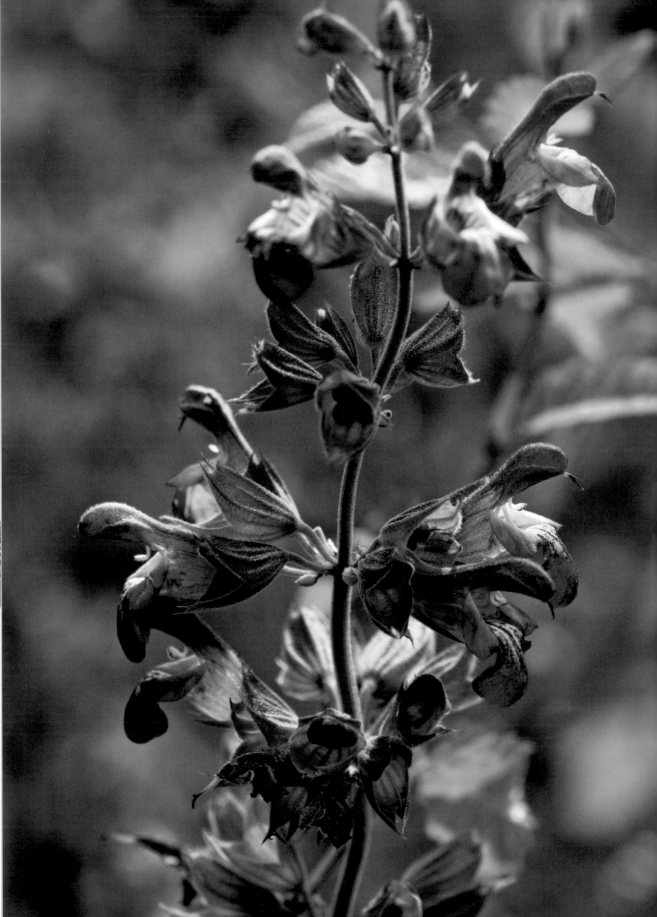

Sage

Salvia officinalis

A classic seasoning herb for poultry and many savory dishes, sage is a highly aromatic, shrubby perennial native to the northern Mediterranean coast. The genus name, *Salvia,* comes from the Latin *salvere,* meaning "to be saved" or "to be healed." Sage was sacred to the ancient Greeks and Romans; they believed it imparted wisdom and mental acuity. The Romans gathered the herb in a solemn ceremony that involved using a knife not made of iron, as sage reacts with iron salts. For many centuries, sage has also been linked with good health and long life.

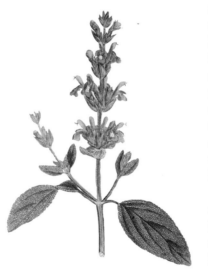

Eighteenth-century herbalist John Evelyn took that one step further, writing that sage "'tis a Plant endu'd with so many and wonderful Properties, as that the assiduous use of it is said to render Men Immortal."

Medicinally, sage has played a role in many healing traditions. The ancient Egyptians believed sage could increase fertility. The Greeks drank preparations of sage to ease coughing and respiratory infections. In India, herbal healers gave patients sage to reduce soreness of the mouth and throat and to relieve indigestion. The Romans probably introduced sage to much of Europe and England, where it has been planted in herb and kitchen gardens since medieval times. Herbals written during the Middle Ages record that sage was used for a wide variety of ailments. In fact, the French called the herb *toute bonne,* which means "all is well." Sage was prescribed for coughs, colds, and headaches, as well as to purify the blood and aid conception. Sage leaves also were chewed to whiten yellowing teeth.

Today, sage-based natural deodorants are sold at most health food stores since sage can reduce perspiration. Many natural mouthwashes contain sage, as it kills bacteria responsible for gum disease. Modern herbal practitioners recommend sage for coughs, colds, and bronchitis. Hot sage tea can soothe sore throats and tonsillitis. Sage is also taken for gastrointestinal disorders and menopausal symptoms and to slow dementia.

Sage's delicate, blue-violet flowers and coarse, woolly, gray-green leaves have been used medicinally for millennia.

TIME LINE OF USAGE AND SPREAD

A.D. 50-70	1597	17TH CENTURY	1772
Greek physician Dioscorides writes of sage's use in stopping bleeding in wounds.	English herbalist John Gerard describes sage as "good for the head and braine."	*Salvia officinalis* is introduced to North America.	*The Virtues of British Herbs* credits regular intake of sage with living to advanced age.

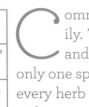

Common garden sage is a member of the largest genus in the mint family. There are 800 to 900 species of *Salvia*, most found in the subtropics and tropics of the New World. Among this great pool of genetic diversity only one species, *Salvia officinalis*, is found in every kitchen spice rack and nearly every herb garden. As the species name *officinalis* signifies, it was once the "official" sage of the apothecary's shop. Sage is a perennial shrub, growing to about 2 feet in height. The erect, branched stems have dense, entangled woolly hairs that give it a silver-gray appearance. Opposite on short stalks, the 3-inch leaves are greenish blue above, with crinkled veins. Beneath, the leaves are white and hairy. The attractive flowers, about an inch long and tall, are usually blue to violet but may also be pink or white.

Growing Habits

Common garden sage is native to dry rocky soils, stony slopes, and dry grasslands from northern and central Spain east through southern France to the Balkan Peninsula. There it is abundant in coastal mountain ranges in Albania, Montenegro, and Croatia.

The common name "sage" is applied to many plants, often with a qualifying term. Some sage found in world markets is not *Salvia officinalis* but *Salvia frutiosa*. When sage is harvested from the wild in Eastern Europe, proper identification is important, as *S. fruticosa* has higher levels of the toxic substance thujone in its **essential oil**.

Cultivation and Harvesting

Sage is propagated from seeds or cuttings. If grown from seeds, resulting plants are highly variable. Germination is also sporadic. Sage is best propagated from new growth stem cuttings taken from the plant's base, then dipped in a rooting hormone to stimulate growth and placed in coarse sand. Before planting outside, young plants should be grown in a protected situation until they become vigorous. Plants should be given a 2-foot spacing. Sage likes a loose, well-drained soil, without too much moisture.

Even though sage is widely cultivated as a garden herb, the majority of the world's sage supply is wild-harvested in coastal mountains in Croatia, Montenegro, and Albania. International sanctions imposed on former Yugoslavian states in the early 1990s resulted in Albania's emergence as the world's major supplier of sage.

Therapeutic Uses

+ *Sore throat*
+ *Colds and coughs*
+ *Memory*
+ *Menopause*
+ *Excessive sweating*

Sage is said to clear the mind and improve memory. In fact, there *may* be a link between the herb and the mind. Researchers have shown that the essential oil of *Salvia officinalis* inhibits acetylcholinesterase, an **enzyme** targeted by Alzheimer's drugs. Animal studies and human trials suggest sage may improve mood and cognition in both healthy adults and those with Alzheimer's dementia.

Sage tea has long been used as a remedy for sore throats, often being used as a gargle, as well as for coughs and colds. Science has confirmed

over the (kitchen) counter SAGE GARGLE

Combine 1 ounce dried sage leaves and 1 ounce dried thyme leaves in a coffee grinder. Grind and place in a quart mason jar. Cover with 16 ounces apple cider vinegar, stir, and close jar with tight-fitting lid. Let sit for 14 days, shaking periodically. Strain and put in a dark-colored bottle. This mouthwash can be safely used for sore throats or also to freshen breath.

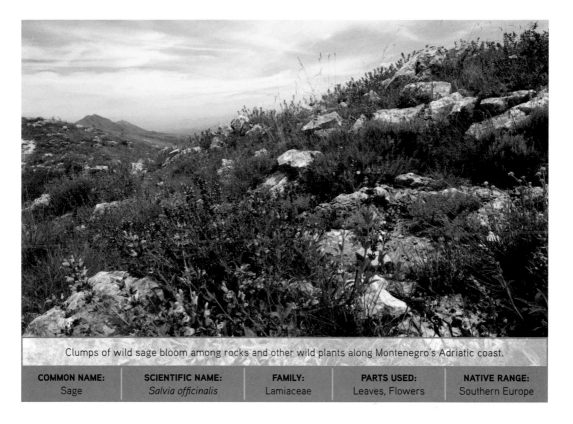

Clumps of wild sage bloom among rocks and other wild plants along Montenegro's Adriatic coast.

COMMON NAME:	SCIENTIFIC NAME:	FAMILY:	PARTS USED:	NATIVE RANGE:
Sage	*Salvia officinalis*	Lamiaceae	Leaves, Flowers	Southern Europe

that sage is highly effective for relieving sore throat. One clinical trial of 286 people with acute sore throat found a 15 percent sage spray given over a period of 3 days to be superior to a **placebo** spray for relief of symptoms. In fact, symptom relief occurred within 2 hours of the first treatment. Similar results were found when an echinacea/sage spray was compared with a chlorhexadine/lidocaine spray in 154 patients with acute sore throat.

Germany's health authorities approve the use of sage as a treatment for excessive sweating based on traditional use and human studies. Sage may also have weak **estrogenic** properties, which may explain why it has been used to relieve night sweats associated with menopause. An 8-week study found that 1 gram fresh sage was superior to **placebo** for relieving night sweats. Sage is often included in combination with other herbs designed to relieve hot flashes and night sweats, and to improve memory and mood.

Sage has been used to aid digestion, stimulate digestive enzymes, and alleviate intestinal cramping; hence its use with beans or other gas-producing foods. Sage exhibits antibacterial activity, which may explain its use for gastroenteritis, or for other minor GI tract infections.

How to Use

TEA: Steep 1 teaspoon chopped sage in 1 cup water for 10 minutes. Strain. Drink or use as a gargle for sore throat.

CAPSULE: 500 mg sage leaf taken twice a day.

TINCTURE: Take 2 ml, twice a day, or follow manufacturer's recommendation. A **tincture** of 5 ml can be added to 1 cup water and used as a gargle 3 times per day.

Precautions

The amount of sage consumed as a culinary herb is safe, but avoid larger amounts because of thujones present in the essential oil. Do not exceed recommended doses. Alcohol **extracts** of sage are higher in thujone than those made with water and should not be used internally for more than 1 to 2 weeks; a tincture diluted in water and used as a rinse or gargle is safe. Do not use sage internally during pregnancy.

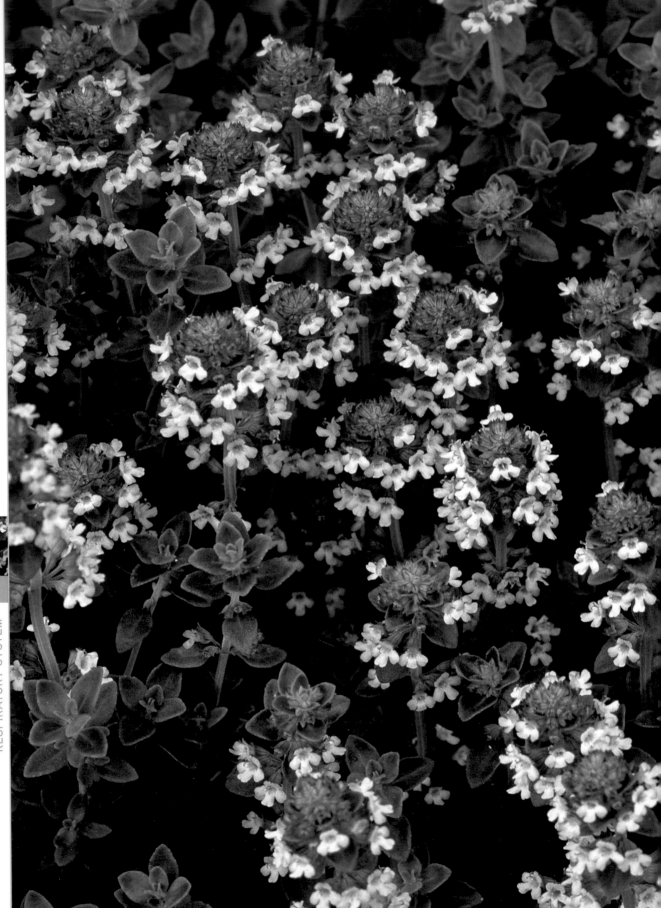

Thyme

Thymus vulgaris

Common thyme is an uncommon herb. Its diminutive leaves give off an invigorating fragrance and impart an agreeable depth of flavor to almost any dish containing meat. Thyme is traditionally bundled together with parsley and bay leaf to form the French bouquet garni and dropped into soups, stews, and other savory dishes while they simmer. Tiny thyme leaves also contain a volatile oil with remarkable antiseptic properties. The ancient Etruscans and Egyptians used thyme oil in embalming their dead. Many early cultures associated thyme with death, and the minute, pale purple flowers were thought to provide a resting place for the souls of those who had died. The ancient Greeks burned thyme as part of funeral rites, as incense in temples, and as a fumigant to chase insects from houses. But they also believed that the herb had the power to instill courage. Thyme's **genus** name may be derived from either the Greek word for "courage" or "to fumigate." The link to courage, however, followed thyme to England, when the Romans introduced it there. During the Middle Ages, ladies of the court presented their brave knights with scarves embroidered with a sprig of thyme.

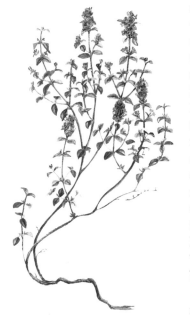

Thyme has been used medicinally since at least the first century A.D. The Greeks considered it a remedy for nervous conditions; the Romans used it to treat melancholy and to revive those who had fainted or suffered an epileptic attack. In medieval Europe and England, it was used to cure everything from digestive upsets to rheumatism and menstrual complaints. Thyme tea was a cure for coughs and flu. In recent centuries, it gained popularity as an effective treatment for digestive problems and lung infections. Until World War I, thyme oil served as a battlefield **antiseptic**.

Today, herbal practitioners recommend thyme for coughs, colds, flu, bronchitis, and asthma. They also give the herb for digestive upsets, as thyme has a relaxing effect on the smooth muscles of the stomach and intestines.

The diminutive size of thyme's flowers and leaves belies its potency as an herb for treating respiratory ailments.

TIME LINE OF USAGE AND SPREAD

50–70 A.D.
Roman physician Pliny the Elder says thyme cures "aberrations of the mind."

1719
German chemist C. Neumann isolates thymol, the active ingredient in thyme oil.

1767
In *The English Physician, Enlarged,* thyme is called "a strengthener of the lungs."

1994
Tobacco firms publish list of substances, including thyme oil, added to cigarettes.

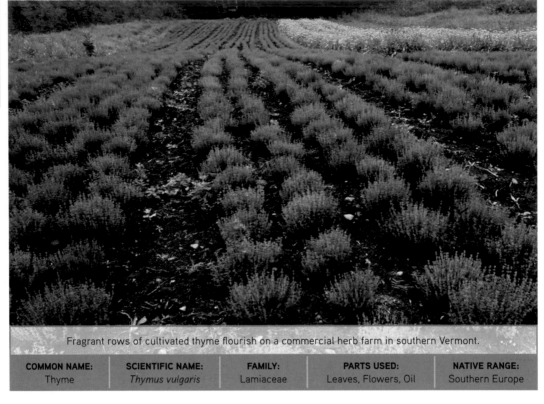

Fragrant rows of cultivated thyme flourish on a commercial herb farm in southern Vermont.

COMMON NAME:	SCIENTIFIC NAME:	FAMILY:	PARTS USED:	NATIVE RANGE:
Thyme	*Thymus vulgaris*	Lamiaceae	Leaves, Flowers, Oil	Southern Europe

There are more than 220 species in the genus *Thymus*, most of which are low-growing, often ground-creeping, small evergreen shrubs native to the Mediterranean region. The most familiar thyme, as suggested by the species name *vulgaris*, meaning "common," is *Thymus vulgaris*. A perennial shrub, often clambering over rocks and dry, gravelly soils, thyme grows to 12 inches. The small, lance-shaped, elliptical or oval leaves, up to ⅜ of an inch long, are arranged opposite on short stalks. Rubbing the leaves releases a pungent lemony scent, the fragrance that we know as thyme. Tiny whitish pink to pale lavender flowers are borne in tight, whorled terminal heads. The upper and lower teeth of the two-lipped calyxes differ in size or shape between the upper and lower segments. Thyme blooms from May through August.

Growing Habits

Native to dry, rocky soils of southern Europe, thyme is particularly associated with Spain, Portugal, southern France, Italy, and the mountains of Greece. It was grown in English gardens by 1548 and known to be cultivated in American gardens by 1806 or earlier. Historically, a form with narrow leaves was grown in gardens on the continent in northern Europe, and referred to as "narrow-leaved thyme." The wider leaf of the form grown in England was called broad-leaf thyme, today sold as English thyme. Whatever its origins, common thyme is highly variable.

Cultivation and Harvesting

Common thyme has been a staple "pot herb" or "sweet herb" of gardens for centuries. Thyme is propagated by seeds, cuttings, layering, or by root divisions. Of course, you can also ask a friend for a division or buy a plant at almost every nursery. To remain true to the plant's desired genetic traits it is best to propagate by cuttings or root divisions. If grown from seed, unexpected variation may occur. Thyme likes room to spread, and should be given at least a 1-foot spacing. After 3 or 4 years it tends to become woody and die out in the center. Clumps can be divided to expand plantings and improve appearance. Thyme likes a light, warm, dry, well-drained soil with a slightly alkaline pH. Most thyme in commercial markets is cultivated in eastern and western Europe.

As a low-growing plant, thyme presents challenges for commercial production. Hand-harvesting is labor-intensive, backbreaking work akin to attempting to mow a lawn with a pair of scissors. A solution developed by foreign specialty producers to reap the crop is a unique mechanical harvester with horizontal rotary blades, something like a weed eater on **steroids**. Much of the thyme consumed in the U.S. was produced here until recently, but like many other commodities and manufacturing processes, thyme production has moved to countries with cheaper labor or innovative technologies for minor specialty crops.

Therapeutic Uses

+ *Coughs*
+ *Colds and flu*

Thyme is one of several fragrant herbs that double as spices and medicines. The aromatic **compounds**, also called **essential** or volatile oils, are the important part of thyme leaves and flowers. The volatile oils in thyme help to relieve coughs, probably in two different ways. Thyme is antispasmodic and an **expectorant**, meaning that the herb not only calms coughs but also helps clear bronchial mucus. It is also antibacterial and antiviral.

Several volatile oils in thyme, including thymol and carvacrol, account for its aroma. Much of the research on carvacrol comes from studies of oregano oil, which is also rich in carvacrol. Carvacrol and thymol are also the oils that account for thyme's expectorant effects and for its inhibition of bacteria, viruses, and fungi. Many bacteria and viruses shown in lab tests to be inhibited by thyme oil are the same ones that cause upper respiratory infections or colds—possible support for its long-standing traditional use.

Few clinical trials have examined the use of thyme for coughs or respiratory infections. One study used a product combining thyme with evening primrose oil in people suffering from bronchitis; the group taking the thyme product showed less coughing than those taking a **placebo** capsule. However, this study, which does not separate out the effects of thyme by itself, or in other types of infections or coughs, does not offer conclusive results.

How to Use

TEA: Steep 1 to 2 teaspoons fresh or dried thyme leaves and flowers in 1 cup of hot water and drink 3 times daily.

CAPSULE/SYRUP: Thyme **extracts** are available as capsules and syrups in a variety of doses and strengths. These products often combine thyme with other herbs thought useful for respiratory conditions; specific use depends on each product.

Precautions

Thyme is safe, especially when consumed as an **infusion**—made by steeping thyme in hot water. Stomach upsets are rare. Consumption of thyme essential oil—as with any essential oils—should be avoided in high doses or for long periods of time.

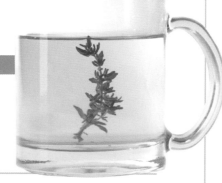

---

over the (kitchen) counter THYME FOR TEA

Steep 1 teaspoon of dried thyme leaf in a cup of hot water. Cover the cup with a saucer so that the important volatile oils do not evaporate. Strain and add honey to taste. Honey complements the expectorant action of thyme by coating the back of the throat. Drink a cup of the tea several times daily for coughs.

CHAPTER THREE

Heart
and
Circulation

Plants *and the* Heart

After Hippocrates, one of the most influential medical personalities of antiquity was Claudius Galen (ca A.D. 129-ca 203), a man of Greek origin with an eclectic education who eventually became the personal physician of the Roman emperor Marcus Aurelius. Galen was familiar with essentially all the medical knowledge of his day—he wrote voluminously about it—and had a particularly inquisitive and experimental mind-set. He was renowned for taking on difficult cases that no other physician would attempt. He also specialized in creating his own preparations of medicinal herbs, and made them with different degrees of potency in order to treat illnesses or dysfunctions of varying severity. Distrustful of the quality, and perhaps identity, of the herbs typically sold in Rome's markets, Galen often gathered his own medicinal plants and personally prepared the prescriptions he gave to his patients. ☜☞ Galen's interest in anatomy also set him apart. In his day, very little was known about how the body's various

systems actually worked. Confusion and myth, for example, surrounded the nature of the heart and the blood. Many of Galen's contemporaries believed that air entered the lungs and then went directly to the heart, where it was changed into a gaseous "vital spirit" that was subsequently taken up by all the body's parts. Galen was an expert surgeon and used his surgical skills to carry out meticulous dissections of animals in order to study in detail many organs, including the heart and blood vessels. He discovered much about the heart's anatomy, the differences between veins and arteries, and the way blood flows into various parts of the body. But he never quite made the connection between the heart's rhythmic beating and the blood's circulation. It wasn't until 1628, more than 14 centuries after Galen's death, that the mystery of the blood's circuitous path through the body was solved by English physician William Harvey.

Today, we know that the cardiovascular system is responsible for transporting oxygen and other gases, together with hormones, nutrients released from the digestive tract, and disease-fighting cells that play a key role in the immune system. There are three major components: the heart; the blood vessels; and blood, which consists of a fluid called plasma, red and white blood cells, and platelets. Generally, we tend to be most aware of the heart, the fist-size, muscular organ that rhythmically contracts to pump blood through a vast and complex network of tubelike vessels. The heart begins beating long before birth, and continues until the final moments of life. During an average lifetime, the human heart will beat more than 2.5 billion times.

Blood vessels form what are essentially two loops in the body. Blood in the pulmonary loop travels from the heart to the lungs, and then back to the heart again. While in the lungs, the blood releases carbon dioxide, a waste gas produced by cells, and picks up oxygen from the air. Upon returning to the heart, this oxygenated blood is pumped out into the systemic loop, the network of arteries, veins, and tiny capillaries that wind their way through the rest of the body. Blood travels through arteries that gradually decrease in size to hair-fine capillaries, where oxygen leaves the blood to be picked up by cells and carbon dioxide enters. Depleted of oxygen but infused with carbon dioxide, the blood travels back to the heart via the veins. Once there, it immediately enters the pulmonary loop to become oxygenated, and the cycle repeats. A special system of coronary arteries supplies blood directly to the heart.

Despite its natural and enduring strength, the cardiovascular system is subject to problems, like every other body system. Some are congenital and present at birth. Some may develop as a result of injury or illness or as a person ages. Several have been strongly linked to diet, lack of exercise, and other lifestyle choices, as well as stress. Common problems of the cardiovascular system include high blood pressure (hypertension), high blood cholesterol (hyperlipidemia or hypercholesterolemia), abnormalities in the body's ability to utilize blood sugar (diabetes), hardening and clogging of the arteries with fatty deposits (atherosclerosis), and coronary heart disease, which involves narrowings or blockages in the coronary arteries that supply the heart with blood. An estimated 80 million American adults, or roughly 1 in 3, have one or more forms of cardiovascular disease.

Cardiovascular problems may be more common today than they were in Galen's day. But they are hardly new. The physicians of antiquity saw evidence of these afflictions in their patients. By and large, they attempted to cure them—or at least ease their symptoms—using medicinal herbs. Modern herbalists still have some of these very old herbs in their armory of plant prescriptions. They've welcomed several newcomers, too. This chapter surveys nine herbs valued for their positive effects on the cardiovascular system.

Bilberry *(Vaccinium myrtillus)* is a close relative of both cranberry and blueberry. Used since the Middle Ages, bilberry fruits and their extracts are widely prescribed in modern herbal practice to treat a variety of circulatory problems. Recent research has shown that chocolate *(Theobroma cacao)* is a heart-healthy food, able to lower blood pressure and cholesterol and help prevent life-threatening blood clots. Another delicious herb, cinnamon *(Cinnamonum verum),* shows promise as a stabilizer of blood sugar levels in people with type 2 diabetes. Ginkgo *(Ginkgo biloba)* is the sole surviving member of a group of ancient plants. Used in traditional Chinese medicine for at least a thousand years, ginkgo has been shown to improve blood flow to the brain and is used to treat dementia.

In vino sanitas—in wine, there is health—is a phrase attributed to the ancient Romans. There is now growing evidence that certain substances in grapes and wine *(Vitis vinifera)* may help protect blood vessels, reduce "bad" cholesterol, and prevent blood clots. Hawthorn *(Crataegus laevigata)* has been valued by herbalists for treating heart conditions for many centuries, and it remains popular today. Herbalists recommend hibiscus *(Hibiscus sabdariffa)* to help control both blood pressure and cholesterol levels and to prevent atherosclerosis, and extracts of horse chestnut *(Aesculus hippocastanum)* for a number of circulatory problems, including chronic venous insufficiency. Finally, green tea *(Camellia sinensis)* is an ancient drink and medicinal herb that research has shown may help prevent atherosclerosis and heart disease.

Bilberry

Vaccinium myrtillus

Cousin of the blueberry, bilberry is the sweet, dark purple fruit of a branching shrub that seldom grows more than knee high. Ripe bilberries are a bonanza for birds and a heavenly treat for hikers to stumble upon in the forest. Most bilberries grow wild because the plants are difficult to cultivate. Given their wonderful flavor, it's no surprise that bilberries have found their way into almost every imaginable culinary delight, from jams, pies, and tarts to sorbets, liqueurs, and wines. One Irish name for bilberry is *fraughan*, from the Gaelic word *fraocháin*. Traditionally,

the berries are picked on the first Sunday in August, called Fraughan Sunday, which corresponds to an ancient Celtic harvest festival. According to legend, the more bilberries collected on that day, the better the harvest. As it is a medicinal herb, bilberry has been used for centuries to control diarrhea and improve circulation.

Bilberry's use as a medicinal herb seems to date from the early Middle Ages in northern Europe. Tea brewed from bilberry leaves was a folk remedy for treating diabetes. The fruits—fresh, dried, or in preparations—were given as a gentle antidiarrheal aid, especially in children; for nausea, vomiting, and stomach cramps; and as a general intestinal tract tonic. By the 1500s, European herbalists, particularly in Germany, were recommending bilberry for bladder infections,

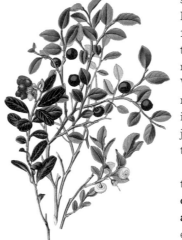

stomach complaints, and more. Herbalists of the 18th and early 19th century used bilberry particularly for dysentery and diarrhea. During the Second World War, English fighter pilots reported that their eyesight improved after they ate bilberry jam. This prompted researchers to investigate.

Bilberry fruits are now known to contain a variety of chemical **compounds** that have potent **antioxidant** properties. In modern herbal medicine, **extracts** of bilberry fruits are used to treat a number of circulatory problems, including varicose veins, **atherosclerosis**, and venous insufficiency. Fruit extracts are effective for treating diarrhea, probably reducing intestinal inflammation. Some take bilberry to maintain healthy eyes, although bilberry's effects on the eye remain uncertain.

Ripe bilberry fruit and leaves are time-honored ingredients in remedies for digestive and circulatory complaints.

TIME LINE OF USAGE AND SPREAD

1539
German physician H. Bock describes bilberry's medicinal properties.

1597
Herbalist J. Gerard writes of "black whortles [bilberries] in creame and milke...."

1878
Bilberries are mentioned in Thomas Hardy's novel *Return of the Native*.

1999
Bilberry sales in the United States top $97 million.

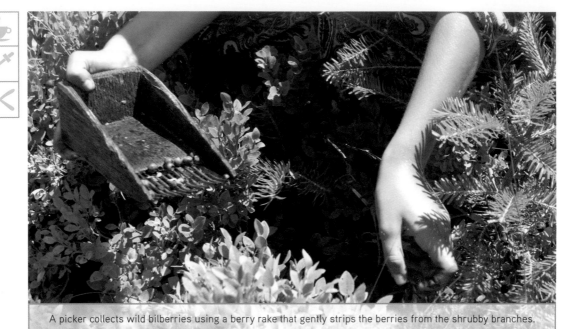

A picker collects wild bilberries using a berry rake that gently strips the berries from the shrubby branches.

COMMON NAME:	SCIENTIFIC NAME:	FAMILY:	PARTS USED:	NATIVE RANGE:
Bilberry	*Vaccinium myrtillus*	Ericaceae	Fruits, Leaves	Northern Hemisphere

Bilberry is one of about 140 species of *Vaccinium* that are primarily found in cooler regions of the Northern Hemisphere. Bilberry is the European equivalent of American blueberries. A major difference between the fruits of the two species, indicated by the familiar blue color of the outer skin, is that the anthocyanadin-rich blue pigment is found throughout the fruit of bilberry; in blueberry, only in the fruit skin. This freely branched shrub, broader than tall, grows to about 18 inches in height, and has **deciduous** leaves, with smooth, green stems. The alternate leaves are flat, mostly oval, with distinctive teeth along the margins. The nodding or drooping, inverted urn-shaped flowers are green to pink-tinged and solitary on leafless stalks. Bilberry blooms from late April through June. The bluish black, sweet fruit ripens mid-July to late August.

Growing Habits

A hike in forests throughout Europe or the mountains of southern Europe (except for Greece) may lead to the chance to pick bilberries in late summer. Bilberry is a common forest understory plant along heaths and moors throughout the continent. Frequently hundreds of plants create large populations. In the mountains of southern Europe, bilberry thrives in open fields and forest margins. It likes soil and subsoil that is rich in humus, common in woods and heaths. Bilberry also occurs in Greenland and mountains of western North America, from British Columbia and Alberta south to Utah, Colorado, northern Arizona, and New Mexico.

The **genus** name *Vaccinium* is the classical Latin name for the plant. The **species** name *myrtillus* refers to myrtle *(Myrtus communis)*, whose leaves resemble those of bilberry.

Cultivation and Harvesting

Wild plants are so common in Europe, bilberry is rarely cultivated. As a specimen plant it is best propagated through layering, taking suckers from the edge of the plant, or by using cuttings of young stems, placed in sand. It likes a slightly acidic, humus-rich, sandy soil and a cool situation. The ripe fruits are available only for a limited 2-week period, so the

Combine 1½ cups fresh or frozen bilberries/blueberries, 1 tablespoon lemon juice, 2 tablespoons dark honey, and a pinch of ground cloves in a saucepan. (Add 2 tablespoons water if using fresh bilberries/blueberries.) Bring to a boil over medium heat, reduce to low heat, and simmer 5 to 10 minutes until juices are slightly thickened. Refrigerate up to 10 days. • Add 2 tablespoons of the juice to sparkling water for a refreshing drink. • Add 2 tablespoons to a yogurt smoothie. • Mix 2 tablespoons with ½ cup olive oil and 1 clove garlic for salad dressing. • Pour over pancakes or waffles.

careful timing of harvest is important for commercial production.

Much of the bilberry supply is wild-harvested in mountains from the Balkans to Scandinavia. Pickers harvest bilberry-rich habitats in late July and early August. Fruits are collected with a berry rake, a small boxlike harvester with long comb teeth that is raked across a plant.

Therapeutic Uses

+ Eye health
+ Antioxidant
+ Diarrhea

Bilberry has long been consumed as both food and medicine. The fruit was enjoyed for its sweet-sour taste and eaten fresh or cooked. Bilberry fruit was also made into syrup and used to treat diarrhea and other digestive problems. This is likely due to the presence of **tannins** that have **astringent** and **anti-inflammatory** activity. Germany's health authorities still approve of the use of the dried, ripe fruit for the treatment of acute diarrhea. However, the majority of research today is focused on the potential use of bilberry fruit for the prevention of age-related diseases.

Bilberry fruit is rich in **anthocyanosides**, plant pigments that have been shown to act as powerful antioxidants in the body. Researchers have found that these powerhouse compounds may help protect the body from heart disease, oxidative stress, and inflammation and help preserve brain function and eye health. A growing body of evidence is linking the relationship of oxidative stress, a condition where there is an increased level of **free radicals** and other oxidation-promoting molecules, to a number of age-related and degenerative diseases. Many fruits and vegetables help reduce oxidative stress, but it is bilberry, and its American cousin, blueberry, that is getting a lot of press. The anthocyanosides seem to have a particular affinity for the eye. Animal studies show that bilberry extracts protect the retina from damage. Two small **double-blind**, **placebo**-controlled studies have shown improvement in patients with diabetes- and hypertension-related retinopathy, serious disorders of the retina that can lead to blindness.

Researchers are also looking at the potential protective effect that bilberry extract may have on colorectal cancer. A study conducted at the University of Leicester in England gave patients with colon cancer a bilberry extract for 7 days and found a 7 percent decrease in cell growth in the tumors when they were surgically removed. This may be due to the ability of the anthocyanadins to prevent the growth of blood vessels in the tissue surrounding a solid tumor. The blood vessels are, in part, what allows the cancer to grow and spread.

How to Use

FRESH BERRIES: 1 cup per day of fresh fruit. American blueberries can be used if bilberries are not available.

TEA: Simmer 1 tablespoon dried berries in 2 cups water for 20 minutes. Strain. Drink ½ cup every 3 to 4 hours for diarrhea.

EXTRACTS: Dosage range is usually 360 to 600 mg per day of an extract standardized to contain 25 percent anthocyanosides (also written as anthocyanadins).

Precautions

There are no known adverse effects. Bilberry may be used as support for the eyes, heart, and gastrointestinal system but should not replace appropriate medical care.

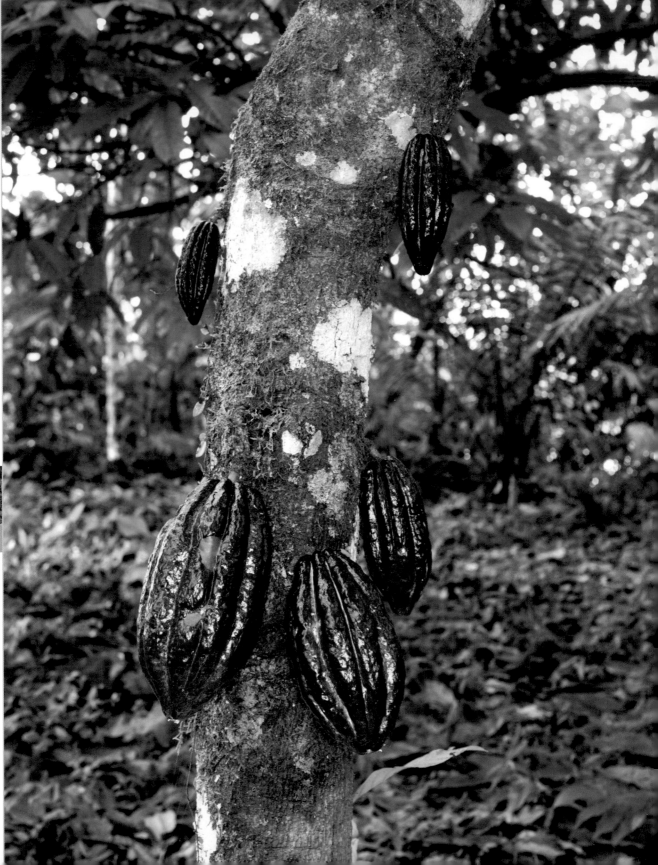

Cacao, Chocolate

Theobroma cacao

For many around the world, life without chocolate would be dismal. Satiny dark or creamy, chocolate is a beloved food intimately linked with celebration, comfort, indulgence, and extravagance. Its source is cacao, a small tree native to Central and South American forests that produces large pods packed with dark brown seeds. From the seeds come fragrant cocoa, luscious chocolate, and creamy cocoa butter. The cultivation of cacao may have originated with the Olmec culture of eastern Mexico more than 3,000 years ago. The Olmec, and later the Maya and Aztec, fermented,

roasted, and then ground cacao seeds into a paste. Mixed with water, chili peppers, cornmeal, and other ingredients, it was whipped into a frothy, spicy chocolate drink. Both the drink, and the seeds from which it was made, were considered sacred. In ancient Mesoamerica, chocolate truly was "the food of the gods," which is what *Theobroma* means.

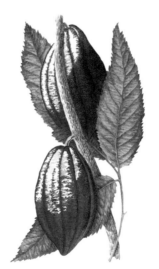

The Spaniards introduced cacao and chocolate into Europe in the early 1500s. They sweetened the bitter brew with sugar, added different spices, and heated it. Before long, hot chocolate had become all the rage, at least among wealthy Europeans who could afford it. As popular as it was as a beverage, however, chocolate was also thought to be a health-promoting drink. From the late 16th century on, European herbals and medical books list dozens of uses for chocolate.

At various times it was considered a remedy for anemia, fever, bronchitis, tuberculosis, fatigue, gout, inflammation, and kidney problems and as an all-around tonic to encourage good health. Cacao butter formed a base for many ointments and salves, and medicines were coated with chocolate to make them more palatable.

Today, chocolate is known to be a rich source of potent **flavonoid antioxidants** (similar to those found in red wine) widely believed to have beneficial cardiovascular effects. Eaten in moderation, pure dark chocolate has been shown to both lower blood pressure and help reduce LDL ("bad") cholesterol in the blood. Chocolate may reduce the risk of heart attack by slowing blood clotting in vessels. Recent research has also shown that eating chocolate may increase a person's chance of surviving a heart attack.

Seeds of colorful cacao fruits, which grow out of the tree's trunk and major branches, are chocolate's source.

TIME LINE OF USAGE AND SPREAD

1500–400 B.C.
The Olmec are believed to be the first to cultivate cacao as a crop.

A.D. 600
Maya establish earliest known cacao plantations in Mexico's Yucatán region.

1753
Swedish naturalist Carolus Linnaeus gives cacao the scientific name *Theobroma*.

1875
The first milk chocolate, made in Switzerland, appears in international marketplace.

Of the 20 South American species of *Theobroma*, only 1 species, *Theobroma cacao,* is the beloved source of chocolate. A small tree, growing to barely 20 feet in height, it has large, alternate, oblong to lance-shaped evergreen, leathery leaves about a foot long. The flowers and fruits are borne on short stalks directly on the trunk or primary branches of the tree. The oblong, 10-ribbed, yellow to purplish fruits ripen to a rich brown and can grow up to a foot long. Inside is a white mucilaginous pulp encasing many seeds—and resembling plump brown lima beans, though they are hard and dense. This is the stuff of chocolate. In the manufacture of chocolate, fatty cocoa butter (an oil) is separated from the cacao "beans" (actually seeds), along with the **alkaloid**-rich, high-protein dry powder, which is cocoa.

Growing Habits

Cultivated in the Americas for millennia, the cacao tree, according to current genetic evidence, originated in the Andean foothills in northern South America and then spread northward into central Mexico through diffusion by humans. Besides *Theobroma cacao,* other **species** of *Theobroma* (or hybrids) are involved in commercial chocolate production, including monkey cacao *(T. angustifolium),* tiger cacao *(T. bicolor),* and cupuacu *(T. grandiflorum).*

Cacao is an understory tree shyly shaded in semidarkness beneath the large rain forest canopy and thriving at elevations of 1,300 to 2,300 feet. It succeeds in a humid climate with little variation in hot temperatures.

The **genus**, *Theobroma,* honors European observations of the sacred position held for cacao in Maya and Aztec cultures. The species name *cacao* (and the word "chocolate") arises in early European literature on the plant as a variation, misprint, or mispronunciation of the Náhuatl (the Aztec language) name *cacahuatl,* a generic designation for cacao-based drinks.

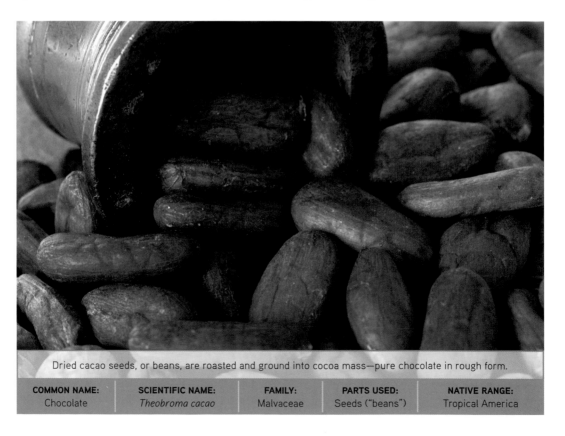

Dried cacao seeds, or beans, are roasted and ground into cocoa mass—pure chocolate in rough form.

COMMON NAME:	SCIENTIFIC NAME:	FAMILY:	PARTS USED:	NATIVE RANGE:
Chocolate	*Theobroma cacao*	Malvaceae	Seeds ("beans")	Tropical America

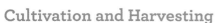
Place ⅔ cup chopped dark chocolatae (or dark chocolate chips) in a microwave-safe bowl and microwave on high for 1 minute. Stir and repeat until chocolate is melted. Sitr ⅛ teaspoon cinnamon into chocolate. Dip the lower half of several dozen strawberries in chocolate, place on plate covered with wax paper. Refrigerate until chocolate is firm. Enjoy several for a heart-healthy dessert!

Cultivation and Harvesting

Chocolate has been cultivated since antiquity by the Maya and earlier civilizations since at least 600 B.C. Widely grown by the Aztec by the time the Spanish arrived, the seeds were still used as currency even in the 1850s. Cacao is produced in many tropical regions as an export for chocolate manufacture. Major producing regions include West Africa, Malaysia, and Brazil, with limited production in Mexico, Central America, and many Caribbean islands. Generally, cacao is cultivated in a band extending 20 degrees above and below the Equator worldwide. A challenging tree to grow, cacao thrives in the understory, not in typical plantation rows. It is therefore planted beneath taller, large-leaved tropicals such as bananas and mangoes.

Therapeutic Uses

+ Antioxidant
+ Heart health (including blood pressure and cholesterol levels)
+ Anti-inflammatory

As more studies emerge linking chocolate consumption to improved cardiovascular health, it is clear that chocolate is both a food and a medicine—not only good but also good for you. Chocolate's main medicinal effects come from a group of **compounds** called **polyphenols** that are strongly antioxidant and **anti-inflammatory**; they also impart to chocolate its dark brown color. Similar compounds are found in green tea, red wine, and many fruits and vegetables. Interestingly, the polyphenols in chocolate seem to act as antioxidants that are stronger than antioxidants in other foods. In humans, these polyphenols are thought to act in several ways. They may stop one of the steps in the development of plaques in coronary arteries by decreasing the oxidation of **low-density lipoprotein (LDL)**, or "bad," cholesterol deposited there; hence LDL plaque does not become as firmly established and is less likely to then rupture and clot, causing a heart attack. The polyphenols also increase the levels of high-density lipoprotein (HDL), or "good," cholesterol protection against cardiovascular disease. These compounds also are mild inhibitors of **platelet** activity, thinning blood in an action similar to that of aspirin.

Another interesting component of chocolate is cocoa butter. By weight, much of chocolate is cocoa butter. Considered a "good" fat, cocoa butter contains oleic acid, a monounsaturated fat also found in olive oil; cocoa butter also contains stearic and palmitic acids, two saturated fats. In combination these fats seem to balance the benefit to the heart and cholesterol levels.

How to Use

Choose a dark chocolate of at least 70 percent cacao to maximize the polyphenol content—and medicinal benefits—of this tasty treat.

Precautions

Due to the small amount of caffeine it contains, along with a related compound, theobromine, chocolate can be stimulating, making it hard to fall asleep after a late-night snack. The fat content of chocolate carries a calorie-heavy punch, so eating too much chocolate can add up. Also, as the percentage of cacao in chocolate drops, it is replaced with milk fats that diminish the benefits of cacao butter and bind healthy polyphenols, making them less absorbable.

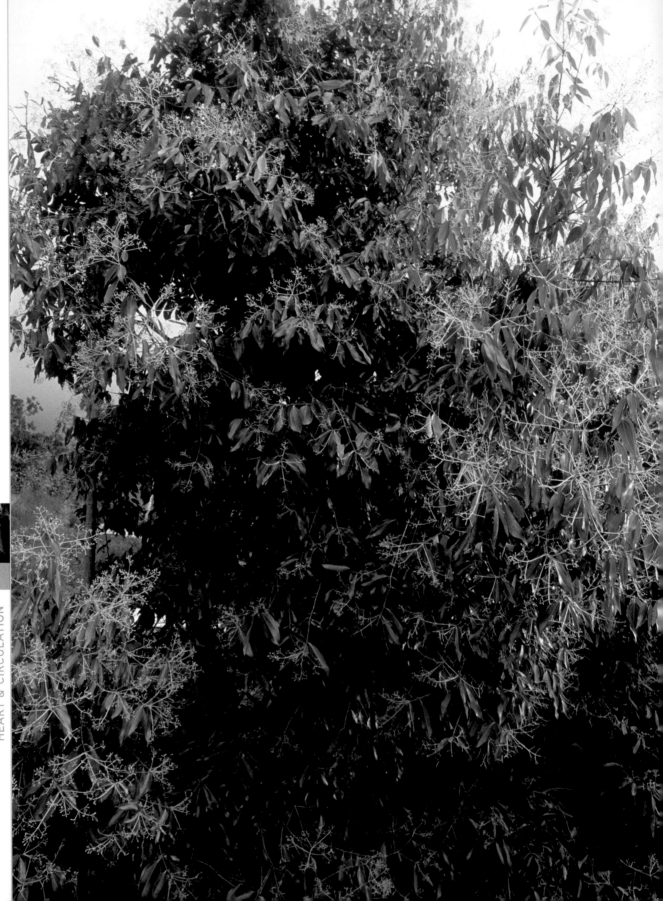

Cinnamon

Cinnamomum verum

The warm, sweet fragrance of cinnamon is unmistakable, evoking visions of hot cinnamon rolls and mulled cider. True cinnamon (*Cinnamomum verum*) is native to the island of Sri Lanka. Cassia, or Chinese cinnamon (*C. cassia*), is a close relative cultivated in Vietnam, China, and Indonesia. Both varieties come from the fragrant inner bark of a tree belonging to the laurel family. Cinnamon was a precious commodity that was traded extensively throughout the ancient world. The Egyptians prized it as an essential ingredient in embalming

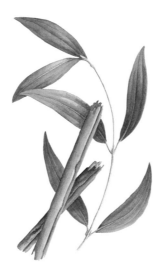

mixtures used to perfume and preserve the dead. Moses of the Old Testament added it to a holy oil for anointing. In Rome during the first century A.D., cinnamon was at least 15 times more expensive than silver, and centuries later, it was still costly. Only the very wealthy in medieval Europe could afford this expensive spice, for which demand was high and supply low. A desire to monopolize the cinnamon trade prompted European expansion into Asia in the 16th and 17th centuries. Eventually, cinnamon became more widely available and affordable.

The first recorded use of cinnamon as a medicinal herb was around 2700 B.C., in China, where it was a treatment for fever, diarrhea, and menstrual problems. In modern Chinese medicine, cinnamon is thought to help circulate vital energy (qi) in the abdomen and

throughout the body. Indian **Ayurvedic** healers used cinnamon primarily for digestive and menstrual complaints. Medieval physicians prescribed cinnamon—for those who could afford it—to relieve coughs, hoarseness, sore throat, and all manner of digestive upsets.

Cinnamon's traditional place in modern herbal medicine has been as a remedy for digestive complaints and a treatment for colds, flu, chest infections, and coughs. The herb is also recommended to improve peripheral circulation, thus increasing blood flow to the hands and feet. More recently, cinnamon has been shown to have an **insulin**-like effect in the blood and may help stabilize blood sugar levels in people with type 2 (adult onset) diabetes. It also may reduce blood cholesterol levels, but more research is needed on both these effects.

Lance-shaped leaves hide the stems of a cinnamon tree, the source of cinnamon bark used as medicine and spice.

TIME LINE OF USAGE AND SPREAD

2000 B.C.
Cinnamon is imported into Egypt.

A.D. 1518
Portuguese traders establish a monopoly on cinnamon that lasts for more than a century.

1650s
The Dutch wrest Ceylon from the Portuguese to control the cinnamon trade.

2006
Sri Lanka produces 90 percent of the world's cinnamon, followed by China.

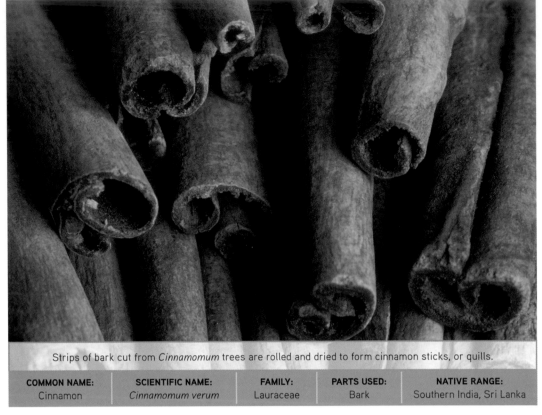

Strips of bark cut from *Cinnamomum* trees are rolled and dried to form cinnamon sticks, or quills.

COMMON NAME:	SCIENTIFIC NAME:	FAMILY:	PARTS USED:	NATIVE RANGE:
Cinnamon	*Cinnamomum verum*	Lauraceae	Bark	Southern India, Sri Lanka

Today about 250 species of *Cinnamomum* are recognized, though more than 450 have been described. Species are distinguished on technical characteristics, which tend to be variable, requiring the knowledge of an expert. *C. verum* is a small evergreen tree up to 35 feet tall, with highly aromatic bark. The smooth leaves are papery to leathery, oval to lance shaped, and up to 6 inches long and 2 inches wide. *C. cassia* (cassia, or Chinese cinnamon) has noticeable leaf hairs above and below (especially when young), with leaf veins fading away from the central leaf axis. *C. burmanni* (Batavia cinnamon) is a larger tree, up to 60 feet, with smooth, leathery ovate to oblong leaves.

The characteristic cinnamon fragrance originates from a **compound** in the **essential oil** known as cinnamaldehyde. Historically, distinguishing the quality of cinnamon bark was as complex as wine tasting. Today however, quality is mainly assessed using chemical analysis.

Growing Habits

The **genus** *Cinnamomum* is primarily concentrated in Southeast Asia, though it also includes **species** from Australia, South Pacific islands, and tropical America. *C. verum* (true cinnamon) is native to and most abundant in Sri Lanka but also produced in the Seychelles, southern India, and Madagascar. *Cassia* is native to southern China and widely cultivated in tropical and subtropical China as well as India, Indonesia, Malaysia, Thailand, and Vietnam. *C. burmanni* is native to sparse or dense forests and thickets, often along streams in southern China, adjacent Vietnam and Myanmar, as well as Indonesia, India, and the Philippines.

Cultivation and Harvesting

Cinnamon and cassia are tropical trees that grow in a range of tropical conditions. The best quality comes from trees grown on white sandy soils, with appropriate amounts of humus. Plants are propagated from seeds or cuttings of young shoots. In the second or third year after planting, trees are coppiced, cut back so as to produce shoots. A half dozen are allowed to grow, and after two years or so, the branches are harvested and cut longitudinally, peeled, and dried to form the cinnamon sticks, or quills, sold commercially. Destructive harvest of wild trees occurs in some regions.

Most imports to the United States come from China, Hong Kong, Indonesia, and Vietnam. Whole cassia and cinnamon bark and ground cassia and cinnamon are considered separate commodities. By the time cinnamon reaches the American consumer, it may be an admixture of several species and grades. Price is a determining factor in quality.

Therapeutic Uses

+ *Diabetes*

Cinnamon may be especially important to people with diabetes. Mainly the bark is used medicinally. A **polyphenol** compound—with the tongue-twisting name methylhydroxychalcone—is found in cassia cinnamon. It is this compound that may be responsible for cinnamon's main medical benefit: lowering blood sugar in people with diabetes. This compound seems to affect insulin receptors and aid in the formation of glycogen, or stored sugar. Cinnamon also has antibacterial effects (from the essential oil) and **antioxidant** effects (from the polyphenols), the latter probably helping with some of the complications of diabetes.

Cassia cinnamon has been studied in clinical trials, primarily by looking at fasting blood sugar

levels in people with diabetes. Although one study found improvements in fasting blood sugar (as much as 29 percent in some cases) and cholesterol levels in people with type 2 diabetes, other studies have found no effect. It may be that cinnamon works better in people whose diabetes is poorly controlled, but there may be other factors, such as genetics and medications, that explain why sometimes cinnamon helps and other times it doesn't.

How to Use

POWDER: For diabetics, powdered cinnamon spice is an option—but for positive effects on blood sugar levels it is necessary to use approximately 1 teaspoon daily. The common spice purchased in grocery stores is not necessarily cassia cinnamon.

CAPSULE: Cinnamon capsules range in dose and suggested use; studies in type 1 and 2 diabetics used 1 to 6 g cinnamon a day, taken in divided doses.

Precautions

Cinnamon is well tolerated, though the volatile oil can cause a skin rash. Cassia and other cinnamons contain small amounts of **coumarin**; blood-thinning and liver problems generally occur with this compound only if large amounts are taken over long periods. To be safe, caution is advised for anyone with liver problems. Due to its blood-thinning effects, cinnamon in quantities greater than use as a spice should end at least one week prior to surgery. Medicinal doses are not recommended during pregnancy. Close monitoring of blood sugar levels in diabetics is warranted to avoid unsafe lowering of blood sugar.

over the (kitchen) counter CINNAMON SPRINKLES

Break a cinnamon stick into several smaller pieces. In a clean spice grinder, grind the chunks into a fine powder. In a small bowl, combine the freshly ground cinnamon with 6 teaspoons of bulk stevia blend (or 12 small packets of stevia blend); mix well. Sprinkle a teaspoon of this mixture on fruit, on plain low-fat yogurt, or add to your morning oatmeal as a delicious treat as well as a digestive and circulatory aid. Better than jimmies on ice cream!

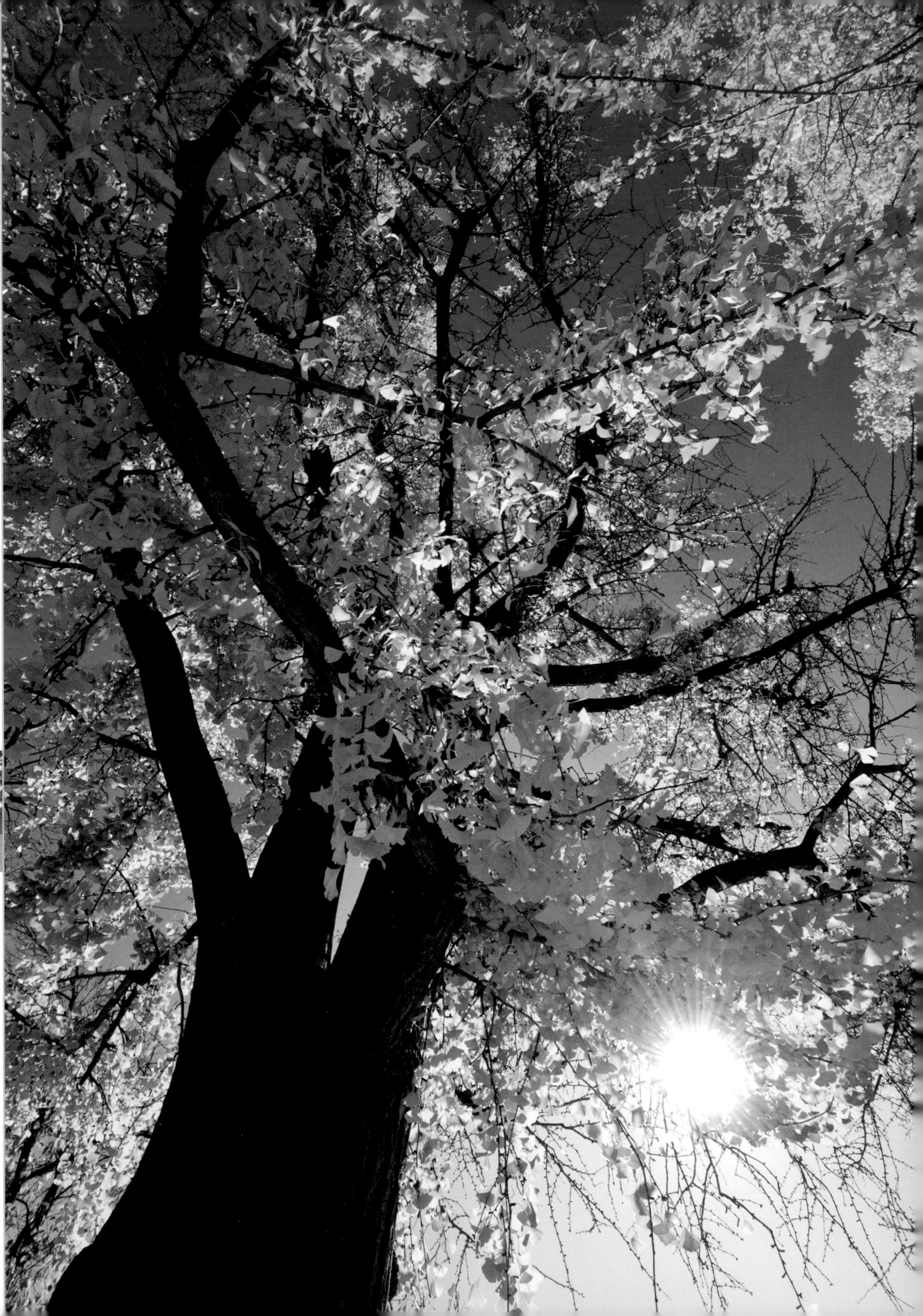

Ginkgo

✦ *Ginkgo biloba* ✦

In rock layers some 270 million years old, scientists have unearthed fossils of ancient trees with delicately veined, fan-shaped leaves that are deeply notched to form two halves, or lobes. Some of these fossils are essentially identical to the leaves of a living tree known as *Ginkgo biloba*. It is the only surviving member of the *Ginkgo* genus, a sort of living fossil that survived into modern times in a remote corner of southeastern China. Buddhist monks began cultivating ginkgo there in the 11th century when ginkgo was revered as a sacred plant and grown for its peculiar fleshy seeds.

The Chinese called these seeds *yinxing*, meaning "silver apricot." In Japan, where ginkgo was introduced, *yin-hsing* is thought to have become corrupted into *gingkyo*. Ginkgo leaves and seeds have been used in traditional Chinese medicine since the 15th century and probably much earlier in folk medicine.

Use of ginkgo leaf is first mentioned in Lan Mao's *Dian Nan Ben Cao (Pharmaceutical Natural History of Southern Yunnan)*, published in 1436. Preparations of the leaves were used externally to treat sores, and internally for diarrhea and as a tonic for the heart and lungs. Ginkgo seed preparations were given for asthma, tuberculosis, coughs, and bronchial conditions. In the early 1700s *Ginkgo biloba* was introduced into Europe, and about 60 years later into North America. Interest

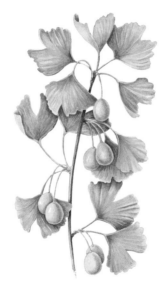

in ginkgo as a medicinal herb began in the West in the late 1900s, when leaf **extracts** were shown to improve circulation, particularly to the brain and extremities. In the United States and Europe, ginkgo leaf supplements are now among the best-selling herbal medications.

Ginkgo supplements contain a standardized extract known as ginkgo biloba extract, or GBE. In Europe, ginkgo is a common treatment for dementia, due to its ability to improve blood flow to the brain. It may improve thinking, learning, and memory in people with Alzheimer's disease. Herbal practitioners and naturopaths also suggest ginkgo for treating age-related macular degeneration, tinnitus (ringing in the ears), and intermittent claudication (cramping and pain caused by poor blood flow in the legs).

The ginkgo is a modern descendant of trees that grew when dinosaurs roamed Earth.

TIME LINE OF USAGE AND SPREAD

1690
German botanist E. Kaempfer is first Westerner to see ginkgo in Japanese gardens.

1730
Ginkgo is introduced to Europe at the botanic garden in Utrecht, Holland.

1784
W. Hamilton brings ginkgos to U.S. and plants them on his estate near Philadelphia.

1945
Ginkgo trees in Hiroshima, Japan, survive atomic blast and are alive today.

There is only one member of the ginkgo family, a survivor for more than 200 million years—*Ginkgo biloba*. The tree that survives today is nearly identical to its ancient ancestors. Six species of ginkgo are known from the fossil record. A large deciduous tree reaching over 120 feet in height, ginkgo is immediately recognizable from its fan-shaped, 2-lobed leaves, with prominent forked veins. The smooth leaves are alternate or borne in clusters, usually 1.5 times broader than long. Male and female flowers are borne on separate trees. The distinctive female "fruits" contain an ovoid seed about an inch long. The seed is covered with a fleshy, buff-orange, foul-smelling coat, which if handled without protection can cause contact dermatitis like poison ivy.

Growing Habits

Ginkgo is native to China, but botanists debate whether small ginkgo populations in remote mountain valleys of Zhejiang province in south-eastern China are truly wild or the remnants of trees once planted around dwellings and monasteries centuries ago. Ginkgo primarily survives in cultivation. Seedlings, naturalized near planted trees in the eastern United States, point to the tree's potential to easily establish itself without cultivation. Birds or small mammals disperse the relatively heavy seeds.

Used as a drug in traditional Chinese medicine for millennia, ginkgo was first described by Western science in 1712. It was introduced in the United States in 1784 in the garden of William Hamilton near Philadelphia.

Cultivation and Harvesting

Ginkgo is commonly cultivated as a street shade tree in many parts of the world. It is extremely resistant to fire, disease, pests, and pollution, and thus commonly planted in city environs where other trees do not survive. Ginkgo can be grown from seed or propagated from cuttings. The vast majority of ginkgo trees available in American horticulture are male branches grafted onto rootstock. The reason for this is that a few decades after the first ginkgos planted in America reached an age where they bore fruit, it became clear that female trees were a nuisance, bearing foul-smelling fruit and also capable of causing allergic skin reactions. So male trees became the tree of choice.

Commercially, for ginkgo leaf harvest ginkgo trees are planted in rows and coppiced—cut back to encourage growth of shoots—to stand at 3 to 6 feet in height. A modified cotton harvester is used to beat the leaves off the branches; leaves are then collected in trailers and immediately transported to a drying facility. Much of the world's ginkgo leaf supply comes from specialized farms in South Carolina, the Bordeaux region of France, and plantations in China.

Therapeutic Uses

+ *Antioxidant*
+ *Mental health*
+ *Circulation*

Perhaps our oldest known tree, ginkgo and its leaves have been an herbal remedy for many centuries. Ginkgo contains potent **antioxidants** called **glycosides**, which protect nerve cells, and **terpene lactones**, which reduce **inflammation**. Ginkgo is used for poor circulation and to reduce the pain of peripheral vascular disease. However, studies investigating these effects show only modest benefit over **placebo.**

over the (kitchen) counter CLARI-TEA

Mix 1 ounce ginkgo leaves and 1 ounce green tea leaves together and store in a glass jar. To prepare tea: Pour 1 cup boiling water over 1 heaping teaspoon of herbs. Steep 5 to 7 minutes. Strain. Add small amount of honey and/or lemon juice. Drink for a delightful afternoon tea.

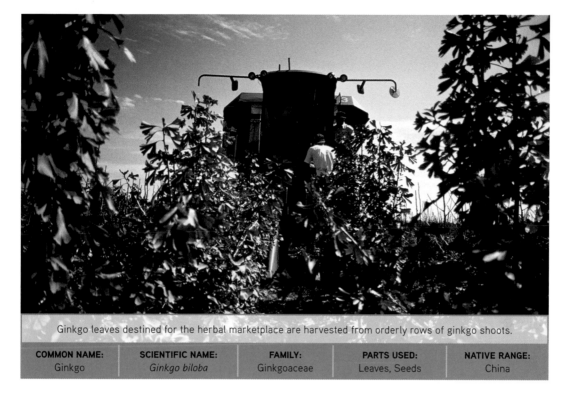
Ginkgo leaves destined for the herbal marketplace are harvested from orderly rows of ginkgo shoots.

COMMON NAME:	SCIENTIFIC NAME:	FAMILY:	PARTS USED:	NATIVE RANGE:
Ginkgo	*Ginkgo biloba*	Ginkgoaceae	Leaves, Seeds	China

Ginkgo is widely used in Europe, Canada, Australia, and the United States for the prevention and treatment of dementia. A number of studies have shown that ginkgo biloba extract (GBE) improves symptoms and stabilizes or slows progression of dementia, including Alzheimer's disease. Studies also show that these extracts modestly improve age-related memory impairment (much less serious than dementia).

Newer studies published in the U.S. have not been as encouraging. A study published in the journal *Neurology* in 2008 did not show that GBE prevented cognitive decline in elderly people with normal cognitive function. However, among the people who actually took ginkgo as directed, memory loss was slowed. A much larger study published in the *Journal of the American Medical Association* in 2008 also failed to demonstrate that taking GBE (120 mg twice a day) prevented dementia in adults ranging in age from 72 to 96 with normal brain function or mild impairment. Likewise, a subsequent analysis published in the same journal in 2009 did not show a significant reduction in cognitive decline.

Nevertheless, studies do show that ginkgo improves arterial function. Several studies noted that extracts improve walking distance in patients with peripheral arterial occlusive disease, a condition in which arterial disease in the legs leads to pain with even minimal exertion.

How to Use

TEA: Steep 1 teaspoon ginkgo leaf in 1 cup water for 5 to 7 minutes. Strain. Drink 1 to 2 cups daily.
TINCTURE: Generally, take 3 to 5 ml twice a day, or follow manufacturer's directions.
EXTRACT: Most research has been conducted on doses of 120 mg taken twice per day of extracts standardized to 24 to 27 percent flavone glycosides and 6 to 7 percent **triterpenes**.

Precautions

Ginkgo leaf is considered safe, as shown in large clinical trials and wide use. But there may be effects on blood clotting. Those taking medications to prevent blood clots should consult a health care professional before using. Stop taking ginkgo at least 3 days before surgery. Use in pregnancy is not recommended due to risk of increased bleeding.

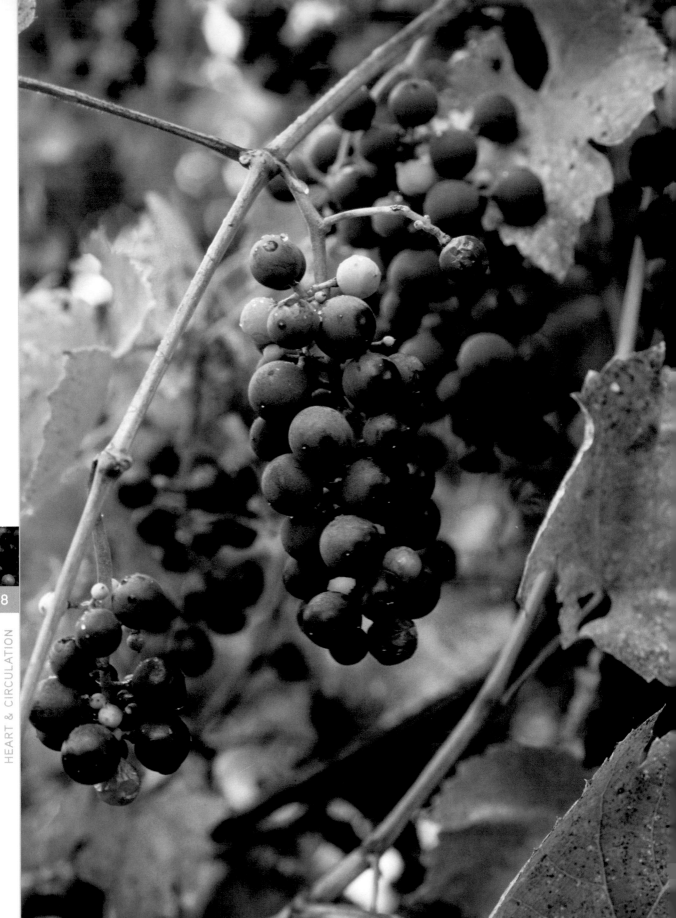

HEART & CIRCULATION

Grapes, Grape Seed

Vitis vinifera

Grapes, and wine made from them, have been part of human culture for a remarkably long time. Archaeologists working at a site in the Democratic Republic of Georgia recently uncovered several pottery jars inside Neolithic ruins dating from around 6000 B.C. The jars contained a reddish residue—the remains of wine. This prehistoric wine was most likely made from wild grapes, as the domestication of grape vines didn't begin until around 5000 B.C. Sumerian texts from 3000 B.C. contain some of the first written accounts of both grapes and wine.

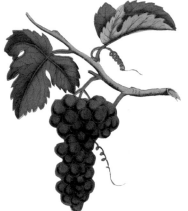

Colorful scenes of grape harvesting and winemaking decorate the walls of many Egyptian tombs, revealing the importance of *Vitis vinifera* in ancient Egypt—and in the afterlife—by at least 2700 B.C. Seven hundred years later, Phoenician sailors were transporting grapevines across the Mediterranean to Greece. From there, grapes and grape growing spread to Europe and the rest of the world.

Both grapes and wine have been lauded as food and medicine for thousands of years. Several ancient Greek philosophers wrote of their healing properties. Roman physician Pliny the Elder (A.D. 23-79) praised the gods for "bestowing healing powers on the vine." Through the ages, almost every part of the plant has been used medicinally. European folk healers made an ointment of grapevine sap to treat diseases of the eyes and skin. Grape leaf **poultices** helped staunch bleeding and reduce inflammation, and the ripe fruit were eaten for kidney and liver diseases, cholera, and cancer.

Research has shown that many health-promoting properties are contained in grape seeds, rich in **antioxidants**. Today, health care professionals recommend standardized grape seed **extract** to lower high cholesterol and high blood pressure and treat a host of circulatory ailments, including coronary heart disease, chronic venous insufficiency, and varicose veins. Chemical **compounds** in red wine may also reduce the risk of developing heart disease. Grape seed extract is given to regulate blood sugar levels, treat certain eye disorders, and relieve symptoms of asthma and allergies.

Prized since prehistoric times, grapes are the source of wine and grape seeds, rich in health-promoting substances.

TIME LINE OF USAGE AND SPREAD

6000 B.C.	2ND CENTURY B.C.	A.D. 500	1869
Wine made from grapes dates at least from this time.	Grape vines are introduced to China and the first Chinese grape wine is produced.	Grape growing and winemaking preserved church after fall of Rome.	Thomas B. Welch introduces unfermented grape juice as a beverage.

Of the 65 species in the genus *Vitis*, the best known is *Vitis vinifera*, source of the common grape from which grape juice, raisins, wine, and a by-product used in herbal preparations, grape seeds, are derived. Grapes grow as a liana or large climbing woody vine. If left to their own habits, grapes will climb high up in a tree, and their trunks may swell to 6 inches in diameter. The stems have forked tendrils, which facilitates climbing. The leaves are simple and conspicuously 5 lobed to 7 lobed and nearly smooth. The leaf blade is oval in outline, 3 to 7 inches broad and 2½ to 6 inches long. The leaf base is heart shaped, with the lobes at the base usually overlapping. Large pointed teeth surround the margins. The flowers are inconspicuous, and the fruits are the familiar grapes of commerce.

Growing Habits

The grape vine is native to southeastern Europe and southwestern Asia. The many varieties now grown around the world have been selected based on fruit color, growing characteristics in various soils and climate, hardiness, resistance to disease and pests, and other factors. This has resulted in a large and diverse genetic pool. The greatest genetic diversity in wild grape **species** appears in eastern North America and in China. During the 19th century, American vines were introduced to Europe for hybridization, confounding determination of the original geographic limits of the cultivated grapes; most likely, cultivation originated in the Caspian Sea region of western Asia. What is clear is that *Vitis vinifera* has been established in cultivation for so long that its exact origins can never be determined.

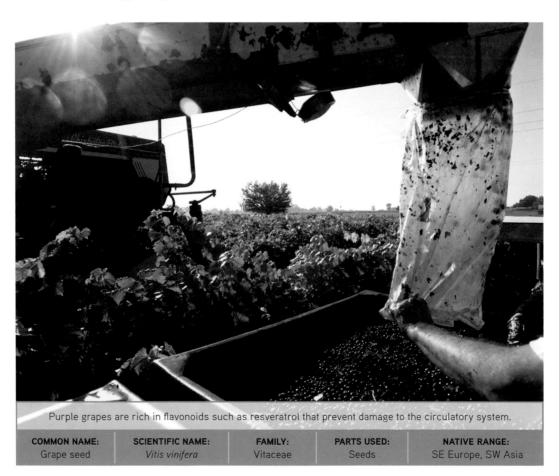

Purple grapes are rich in flavonoids such as resveratrol that prevent damage to the circulatory system.

COMMON NAME:	SCIENTIFIC NAME:	FAMILY:	PARTS USED:	NATIVE RANGE:
Grape seed	*Vitis vinifera*	Vitaceae	Seeds	SE Europe, SW Asia

over the (kitchen) counter GRAPE SHAKE

In a blender, combine 4 ounces of dark purple grape juice, 4 ounces milk (dairy or soy), and ½ cup nonfat vanilla yogurt. Add ½ cup ice. Mix in blender for 5 to 10 seconds, until smooth. Garnish with fruit. Enjoy your heart-healthy treat!

Grapes are among the oldest cultivated fruits and are frequently mentioned in the Bible. Noah himself is said to have planted grapes. They were grown in Egypt at least 6,000 years ago. Some have estimated that grapes were introduced to Greece between the 18th and 16th centuries B.C. The common cultivated grape is represented by more than 8,000 named varieties. Only about 20 percent of those variations are currently grown—still a mind-boggling number of cultivated varieties for one plant species.

Cultivation and Harvesting

Volumes have been written about the cultivation of grapes, an agricultural activity stretching back to the dawn of history. Agricultural research stations and entire university departments are devoted solely to the subject of grape growing, a branch of horticulture that has garnered its own designation—viticulture.

Therapeutic Uses

+ *Heart health*
+ *Antioxidant*

Scientists have looked at the juice, seed, and skin of grapes collectively and separately. While there are a number of health-enhancing compounds in grapes, it is the **flavonoids**, particularly resveratrol, which has gained international attention as a powerhouse antioxidant. Resveratrol is concentrated in the skin, seeds, and stems of grapes and may be a key ingredient in dark purple grape juice and red wine that helps prevent damage to blood vessels, reduces "bad" cholesterol and inflammation, and prevents blood clots. In general, purple and other dark-colored grapes contain greater concentrations of flavonoid compounds than light-colored grapes.

So is red wine better than white wine for your heart? Some studies do indeed show that red wine is superior to other types of alcohol, but others show that red wine isn't any better than beer, white wine, or liquor for heart health. Thus, it is good news that researchers at Georgetown University have shown that grape juice, similar to red wine, lowers the risk of developing blood clots that may lead to heart attacks. Further, grape juice is a good alternative for those who do not drink alcohol or want to limit its consumption. Another benefit to drinking grape juice is the "antioxidant advantage." Researchers at the University of California, Davis, found that **catechin**, another key antioxidant in grapes, remains in the blood for more than four hours after grape juice is drunk, compared with only 3.2 hours for full-strength cabernet, suggesting that alcohol likely hastens the breakdown of catechin.

A growing body of research is showing that extracts from grape seeds are beneficial for your health. Grape seeds contain powerful antioxidants known as **proanthocyanidins**, which science is finding may help prevent heart disease, diabetes, and cataracts. Human studies have found grape seed extract can lower blood pressure and cholesterol and reduce inflammation.

How to Use

WINE: 1 serving a day for women, 1 to 2 for men.
GRAPE JUICE: 4 to 6 ounces of dark purple grape juice per day.
GRAPE SEED EXTRACT: 300 to 600 mg per day.

Precautions

Grapes are one of the more highly pesticide-ridden fruits, so it may be advisable to purchase organic when possible. Women should limit alcohol intake to one serving per day, as higher amounts can increase the risk of breast cancer. Alcohol should not be consumed during pregnancy.

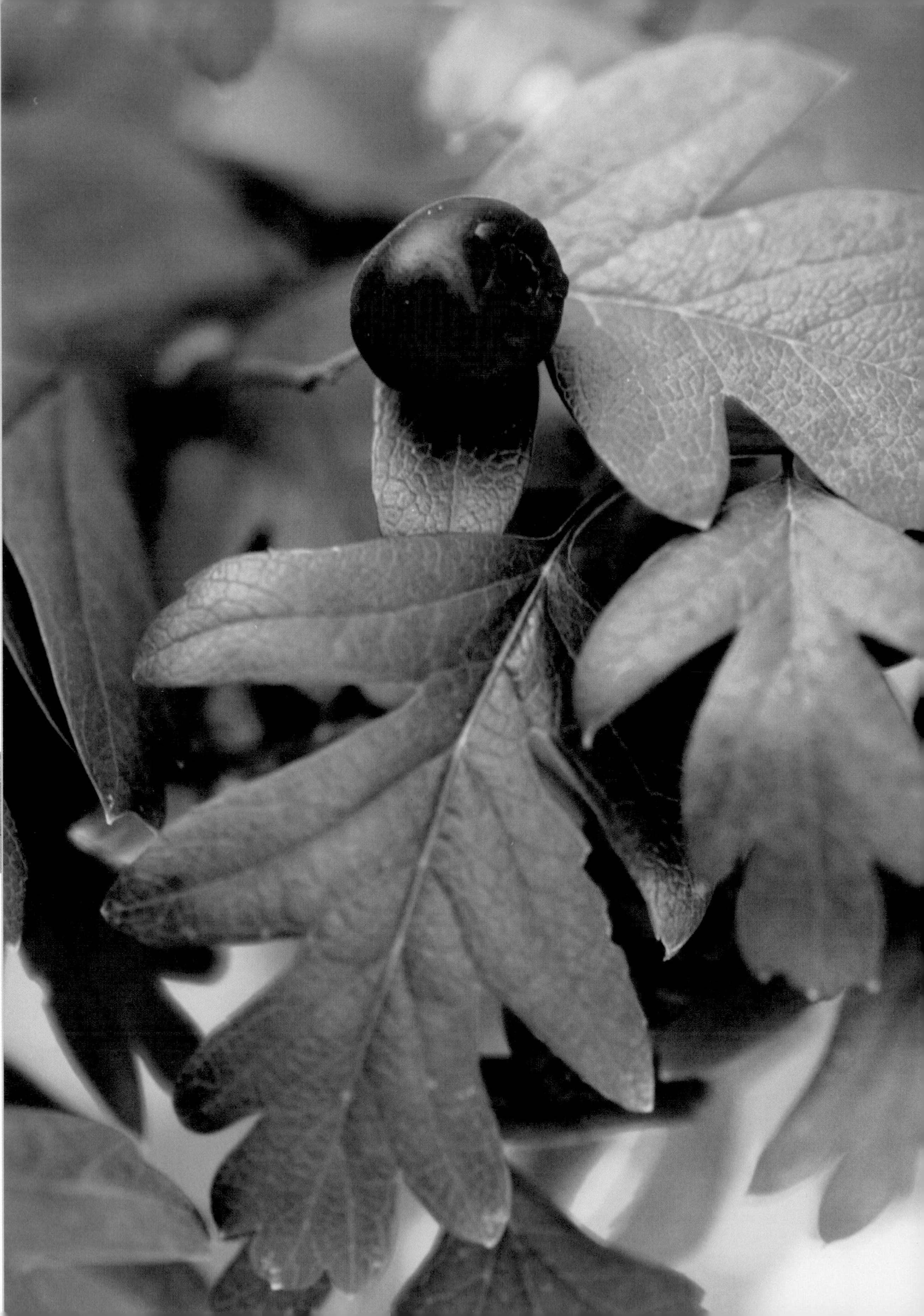

Hawthorn

Crataegus laevigata

The *haw* in hawthorn comes from an old Anglo-Saxon word for "hedge." Since medieval times, spiny-limbed hawthorn has been used to keep cattle in pastures and people out of private properties. In England and parts of Germany today, dense hedges of hawthorn are still commonly planted as fences. Hawthorn's genus name, *Crataegus*, comes from the Greek *kratos*, meaning "hardness" or "strength"—a reference to the plant's extremely hard and durable wood. Many somewhat conflicting superstitions surround hawthorn. On one hand, the tree was associated with

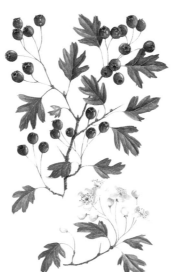

new life and renewal. Maypoles—the focus of many pagan celebrations of spring—were often made of hawthorn, and its white, roselike blossoms woven into the garlands that decorated it. Hung over a doorway, hawthorn branches were thought to prevent evil spirits from entering a dwelling. In medieval England, however, hawthorn was associated with death, as its fetid-smelling flowers seemed to reek of decay.

For many centuries, hawthorn has been a valued herb in both Western and Eastern herbal medicine traditions. The Greek physician Dioscorides recommended hawthorn for heart problems. By at least the seventh century, the Chinese were using a closely related **species**, *Crataegus pinnatifida*, as a remedy for high blood pressure, arteriosclerosis, heart pain,

and other heart-related conditions. During the Middle Ages, hawthorn was prized more as a **diuretic** and to treat insomnia and sore throat. By the 19th century, hawthorn's popularity as a remedy for heart conditions had resurfaced in Europe, and later in the U.S.

Today in herbal medicine hawthorn is used for a variety of heart-related conditions. In those suffering from congestive heart failure, hawthorn can help improve heart function and relieve shortness of breath and fatigue. It may also help relieve chest pain (angina) caused by restricted blood flow to the heart. Herbal practitioners also recommend hawthorn for reducing high blood pressure, high cholesterol, and the buildup of fatty plaques in blood vessels that can lead to **atherosclerosis**.

Hawthorn fruits have been used since the first century for the heart; modern herbalists also use leaves and flowers.

TIME LINE OF USAGE AND SPREAD

659
Chinese herbal *Tang Ben Cao* mentions hawthorn's use in treating heart problems.

1633
English herbalist J. Gerard notes hawthorn berries "stay fluxes of bloud."

1753
Linnaeus introduces botanical name *Crataegus oxyacantha*, later changed to *C. laevigata*.

1845
British Enclosures Act allows hawthorn to be used for hedges across Britain.

The initial charm of hawthorn's delicate flowers fades quickly after one gets a whiff of their offensive fragrance.

COMMON NAME:	SCIENTIFIC NAME:	FAMILY:	PARTS USED:	NATIVE RANGE:
Hawthorn	*Crataegus laevigata*	Rosaceae	Leaves, Flowers, Fruits	Europe

Hawthorn is an extremely complex and confusing plant group for botanists, with more than a thousand species described, most from northern temperate regions, especially North America, and about 20 species from Europe and 18 species in China. There are numerous wild races in North America produced through hybridization, confounding identity. The current understanding of the genus *Crataegus* includes about 140 species.

Hawthorns are small trees or shrubs, mostly **deciduous** and usually with spines. The leaves are lobed and have serrated teeth. The 5-petaled, usually white flowers come at the end of branches. The small reddish, mostly dry fruits are used, along with the flowers and leaves. The lateral-veined leaves are sharply toothed, and the flower group usually has 5 to 10 flowers in each group.

One-seeded hawthorn (*C. monogyna*), as the name implies, has only a single seed and leaf lobes without teeth. At least 8 **subspecies** are recognized. Chinese hawthorn (*C. pinnatifida*) has broadly wedge-shaped leaves with several pairs of lobes. It produces a dark red fruit.

Growing Habits

Native to northern and central Europe from England to Sweden, east to Latvia, and south to the Pyrenees and northern Italy, English hawthorn (*C. laevigata*) has long been cultivated as an ornamental shrub. It is found in fields and along roadsides, fencerows, and hedgerows. One-seeded hawthorn is widespread across most of Europe. Chinese hawthorn occurs in shrubby thickets and slopes of mountains and hills of central and northern China. It is so similar in appearance to English hawthorn that Carolus Linnaeus, the father of the modern scientific biological naming system, classified it as a **variety** of English hawthorn. Chinese hawthorn has been cultivated for many centuries in China both as a fruit tree and for its uses in traditional Chinese medicine.

Cultivation and Harvesting

More than 60 species of *Crataegus* are grown in American horticulture. Most are hardy and are readily transplanted. They prefer limey, rich loam and a sunny situation. Propagation is by seeds moist-stratified at 41°F, for 3 or 4 months, after which they may take 2 years to germinate.

Propagation can also be achieved by hardwood cuttings, budding, or grafting. Their ornamental effect in flower and fruit makes them excellent subjects for lawn plantings.

Most of the world's supply of European hawthorn species is wild-harvested in Eastern Europe. Chinese hawthorn comes primarily from cultivated supplies in China.

Therapeutic Uses

+ *Heart health*

Hawthorn is considered by Western herbalists to be the premier tonic to gently support the healthy functioning of the heart. It appears to do this by strengthening the force of the heart muscle and maintaining a normal heart rhythm and healthy blood pressure. Research also shows that hawthorn improves blood flow through the heart itself, ensuring that muscle cells are well oxygenated. In addition to these benefits, the **flavonoids** found in the fruit, leaves, and flowers act as potent **antioxidants**, helping to protect cells from damage.

Hawthorn is widely accepted in Europe as a treatment for mild cases of congestive heart failure and minor heart arrhythmias. While there have been many clinical studies, the largest was the large SPICE trial conducted in 13 European countries. Researchers randomized 2,681 patients with heart failure to receive either a proprietary hawthorn **extract** or a **placebo** for 2 years, in addition to standard congestive heart failure therapy. Overall, no beneficial effect was noted except in those patients who had evidence of moderately reduced function of the left ventricle muscles of the heart. (The left ventricle of the heart is one of the body's hardest working muscles, as it has to pump the blood out of the heart into the aorta and then throughout the body.) This group was shown to have a significantly reduced risk of sudden cardiac death from month 12 to month 24. This effect was not seen in those who had normal left ventricular function or in those who had severely reduced muscle function. Interestingly, this is consistent with the traditional notion that hawthorn is a tonic and most beneficial for those with milder forms of heart disease. Hawthorn gently strengthens the contractile force of the heart muscle and maintains a healthy rhythm. Importantly, the SPICE trial failed to find any evidence of herb-drug interactions with any of the drugs taken by the participants.

International reviewers concluded, after looking at all clinical trials conducted on hawthorn, that the evidence suggests "a significant benefit in symptom control and physiologic outcomes from hawthorn extract as an adjunctive treatment for chronic heart failure."

How to Use

TEA: Steep 2 teaspoons of hawthorn leaves and flowers in 12 ounces of water for 10 minutes. Strain and drink 1 to 2 cups per day.

TINCTURE: Generally, 5 ml taken twice daily.

STANDARDIZED EXTRACT: HeartCare is a product standardized to the same specification as the proprietary hawthorn product used in the large SPICE trial (of extract WS-1442).

Precautions

Hawthorn appears to be very safe and well tolerated. Hawthorn is best used under the supervision of a medical professional, for anyone who suffers from congestive heart failure or is being treated for heart disease.

---

over the (kitchen) counter HAWTHORN SYRUP

Combine 1 cup fresh or ½ cup dried hawthorn berries and 3 cups water in a medium-size saucepan. Simmer for 10 minutes. Remove from heat and cool. Mash berries with potato masher and simmer again for 10 minutes. Strain liquid and pour back into pan. Add 1 cup of honey or agave nectar. Heat gently until sweetener dissolves. Store in refrigerator for up to 3 weeks. Enjoy 1 to 2 tablespoons of syrup daily as part of a heart-healthy diet.

Hibiscus

Hibiscus sabdariffa

On many Caribbean islands, it's not uncommon to see roadside stands selling what appear to be stubby, wine-red flower buds. The "buds" are actually the fruits of *Hibiscus sabdariffa,* a robustly bushy plant with striking crimson stems and pale yellow flowers reminiscent of hollyhocks. Native to India and Malaysia but cultivated in tropical and subtropical regions worldwide, *H. sabdariffa* goes by many names: hibiscus, roselle, red sorrel, Jamaican sorrel, Queensland jelly plant, sour-sour, and Florida cranberry. The nutritious fruits of hibiscus are made into jams and jellies, tossed in fruit salads, turned into sauces for ice cream and fillings for pies and tarts, processed into chutneys and relishes, and added to many herbal tea blends. In parts of Africa, hibiscus fruits are a favorite side dish, often served with ground peanuts. Hibiscus is probably most prized, however, for the refreshing, slightly **astringent** beverage made by brewing its fruits in hot water and sweetening the resulting cranberry-colored liquid with sugar. Flavored with ginger or other spices, the drink is very popular from the West Indies to West Africa.

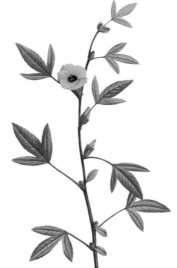

All the aboveground parts of hibiscus have been used in the folk medicine traditions of India, Africa, Mexico, and parts of Central America. The fruits and seeds are valued for their mild **diuretic** and laxative effects. Both the leaves and flowers are used to make a tea drunk to improve digestion and kidney function. An **infusion** of the ripe fruits can be drunk to relieve coughs and liver and gallbladder problems—and hangovers. Infusions of leaves or fruits are also used to treat fevers, lower blood pressure, and improve circulation. A lotion made from hibiscus leaves is a remedy for sores and wounds.

Modern herbal practitioners recommend hibiscus to help lower blood pressure and levels of harmful **low-density lipoprotein** (LDL) cholesterol. It is also suggested for improving circulatory health by preventing **atherosclerosis**, as hibiscus has been shown to slow or reverse changes in blood and blood vessels that can lead to the development of this condition. Rich in **antioxidants**, hibiscus may be helpful in cancer prevention.

The crimson fruits of hibiscus, known as calyxes, are the part of this tropical native mainly used in herbal medicine.

TIME LINE OF USAGE AND SPREAD

1576
Flemish botanist M. de L'Obel publishes first written observations of *H. sabdariffa.*

1707
Cultivation of hibiscus begins in Jamaica.

1887
Hibiscus is introduced to Florida and grown as an ornamental until the 1950s.

1892
Two roselle jam factories in Queensland, Australia, export large quantities to Europe.

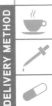
Hibiscus is a large plant group with more than 675 species, the vast majority of which are native to warm temperate and tropical regions of the world. *H. sabdariffa* is often called roselle. It is grown not only for herbal teas but also as a fiber plant, its leaves eaten like spinach and its fleshy, slightly sour calyx (the floral envelope at the base of the flower) as a fruit. The most commonly grown variety of *H. sabdariffa* is an erect, bushy annual growing to 8 feet.

The stems are smooth and usually purple-tinged or completely reddish purple. The alternate, lobed leaves are 3 to 5 inches long and usually have reddish veins. The yellow or buff showy flowers have a prominent rose or maroon eye in the center. At the base of the flowers is a large red calyx, a structure that is a curious cross between leaf and flower. It envelops the base of the flower and holds all the flower structures intact. It is this fleshy, crisp, juicy structure, the calyx, 1 to 2 inches long, that is used in Western herbal medicine and herbal teas.

Growing Habits

Widely cultivated in the tropics, some writers place the origins of hibiscus in southern Asia from India to Malaysia. From there it was brought to Africa at an unknown early date. Others believe it originated in East Africa. Like its close relative okra, hibiscus was brought to the Americas by African slaves. It was quickly adopted in the New World, cultivated in Brazil in the 17th century, and in the following decades became a staple offering in every market in the Caribbean as well as in Central and South America.

The **genus** name *Hibiscus* is most likely derived from the Latin *ibis,* meaning "stork," in reference to the striking similarity of a stork's beak to the shape and appearance of the pointed seed capsules of many varieties of hibiscus.

Cultivation and Harvesting

Hibiscus is grown from seed but also can be propagated from cuttings. Seeds are sown March to May, usually at the beginning of the rainy season in tropical climates. The buds usually set in October or November. The plant likes hot weather and full sun and is sensitive to frost. It does well in a deep, fertile sandy loam.

The calyxes (fruits) are harvested just after flowering, when they are fully plump but still tender. They are harvested by hand, snapped off in the early morning. If they are slightly older, fibers develop in the structure, requiring harvesting with clippers, as they will not easily snap off by hand. Most world production is for local fresh markets. For herb tea use, the calyxes are dried. The material used for tea imparts a rich red color to hot water. It is primarily produced in tropical regions with ready supply of inexpensive labor for the intensive hand harvesting.

Therapeutic Uses

+ *Diuretic*
+ *Heart health*
+ *Colds and sore throat*

Hibiscus is widely used in the traditional medicines of India, Africa, Mexico, South America, and some Caribbean islands, where it is valued as a diuretic or mild laxative and used to treat colds, coughs, and

over the (kitchen) counter AGUA DE JAMAICA

Make your own delicious, refreshing, easy-to-prepare hibiscus drink. Bring 4 cups water to boil, remove from heat. Add ½ cup natural cane sugar and ½ cup chopped hibiscus calyxes (often sold as hibiscus "flowers"). Steep covered for 15 minutes. Strain well, pour into a pitcher. Add 3 cups cold water and orange slices.

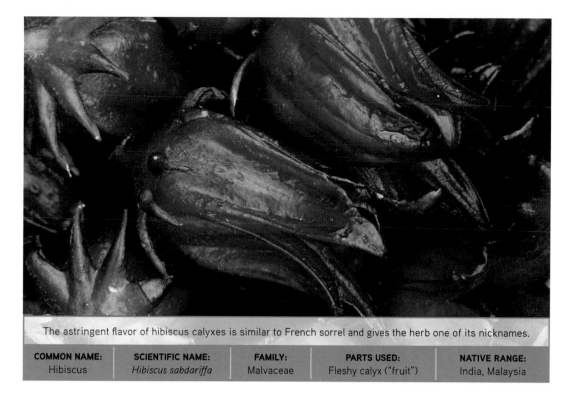

The astringent flavor of hibiscus calyxes is similar to French sorrel and gives the herb one of its nicknames.

COMMON NAME:	SCIENTIFIC NAME:	FAMILY:	PARTS USED:	NATIVE RANGE:
Hibiscus	*Hibiscus sabdariffa*	Malvaceae	Fleshy calyx ("fruit")	India, Malaysia

heart disorders. Delicious, refreshing hibiscus tea is loaded with vitamin C, as well as **mucilage**, **pectins**, and **anthocyanins**, antioxidant **compounds** that work to protect the body's cell membranes. The mucilage is a complex mixture of **polysaccharides** that produce a soothing gelatinous layer when mixed with water and soothe irritated tissues of the mouth, throat, and gastrointestinal tract. Both the mucilage and the vitamin C likely explain the plant's historical use in treating colds and sore throats. Hibiscus tea is still used in many parts of the world to relieve coughs and mild fevers in both children and adults.

One of the most promising areas of recent research is the potential role for hibiscus in cardiovascular health. Scientists have confirmed that constituents in the deep red calyxes of hibiscus exhibit potent antioxidant activity and exert beneficial effects on blood pressure and cholesterol. Hibiscus appears to lower blood pressure in part because of its diuretic effect and by inhibiting angiotensin-converting **enzyme** (ACE), a compound that increases blood pressure. Human studies show that it reduces blood pressure to the same degree as two commonly prescribed ACE inhibitors, captopril and lisinopril. A clinical trial with type 2 diabetics found that it lowered blood pressure and increased **high-density lipoprotein** (HDL), or "good" cholesterol.

Hibiscus is used in a number of weight-loss teas, for flavor and also for its diuretic activity. Preliminary evidence suggests that compounds in hibiscus may mildly inhibit the absorption of carbohydrates.

How to Use

TEA: Pour 1 cup boiling water over 2 teaspoons chopped hibiscus. Steep for 15 minutes. Strain and add sugar or honey. Serve chilled or hot.

TINCTURE: Take 1 teaspoon twice daily.

CAPSULES: Take 1,000 mg dried hibiscus 2 to 3 times per day.

Precautions

There are no known adverse effects of hibiscus; however, those taking prescription diuretics should use sparingly. High blood pressure or heart disease patients should consult a health care provider before using natural remedies for treatment.

Horse Chestnut

Aesculus hippocastanum

In England, the hard, dark brown seeds of *Aesculus hippocastanum* are called conkers. In the United States and Canada, they're horse chestnuts. The seeds are contained inside prickly green casings that turn brown as they ripen, and eventually split open to reveal the shiny seeds inside. (Horse chestnuts are not to be confused with sweet, edible chestnuts, which come from the tree *Castanea sativa*.) Believing conkers were lucky, English children—and superstitious adults—would chant "Oddly, oddly, onker, my first conker" upon finding their first seed of the season in order to ensure good

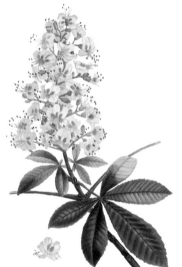

fortune for the rest of the year. Native to western Asia, horse chestnut was introduced to Europe in the late 1500s. The trees were widely planted for their dense shade, spectacular flowers, and abundant seeds. When horse chestnut was introduced into North America in the 1700s, it was already well established in European folk medicine as a healing plant.

A number of Native American tribes in North America used parts of *A. glabra*, a tree closely related to *A. hippocastanum*, as medicine. After several centuries of use in traditional medicine, European doctors began prescribing an **extract** of horse chestnut seeds in the 1800s to treat varicose veins, hemorrhoids, nerve pain, and poor circulation. Since the 1960s, horse chestnut has been the subject of considerable research,

especially in Germany, that has led to the development of horse chestnut seed extracts used primarily for circulatory disorders. Currently, horse chestnut is the third most popular herb in the German market after ginkgo and St. John's wort.

In Europe today, horse chestnut seed extract (HCSE) is widely used for treating many vascular conditions, as well as sports injuries. Interest in the extract's medicinal applications is growing in the United States. Herbal practitioners and physicians most commonly suggest HCSE for cases of chronic venous insufficiency, a condition characterized by leg swelling, varicose veins, leg pain, and skin ulcers. The herb is also recommended for nocturnal leg cramps, phlebitis, joint pains, and diarrhea.

Though nearly every part of horse chestnut was once used, modern herbalists use extracts from the tree's seeds.

TIME LINE OF USAGE AND SPREAD

1563
First printed illustration of horse chestnut published by Italian botanist Pietro Mattioli.

1576
Horse chestnut trees are introduced to Europe from Asia.

1848
First recorded conkers game, using horse chestnuts, occurs on Isle of Wight.

1944
Anne Frank's diary mentions a horse chestnut tree visible from her hiding place.

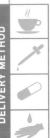
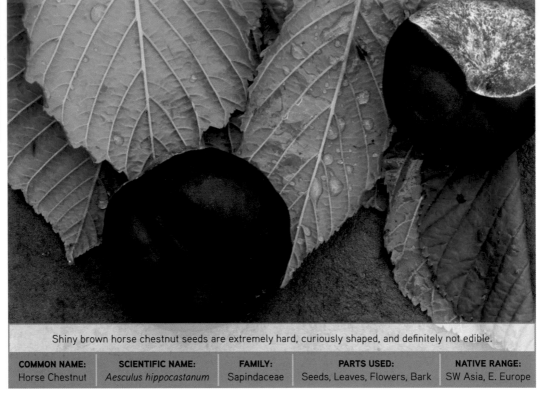

Shiny brown horse chestnut seeds are extremely hard, curiously shaped, and definitely not edible.

COMMON NAME:	SCIENTIFIC NAME:	FAMILY:	PARTS USED:	NATIVE RANGE:
Horse Chestnut	*Aesculus hippocastanum*	Sapindaceae	Seeds, Leaves, Flowers, Bark	SW Asia, E. Europe

There are only 13 species in this small plant group. Seven are native to North America, including buckeye, *A. glabra*, perhaps more famously associated today with a college sports program (the Ohio Buckeyes) than its namesake tree. A stately tree with an umbrella-like crown, horse chestnut grows to about 60 feet. The opposite leaves have 7 leaflets radiating from a central point. The middle leaflets are the longest, with serrated margins. This deciduous tree is among the first to lose its leaves in autumn. The showy flowers, borne in a pyramid-shaped cluster, are white with yellow and red markings. As they age, they turn from yellowish to reddish. The fruit is a spiny ball about the size of a golf ball, holding large, shiny brown seeds.

Growing Habits

Horse chestnut is native to dry soils of Asia Minor from the Himalaya through the Caucasus, and west to the central Balkans. Although generally associated with European traditions, it did not reach western Europe until its introduction to Vienna, Austria, in 1576. A favorite shade tree throughout Europe, it was brought to America by early settlers. It is commonly planted as a shade tree along streets throughout the U.S.

The name *Aesculus* was applied by classical authors to a type of oak with edible nuts; *esca*, the Latin root, means "food or nourishment." In this sense, the name is misapplied, as the fruits of horse chestnut are not edible; in fact, they are considered toxic. The name "horse chestnut" may derive from an observation of Turks grinding the fruits and adding the meal to horse feed. Many farm animals readily eat the seeds.

Cultivation and Harvesting

Horse chestnut trees were often planted around Early American homes to beautify the landscape, and as a reminder of Europe. Horse chestnut is propagated by seeds, budding, or grafting. The seeds have dormant embryos and must have a pretreatment mimicking winter before they will germinate. This is achieved by putting the seeds in moist sand in a refrigerator for about 4 months before planting. This can also be done simply by planting the seeds outdoors in autumn for germination the following spring. Horse chestnuts do best in a fairly rich, moderately moist soil but are tolerant of dry conditions.

It is the seeds of horse chestnut that are used today in modern herbal preparations. Horse chestnut commercial production for the medicinal herb market occurs in Poland and elsewhere in Eastern Europe.

Therapeutic Uses

+ *Varicose veins*
+ *Chronic venous insufficiency*
+ *Hemorrhoids*

In folk tradition, horse chestnut bark and fruit were used to prepare topical ointments that could be used to relieve hemorrhoids and swelling from sprains and strains. Today, horse chestnut seed extracts are widely used in Europe for the treatment of varicose veins and chronic venous insufficiency (CVI), a condition in which blood pools in the veins of the lower legs, especially after standing or sitting. It is associated with varicose veins, pain, swelling in the ankles, feelings of heaviness in the lower legs, itching, and nighttime leg cramping. Compression stockings are one of the primary treatments, though many object to wearing them.

There is evidence from laboratory, animal, and human research that horse chestnut seed extracts (HCSE) are effective for relieving the symptoms of CVI. The **compound** most responsible for this beneficial effect is aescin. It blocks the release of **enzymes** that break down **collagen** and cause capillaries to leak fluid; it improves the elastic strength of veins, leading to a reduction in inflammation and swelling. A review of 13 clinical trials of HCE for chronic venous insufficiency found it was superior to **placebo** and as effective as compression stockings. Participants in the studies had a reduction in leg circumference at calf and ankle, as well as less pain, itching, and leg fatigue. The German health authorities approve the use of HCE for the treatment of varicose veins and CVI.

Hemorrhoids are a form of varicose veins. One controlled study of 80 people with symptomatic hemorrhoids found that HCE providing 120 mg of aescin per day reduced pain, swelling, and bleeding within 1 week.

Horse chestnut was traditionally used topically to reduce swelling after injury. A **double-blind** study of 70 people found that when horse chestnut gel, containing 2 percent aescin, was applied within 5 minutes of injury, it reduced tenderness, tendency to bruise, and swelling.

How to Use

STANDARDIZED EXTRACT: Given the toxicity with unprocessed horse chestnut seeds, only appropriately prepared seed extracts should be used. Most studies used a daily dose of 600 mg per day of HCE containing 100 to 150 mg of aescin. **TOPICAL:** Gel preparations of horse chestnut containing 2 percent aescin are commercially available. Use as directed.

Precautions

Horse chestnuts are poisonous to humans (though some animals can eat them). Properly prepared standardized extracts of horse chestnut seed appear to be safe and well tolerated. Unprocessed horse chestnuts should not be eaten or used as herbal medicine as they are associated with serious toxicity. Do not apply gel to broken or ulcerated skin.

over the (kitchen) counter GEL FOR LEGS

Purchase a high-quality horse chestnut gel and store in the refrigerator. Apply the cool gel to the lower legs each evening and elevate the legs to heart level for at least 15 minutes. This will reduce the swelling and ease the aches and pain associated with chronic venous insufficiency.

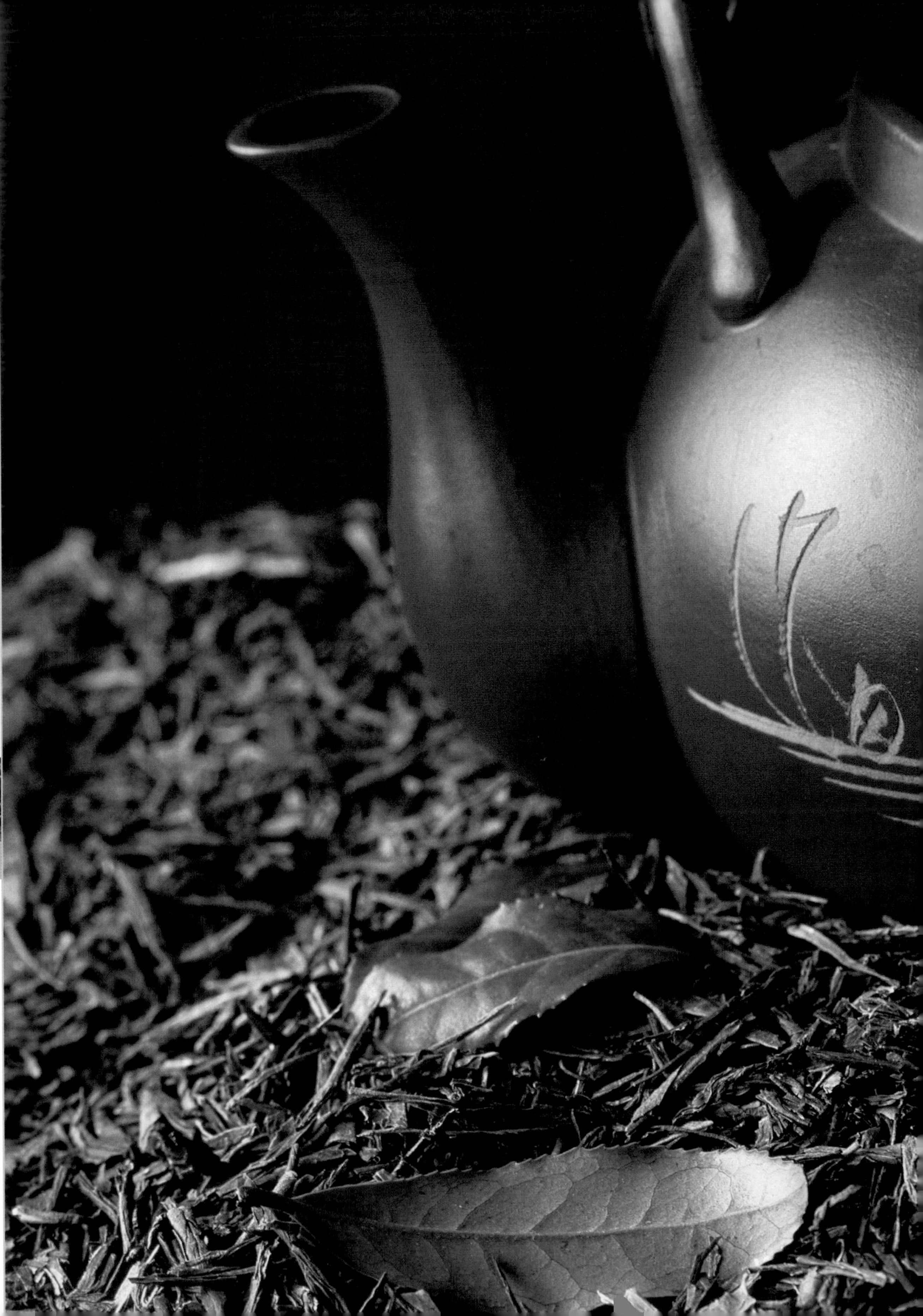

Tea

✑ *Camellia sinensis* ✑

Tea is second only to water as the world's most popular beverage. Using the dried leaves of *Camellia sinensis* to brew a steaming, soothing drink is an activity that has been going on for thousands of years. Tea's species name, *sinensis,* is a reference to China, where both this bushy shrub and tea culture got their start. Precisely when that occurred, however, is unclear, as tea's historical origins are intertwined with considerable legend and myth. According to one of those legends, the fabled Chinese emperor Shen Nong took the first sip of tea by chance in 2737 B.C.

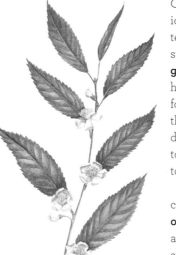

when dried leaves of the tea bush accidentally fell into a pot of boiling water, tinting it a light brown and transforming it into a refreshing drink. By the fourth century Chinese texts were consistently mentioning tea in their pages, and within several hundred years it had become the national drink. Tea spread from China to Japan in the 12th century. The Dutch East India Company brought the first tea to Europe in the early 1600s. Tea drinking soon became firmly entrenched in England and its North American colonies, where struggles over tea's taxation and control of its trade helped ignite the American Revolution.

The three main varieties of tea—green, oolong, and black—owe their differences to variations in processing the leaves. It is primarily green tea that has been used in traditional Chinese and Indian herbal medicine for many centuries. Green tea has long been valued as a stimulant, a **diuretic**, an **astringent** to control bleeding and help heal wounds, and a tonic for improving the condition of the heart and blood vessels. Traditionally, green tea was given to promote digestive health and to regulate blood sugar..

Green tea contains high concentrations of powerful **antioxidants**. Results from human, animal, and laboratory research suggest green tea may help prevent coronary heart disease. It aids in reducing cholesterol and may thwart diabetes by regulating blood sugar levels. Green tea also may reduce **inflammation** associated with inflammatory bowel diseases, promote weight loss, and inhibit or even prevent the growth of many types of cancer.

Integral to Far Eastern cultures, tea is drunk worldwide and prized for the compounds in its leaves and tender buds.

TIME LINE OF USAGE AND SPREAD

780	815	1610	1650
Taoist poet Lu Yu's "Cha Jing" describes the tea ceremony.	Buddhist monks bring the first tea seeds from China to Japan.	The Dutch East India Company imports the first tea to Europe.	Tea arrives in New Amsterdam, later to be renamed New York.

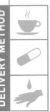
If you are a Southerner and you hear the word "camellia" you might envision the voluptuous creamy white or flamingo pink blooms that botanists label *Camellia japonica*. But the botanical definition of the genus *Camellia* describes a plant of even greater fame, known by its common name—tea. *Camellia sinensis* is by far the most widely used of the 120 species of *Camellia*. The tea plant has been cultivated in China for almost 5,000 years. It is a highly variable evergreen shrub growing from 3 to 50 feet in height. The elliptical, leathery leaves, 2 to 5 inches long and up to 2 inches wide, are dark green and glossy. Its nodding flower, about an inch across, is white, with 7 to 8 petals growing solitary or in clusters. Chinese botanists recognize 4 distinct **varieties** of the plant from collections in wild areas.

Growing Habits

The tea plant is found in warm temperate, subtropical, and tropical mountain evergreen forests in much of central and southern China, as well as northeastern India, southern Japan, South Korea, Laos, Myanmar, Thailand, and Vietnam. It is the most widely used beverage plant in the world. Since it has been grown for millennia, it is unclear whether wild-growing plants are truly wild or escaped from cultivation at some point in the distant past.

Commercial cultivation in India began with the British East India Company in the mid-19th century. In China and Japan, the selection and use of tea has evolved beyond a mere agricultural pursuit to a high art. The familiar beverage is made from the young leaves and buds of the tea plant. Fermenting wilted leaves before final drying produces black tea. Green tea leaves are simply wilted before drying. Different processing methods produce tea with varying chemical profiles, and therefore flavors, as well as various medicinal attributes.

Cultivation and Harvesting

Tea is commercially cultivated in the subtropics and tropical mountains in East Asia, where it has been grown on a large scale for many centuries. Seldom seen in American horticulture except as a specimen plant, the tea plant can be grown as a container plant, though it is finicky about soil, moisture, and light. It likes slightly acidic to neutral soils—in full sun in cooler areas, but in dappled shade in hotter areas. Soil should be moist in summer, but well drained, and relatively dry in winter. A soil mix with peat, about ⅓ sand, and high amounts of humus is suitable. In the United States limited commercial production occurs in South Carolina.

Therapeutic Uses

+ *Heart health*
+ *Cholesterol*
+ *Anti-inflammatory and antioxidant*
+ *Weight loss*
+ *Cancer prevention*

There are numerous health benefits to drinking tea. Even though black and green tea come from the same plant, much of the current press

over the (kitchen) counter EYE RELIEF

Soak 2 tea bags in cool water, wringing them out, and then chilling them well in the refrigerator. (You can also save two tea bags after having made cups of green or herbal tea.) Once the bags are chilled, lie down and place them on closed eyelids for 5 to 10 minutes. This is an easy and effective remedy to reduce puffiness around tired eyes—and seize a chance for a quiet moment or two as well.

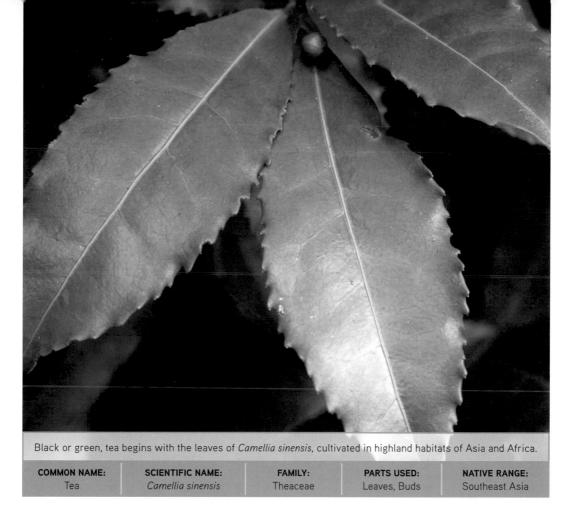

Black or green, tea begins with the leaves of *Camellia sinensis*, cultivated in highland habitats of Asia and Africa.

COMMON NAME:	SCIENTIFIC NAME:	FAMILY:	PARTS USED:	NATIVE RANGE:
Tea	*Camellia sinensis*	Theaceae	Leaves, Buds	Southeast Asia

revolves around green tea, mainly because it contains more of the **polyphenol compounds** credited with many medicinal benefits. Polyphenols are strongly antioxidant and **anti-inflammatory** and are thought to combat **atherosclerosis**, to increase HDL, or "good," cholesterol, and to weakly thin the blood. Some research has shown a decrease in risk of stroke or heart attack in people who drink 5 or more cups of green tea daily.

Tea also contains small amounts of caffeine and theophylline, compounds with a stimulating effect. The combined effect of these and polyphenols may help people to lose weight by shifting metabolism and burning fat. One study in 240 overweight people in Japan showed that a green tea **extract** lowered body weight and fat mass over a 3-month period.

Green tea also is thought to be beneficial in cancer prevention. Those who regularly drink green tea may have lower rates of some cancers, such as breast or colorectal cancer.

How to Use

INFUSION: Steep 1 teaspoon of tea leaves in a cup of hot water (steeping time depends partly on desired strength). For weight loss, weight loss maintenance, and cancer and heart attack prevention, 4 to 6 cups daily may be necessary. Decaffeinated products are an option and provide most medicinal benefits; however, caffeine and theophylline are part of how tea helps with weight loss. Adding milk to tea may decrease the absorption of polyphenols; the most medicinally effective cup of tea is made with just water, perhaps with a bit of sweetener to taste.

CAPSULE: Capsules of dried tea leaves standardized to polyphenol content are available; generally, dosage is 500 mg once or twice daily.

Precautions

There are few problems with tea, though some people feel restless and anxious as a result of the caffeine. Green tea extracts have been associated with a few reports of liver toxicity.

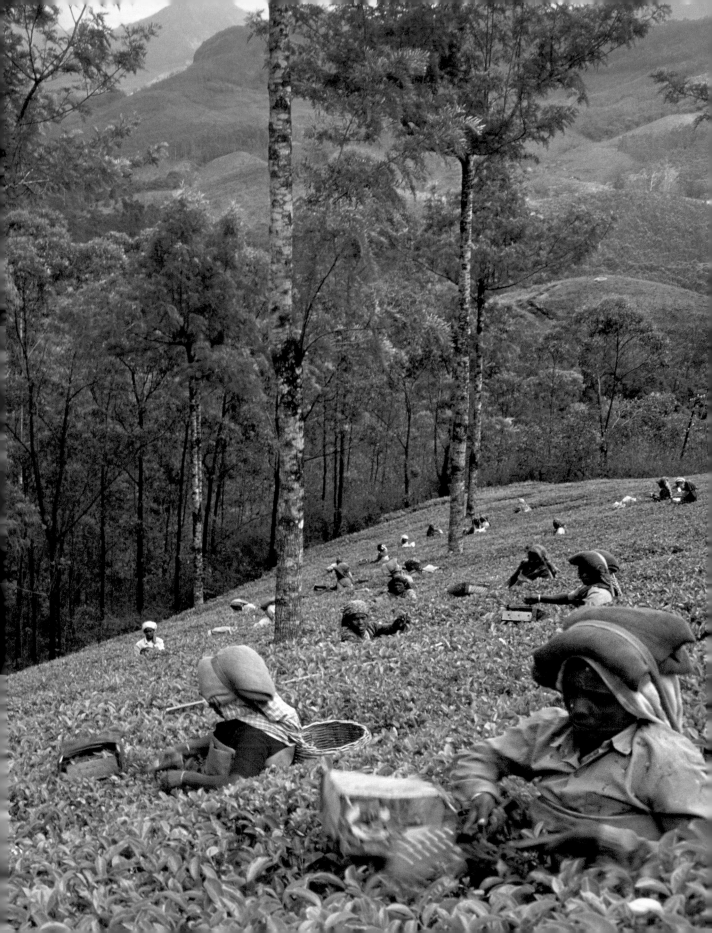

Tea Harvest

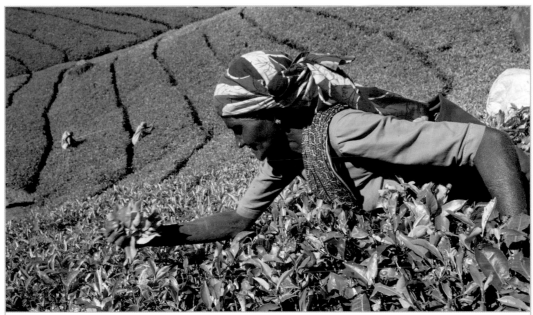

Moving slowly between verdant rows of tea plants, Tamil workers (left) harvest tea leaves on the high slopes of the Western Ghats in the Indian state of Kerala. Only the youngest shoots are plucked, typically the last 2 or 3 leaves plus the bud on a branch. Intent on her task, a Tamil woman (above) picks leaves for prized Ceylon tea on a plantation in Sri Lanka. Tea harvesting is highly labor intensive, and a deft hand is essential in order to avoid bruising the tender leaves. Sri Lankan tea harvesters (below) come in from the fields to weigh their baskets. Renowned for its high-quality tea, Sri Lanka is one of the world's largest tea-producing countries.

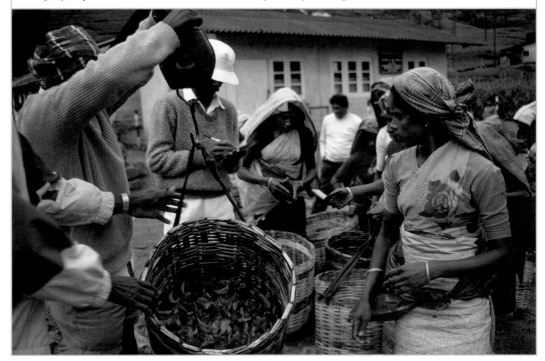

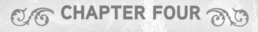

CHAPTER FOUR

Digestive System

Plants *and* Digestion

❧⟜◉⟜❧

Throughout human history, people have relied primarily on medicinal herbs to treat digestive disorders. Some of these plant remedies were probably discovered by trial and error. Others began as foods or as flavorings that, in addition to spicing up a dish, helped in digesting it. Ginger *(Zingiber officinale)* is a good example. Grown in tropical Asia since before recorded history, ginger has been used as a spice, beginning probably in South Asia, since at least 2000 B.C. One of the first known references to the herb's use in cooking is in the Hindu epic *Mahabharata*, written around the fourth century B.C., which describes a meal that includes a meat dish stewed with ginger and other spices. About this time, references to ginger had begun to appear in ancient medical works in both India and China. As trade spread ginger throughout the ancient world, its dual nature—part food, part medicine—followed it everywhere. Ginger was one of the most widely traded spices during the latter part of the Middle Ages, and it remained

particularly popular in England, where it became a common ingredient in meat dishes and sweets yet was equally valued as a digestive aid. The renowned English herbalist John Gerard summed up the English view of ginger perfectly in his 16th-century *Herball or Generall Historie of Plantes* (1597). "Ginger," he wrote, ". . . is right good with meate in sauces, or otherwise in conditures; for it is of an heating and digesting qualitie, it gently looseth the bellie, and is profitable for the stomacke."

The stomach, of course, is one of several essentially hollow organs, including the mouth, esophagus, and intestines, that together make up the digestive tract. They all connect to form a long, twisting tube that runs completely through the body. The inner walls of all these structures are lined with a type of moist, slippery tissue. Embedded in this lining are tiny glands that produce acids and enzymes essential to the process of digestion. Two adjunct organs, the liver and the pancreas, produce additional digestive juices that enter the small intestine via tiny ducts. The task of the

digestive tract is to break down and chemically convert food into small molecules of nutrients. These pass through the lining of the digestive tract (primarily in the small intestine) and ultimately enter the blood, which carries them to cells throughout the body.

It sounds so simple and straightforward. Yet digestive complaints are some of the most universal and common health concerns, and probably have been since prehistoric times. While eating is essential for survival—not to mention being one of life's great pleasures—it isn't without risks. Before proper refrigeration, food kept too long became an intestinal upset in the making, if not food poisoning. Improperly cooked meat and unwashed produce can harbor bacteria and parasites. Eating too fast or too much or failing to eat a balanced diet can cause a host of digestive problems. Left untreated, prolonged lack of appetite can harm many body systems. Illnesses, such as stomach flu, can wreak havoc with the digestive tract as well. So can stress.

Faced with these problems in their patients, the herbalists of antiquity sought plants that could remedy digestive complaints. Over time, they found many herbs that could bring about certain desired effects. Purgatives—violently powerful laxatives—were an important feature of herbal medicine in past centuries. The ancient Egyptians believed that putrefying food in the bowels would release gases that could lead to disease. Egyptians typically underwent three-day purges every month, hoping to avoid illness by cleansing their digestive tracts. Use of strong purgatives remained common in herbal and conventional medicine up until the early 19th century.

Some very bitter herbs, often simply called bitters, have also been used for millennia as digestive aids. Bitters stimulate the secretion of digestive juices in the pancreas and liver and can also spark a poor appetite and relax muscle spasms in the digestive tract. Unlike purgatives, bitters are still employed in herbal medicine.

This chapter takes a close look at 10 digestive-health-promoting medicinal plants currently widely prescribed and readily available, and whose actions are gentle, effective, and in some cases, also well documented by scientific research. Although both over-the-counter and prescription medications are widely available for most digestive problems, many people prefer medicinal herbs because they usually have fewer side effects.

The ancient Egyptians so revered chamomile (*Matricaria recutita*) for its healing powers that they dedicated it to their gods. Its popularity has hardly diminished through the centuries, and it is recommended by herbalists today for a host of problems, including indigestion, diarrhea, and inflammatory bowel conditions. Chamomile is often classified as a bitter herb.

Fennel (*Foeniculum vulgare*) has been used to treat digestive ailments for several thousand years. Most good Indian restaurants keep a small dish of fennel seeds and other digestion-aiding herbs by the door for departing patrons. Garlic (*Allium sativum*), like ginger, was probably eaten first as food and seasoning before being used medicinally. Research strongly supports garlic's role as a preventative and treatment for heart disease and atherosclerosis, and more recently as a stomach-protecting herb for warding off ulcer-causing bacteria. Ginger's popularity is growing as an herb that can combat nausea. Herbalists also recommend goldenseal (*Hydrastis canadensis*) for many of the same complaints for which Native Americans made use of it, including stomach upsets and problems with digestion.

Milk thistle (*Silybum marianum*) and peppermint (*Mentha x piperita*) trace their introduction into herbal medicine to ancient Greece and Rome and were popular herbs in medieval Europe. Milk thistle exhibits significant liver-protect- ing properties, while peppermint remains a classic calming herb for digestive tract upset and inflammation. Both milk thistle and peppermint are classified as bitters.

Another Native American herb used by indigenous tribes and later by European settlers, slippery elm (*Ulmus rubra*), is such an effective soothing agent for irritated digestive tract linings that it has been approved as an over-the-counter drug in the United States. Finally, both psyllium (*Plantago ovata, P. afra*) and turmeric (*Curcuma longa*) have been used in Indian Ayurvedic medicine for many centuries and today are highly respected herbal remedies for constipation and inflammatory bowel diseases, respectively.

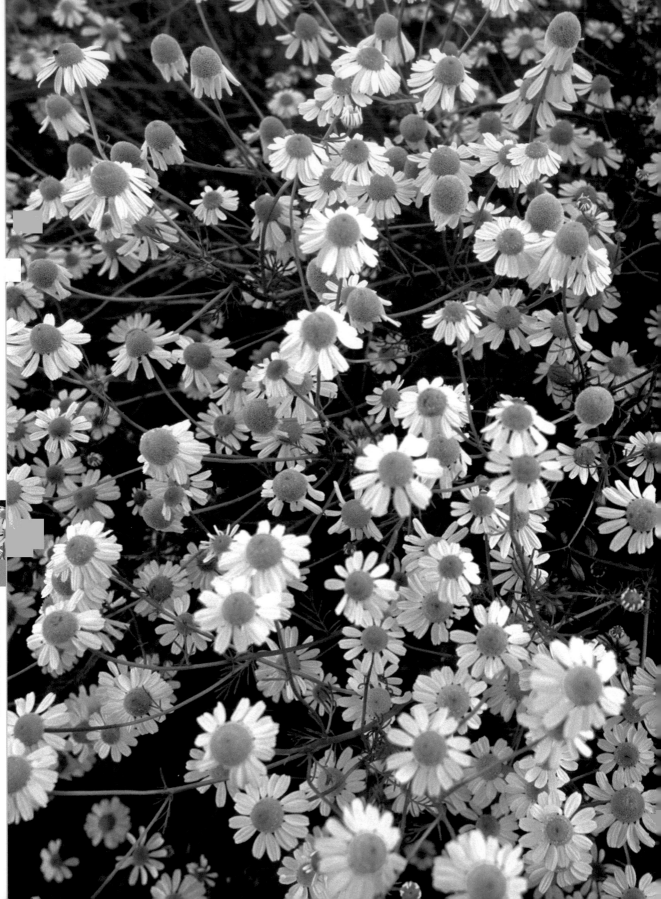

Chamomile

Matricaria recutita

After a rain, or when lightly bruised, chamomile's lacy green leaves and small, daisylike flowers give off the distinct scent of apple. That may explain the Spanish name for this herb, *manzanilla,* which means "little apple," as well as the medieval habit of strewing chamomile stems and flowers across the floors to freshen the air indoors. Two very closely related species of chamomile have earned a time-honored place in herbal medicine. German chamomile *(Matricaria recutita)* has similar effects to Roman or English chamomile *(Chamaemelum nobile)* but a

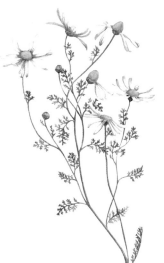

less pronounced aroma. Both varieties of this herb have been prized for many centuries—especially brewed as a pleasant-tasting tea—as a remedy for nervous tension, muscle cramps, skin conditions, and digestive upsets in babies, children, and adults. Chamomile is perhaps the most commonly used European herb in herbal medicine today.

The ancient Egyptians revered chamomile for its healing properties, believing it to be a sacred gift from the sun god, Ra. It was used medicinally, cosmetically, and in mummifying the dead. Greek physicians prescribed chamomile for fevers and gynecological problems. Chamomile found its way into European herbal medicine as early as the first century A.D. During the Middle Ages, it was an essential plant in monastery gardens; herbals of the time comment on its use to ease digestive complaints and tension, aid sleep, and dissolve kidney stones and gallstones. Introduced to North America by European colonists in the 16th century, it was prescribed in the 1800s to treat digestive problems and skin conditions.

Chamomile remains a popular treatment for digestive and inflammatory conditions. In modern herbal medicine, it is suggested for indigestion, heartburn, flatulence, diarrhea, gastritis, infant colic, Crohn's disease, and irritable bowel syndrome. It is recommended to relieve muscle tension and to ease anxiety. Applied externally, chamomile soothes irritated or inflamed skin, including eczema. Used as a mouthwash, chamomile has been found to prevent mouth sores associated with chemotherapy and radiation.

Treasured for centuries, chamomile's daisylike blooms are the source of its power to soothe the digestive tract.

TIME LINE OF USAGE AND SPREAD

CA 1550 B.C.	A.D. 1500s	1653	1987
Chamomile's medicinal use first recorded in *Codex Ebers* in ancient Egypt.	European colonists introduce chamomile to North America.	Herbalist N. Culpeper touts chamomile as a digestive aid in *The English Physician.*	Germans name chamomile medicinal "plant of the year."

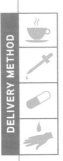
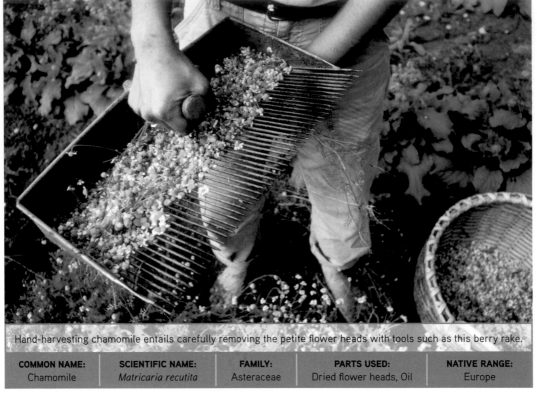

Hand-harvesting chamomile entails carefully removing the petite flower heads with tools such as this berry rake.

COMMON NAME:	SCIENTIFIC NAME:	FAMILY:	PARTS USED:	NATIVE RANGE:
Chamomile	*Matricaria recutita*	Asteraceae	Dried flower heads, Oil	Europe

DIGESTIVE SYSTEM

There are six species in the genus *Matricaria*. In many herb guides, German chamomile is designated *Matricaria chamomilla* and *Matricaria recutita*, causing some confusion. German chamomile is an erect, smooth-stemmed annual from 4 to 16 inches tall, and much branched above. The feathery leaves have narrow, divided segments The flowers look like small daisies, about an inch or less across. Chamomile is one of numerous small flowers in the aster **family** distinguished by their technical characteristics.

Slovak chamomile specialist Ivan Salamon has identified four basic chemical types of German chamomile. The categories are based on chemotypes, or distinct chemical groups containing certain constituents in their **essential oils**. Commercial producers select these variations based on the specifications for a final product. Selection and breeding programs have resulted in producing higher quality chamomile with more stable, predictable components and higher levels of active ingredients. In addition to genetic differences, quality and quantity of essential oils depend on variables such as environmental factors, cultivation practices, plant parts and age, and post-harvest handling.

Growing Habits

Chamomile has been cultivated for centuries, probably originating in southeastern Europe, but today grows throughout Europe. Introduced to North America by European settlers, it is found throughout eastern North America.

Another **species** of chamomile, known as English or Roman chamomile (*Chamaemelum nobile* or *Anthemis nobilis*) is a perennial that is primarily grown in England and popular among herb gardeners for its foliage.

In dried chamomile flowers it is easy to tell the difference between German and English chamomile by cutting a flower head in half longitudinally. The receptacle, the end of the stalk bearing flowers, in German chamomile is hollow within; in English chamomile, it is solid.

Cultivation and Harvesting

Chamomile is easily grown from seed and self-sows freely. If allowed to go to seed, chamomile will be found at garden's edge the following spring, growing on its own. From sowing seed to flowering, chamomile is a short-lived annual, lasting about 8 weeks, germinating in early spring, and completing its growing cycle by the end of June. German chamomile likes full sun and will grow in almost any soil. It does well in sandy loam with good drainage. Chamomile is a cool weather plant that does best in spring and early summer, wilting under summer heat.

It is grown commercially in Eastern Europe, particularly Slovakia, Czech Republic, and Hungary. Argentina and Egypt are also major producers of chamomile flowers. Specialized, modified combines that comb flowers from row plantings are used for flower harvest.

Therapeutic Uses

+ *Digestive aid*
+ *Colic*
+ *Mouth ulcers*
+ *Eczema*

A treasured herbal medicine, chamomile has soothed digestive systems and calmed people of all ages for centuries. But not until the 1970s were scientists able to document and verify chamomile's healing and protective effects on the gastrointestinal mucosa (lining). Germany's health authorities recognize the effectiveness of chamomile for relieving digestive spasms and inflammation when taken internally. Chamomile eases bloating and indigestion when taken after meals and can soothe occasional heartburn. Many herbalists consider chamomile the premier children's herb for easing upset tummies and calming frayed nerves after an exhausting day. Remember Peter Rabbit? His mother gave him a dose of chamomile tea ("One tablespoonful to be taken at bed-time.") after his escapade sampling all the vegetables in Mr. McGregor's garden left him with a tummy that needed soothing. A study of colicky babies found that chamomile, in combination with other herbs, was highly effective in reducing crying times when the babies were compared with those in the control group.

Chamomile is also popular for alleviating inflammation of the mouth and skin. A study of patients with chronic mouth ulcers found a remarkable 82 percent rated chamomile **extract** as excellent for relieving pain. **Compounds** in chamomile have been shown to enhance skin healing and help prevent infection.

Applied topically, a proprietary chamomile cream was shown to be as effective as low-dose, over-the-counter hydrocortisone cream for relieving eczema. Chamomile is also found in creams designed to soothe and heal diaper rash, skin irritations, and minor wounds. Germany's health commission also recognizes the effectiveness of using chamomile externally for inflammation of the skin and mucous membranes, including those of the mouth and gums.

How to Use

TEA: Pour 1 cup boiling water over 1 teaspoon of herb. Steep for 5 to 7 minutes. The longer it steeps, the more powerful its calming effects.
CAPSULES: 500 to 1,000 mg dried chamomile flowers taken 2 to 3 times per day.
TINCTURE: 3 to 5 ml taken 2 to 3 times per day.
TOPICAL: Creams are available. Use as directed.

Precautions

Chamomile is very safe. In rare cases, allergic reactions occur, especially in those with severe ragweed allergies.

over the (kitchen) counter CHAMOMILE COMFORT

For a nice soothing pick-me-up in the afternoon, pour 2 cups boiling water over 1 tea bag chamomile, 1 tea bag peppermint, and 1 tea bag green tea. Let the tea bags steep for 5 to 7 minutes. Strain. Drink warm and share with a friend.

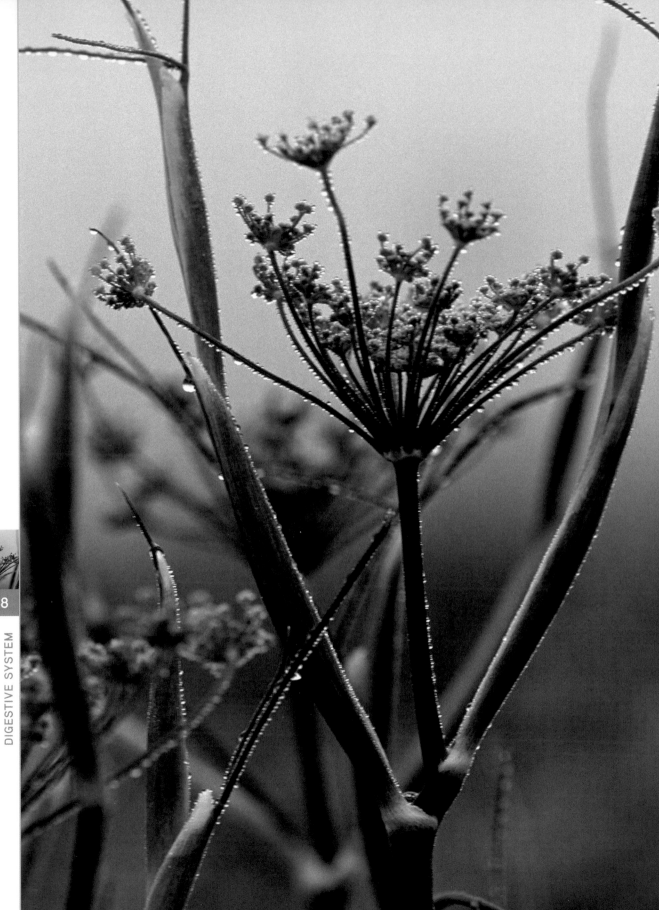

DIGESTIVE SYSTEM

Fennel

Foeniculum vulgare

A close cousin to parsley, caraway, and dill, fennel is a statuesque plant with graceful, feathery stems that can easily reach 4 or 5 feet tall. The stems arise from a white or pale green bulb that is crunchy and sweet. All parts of fennel, in fact, are edible and possess a mild flavor similar to anise or licorice. The word "fennel" came from the Old English *fenol* or *finol*, which in turn is likely a corruption of the name the Romans gave the plant: *foeniculum* (now its genus name). In ancient Greece, however, it was called *marathron*, from *maraino*, which means "to grow thin"—a reference to fennel's use as an appetite suppressant. Centuries later, the American Puritans used fennel seeds in the same way. Called meeting seeds, small dry fennel seeds were chewed to dull hunger pangs during church services.

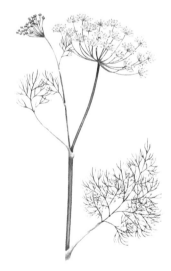

Fennel has been a medicinal herb, as well as a culinary plant, for more than 2,000 years. The Greek physicians Hippocrates (460-377 B.C.) and Dioscorides (A.D. 40-90) recommended fennel to soothe colicky infants and to stimulate the flow of breast milk in nursing mothers. Roman physician and naturalist Pliny the Elder (A.D. 23-79) included fennel in more than 20 different medicinal remedies. In India, fennel was considered a digestive aid by **Ayurvedic** practitioners. Impressed by fennel, the emperor Charlemagne (A.D. 742-814) is credited with introducing the herb to central and northern Europe. In England, fennel became one of the 9 sacred herbs—described in a tenth-century herbal—believed to cure all illness. European colonists brought fennel to the United States, where it was used to aid digestion, freshen breath, soothe sore throats and heal infected gums, promote milk production in nursing mothers, and flavor medicines.

Contemporary herbalists, like their earlier counterparts, recommend fennel for digestive health: to relieve bloating, gas, and diarrhea; settle upset stomachs; improve appetite or reduce food cravings; and buffer cramping effects of laxatives. And fennel is still given to infants to relieve colic, gas, and bloating and increase the flow of breast milk. As a gargle, it relieves coughs and sore throats.

Elegant flower stalks of fennel develop as airy clusters that ultimately produce tiny fruits used in herbal medicine.

TIME LINE OF USAGE AND SPREAD

50-70	CA 1145	1797	1842
Greek physician Dioscorides mentions fennel in medical text *De Materia Medica*.	Benedictine Abbess Hildegard von Bingen touts fennel for flu and digestion.	First distillery to make absinthe, from wormwood and fennel, opens in France.	Poet H. W Longfellow in "Goblet of Life" writes that fennel imparts courage.

The genus *Foeniculum* is a small plant group with 4 or 5 species from Eurasia. Two varieties are commonly grown in gardens. Finocchio, or Florence fennel, is a well-known annual that is grown as a vegetable for its swollen leaf bases, often blanched and sold wherever specialty vegetables are offered. Variety "Dulce" is primarily grown for its seeds as a flavoring herb and for its essential oil content. Depending upon the flavor and fragrance of components in the fruit, varieties are deemed either sweet fennel or bitter fennel. These are the fennel seeds of commerce, also used in herbal preparations.

Mostly annual in habit, fennel may also be **biennial** or a short-lived perennial. Once it goes to seed, the plant's life cycle ends. A tall, erect plant, fennel grows from 3 to 8 feet tall, depending on the cultivar and growing conditions. The branching stems are light to dark green, polished in appearance, finely furrowed, and filled with a nearly solid pith. The fine, filament-like, many-branched leaves have a wispy appearance. The flowers are yellow, borne in numerous umbels (umbrella-like structures) at the top of the plant. It flowers from July to September.

The anise-flavored seeds (technically fruits) are oblong or ellipsoid, greenish yellow, and 5-ribbed.

Growing Habits

Common fennel was cultivated in Greece at least 5,000 years ago. It is believed native to Asia from western China to the Caspian Sea, but is now so widely naturalized throughout Europe that its origins are obscured in history. It spread across central and northern Europe during the Middle Ages and was grown in Spain as early as 961.

Fennel undoubtedly arrived in North America with early European settlers. It has become naturalized, even weedy, along the West Coast

DIGESTIVE SYSTEM

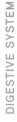

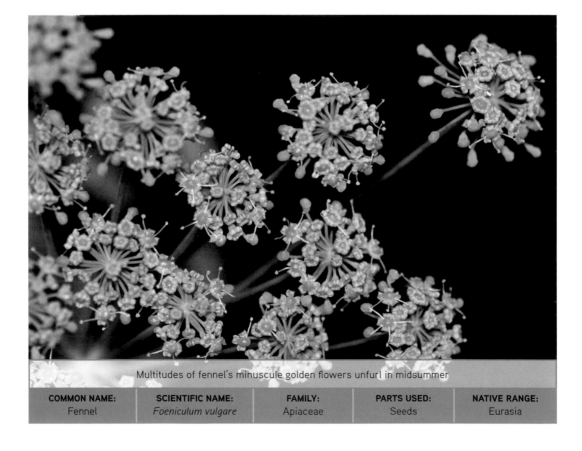

Multitudes of fennel's minuscule golden flowers unfurl in midsummer

COMMON NAME:	SCIENTIFIC NAME:	FAMILY:	PARTS USED:	NATIVE RANGE:
Fennel	*Foeniculum vulgare*	Apiaceae	Seeds	Eurasia

Combine in a saucepan, ½ tablespoon fennel seed, 3 tablespoons organic honey, and 1 cup water. Bring ingredients to a boil. Turn down the heat and simmer on low for approximately 20 minutes. Remove from heat and strain. Store in refrigerator for up to 1 week. Take 1 tablespoon syrup every 3 to 4 hours as needed for a cough or cold.

from California to Washington State. It is commonly seen along roadsides in the western reaches of those states. It is also naturalized in much of eastern North America but is not as common as it is on the West Coast. In the Mediterranean region, northern Europe, and the western United States, it is often associated with coastal habitats.

Its **genus** name, *Foeniculum,* is the ancient classical name for the plant, from the Latin *foen,* meaning "hay"; the fragrance of the freshly dried leaves is like that of hay.

Cultivation and Harvesting

Fennel is easily grown from seed sown directly in the garden after danger of frost has passed. Seed usually germinates in 14 days. It is a cool season crop that can be planted early in the year. Fennel thrives in full sun and likes a light, dry, limey soil with a pH from 7 to 8.5. Finocchio fennel, grown for its fleshy stalks, needs a rich soil with plenty of moisture to produce succulent, delicious stems.

Fennel seed is harvested once the plants ripen. Finocchio fennel is usually grown locally for nearby markets. The largest suppliers to world markets are China, Egypt, and India.

Therapeutic Uses

+ *Digestive aid*
+ *Colic*
+ *Menstrual cramps*
+ *Coughs and colds*

Fennel has a rich history as a medicinal and culinary herb. Fennel seeds have a flavor similar to anise or licorice and are baked into breads, stuffed into Italian sausages, and often added to sauerkraut. As a medicine, fennel seeds are considered to be a premier **carminative**, or herb that aids digestion and alleviates cramping

by relaxing the muscles of the digestive and reproductive systems. Two studies in infants have shown that fennel seed reduces colic when used alone or in combination with chamomile and lemon balm. Carminatives are often added to laxatives to prevent intestinal cramping. A 28-day study of nursing home patients with chronic constipation found that an herbal tea that included fennel was effective and well tolerated. Chewing fennel seeds to improve the breath and aid digestion is common in India, and candied fennel can be found in many Indian restaurants.

Fennel seeds may help women suffering with menstrual cramps. One study found that fennel eased cramping to roughly the same degree as mefenamic acid, a commonly prescribed **anti-inflammatory** medication. Historically fennel was used as a lactagogue, or herb that can increase breast milk production, though there is no modern evidence to confirm this effect.

Fennel seeds are sometimes added to cough and cold syrups both for flavor and medicinal purposes. Animal studies show that fennel helps thin mucus and aid **expectoration**. German health authorities recognize fennel seed to treat gas, indigestion, and upper respiratory congestion. Fennel seed makes an excellent gargle for sore throats and bad breath.

How to Use

TEA: Pour 1 cup boiling water over ½ teaspoon crushed seeds and steep for 10 minutes and strain. Cool thoroughly if giving to a child.

Precautions

Fennel is included on the Food and Drug Administration's list of herbs generally regarded as safe (GRAS). Use in pregnancy should be limited to what is found in food.

Garlic

❧ *Allium sativum* ❧

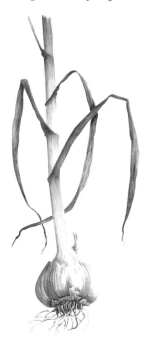

Garlic's slender green leaves, bulbous white roots, and pungent flavor and aroma mark it as a member of the genus *Allium*, along with onions, leeks, and chives. Prized as a vegetable, a condiment, and a medicine, garlic has been part of human culture since ancient times, in both East and West. First cultivated perhaps more than 7,000 years ago, this herb was long thought to impart strength and stamina. The legions of slaves who built Egypt's great pyramids were given garlic and onions as part of their daily diet. The original Olympic athletes in Greece ate garlic before competitions, possibly making it one of the earliest performance-enhancing substances. Widely used in spells and charms, garlic was believed to protect against all forms of evil, including witches and, more famously, vampires. Medicinally, garlic has long been revered for its powers, particularly in treating infections.

In China—by or even before 2000 B.C.—garlic was prescribed for digestive and respiratory ailments, diarrhea, and worm infestations. The **Ayurvedic** medical tradition of India also used garlic medicinally. No fewer than 23 prescriptions that include garlic are found in the writings of the Greek physician Pliny the Elder. During the Middle Ages, garlic was grown in monastery gardens throughout Europe, where it was used for digestive, kidney, and breathing disorders. European explorers and colonists introduced garlic to the New World, and by the 1800s it had found a home in American traditional medicine. Even in the 20th century, garlic's properties were so respected that it was given to wounded soldiers to fight infection and prevent gangrene during World War I and even later, when antibiotics were unavailable.

Today, garlic is used to prevent and treat heart disease, regulate cholesterol levels, reduce high blood pressure, and strengthen the immune system. It is suggested to ease cold symptoms and respiratory infections. Herbal practitioners also recommend it for digestive complaints, as it may help inhibit gut bacteria, including *Helicobacter pylori*, implicated in ulcers and stomach cancer.

Layers of papery skin cover the cloves of a garlic bulb, a source of time-tested remedies in the herbal apothecary.

TIME LINE OF USAGE AND SPREAD

1550 B.C.	**A.D.50-70**	**1665**	**1858**
The *Codex Ebers*, a medical text from ancient Egypt, mentions garlic's value.	Greek physician Dioscorides praises garlic in his medical treatise *De Materia Medica*.	The London College of Physicians recommends garlic to prevent plague.	French microbiologist Louis Pasteur shows garlic juice can kill infectious bacteria.

Garlic comes from the large genus *Allium*, the same genus to which onions and chives belong. Garlic is a perennial usually grown as an annual. It has several flat, grayish-green leaves about a foot long and a half inch wide. The flower stalk, arising from the base of the plant, may reach 3 feet in height. Globular clusters of white flowers unfold from a papery beak-like envelope; bulbels—miniature seed bulbs—often develop in place of flowers.

If planted in early spring, flowers emerge in midsummer. The root is a fleshy bulb, one or more inches broad. A thin white, pink, or reddish papery sheathing encases a half dozen or more pointed oblong cloves. Numerous **varieties** are grown commercially.

Growing Habits

Garlic is not known in the wild. Rather it is deemed a cultigen, evolved over millennia of human interaction with the plant. Garlic's closest wild relatives grow in the Asian steppes and have been cultivated for perhaps 7,000 years. Two thousand years ago, Pliny (A.D. 23-79) described 6 varieties of garlic grown in ancient Rome. In China large-scale cultivation is recorded in the Tang dynasty (618-907).

Allium is the ancient Latin name for garlic, derived from the Celtic *all*, signifying "hot or burning." The **species** name *sativum* means "cultivated" or "planted." *Gar-leac*, or "spear-plant" is an Anglo-Saxon designation from which "garlic" is derived.

Cultivation and Harvesting

Garlic grows well in any good soil suitable for a vegetable garden. It prefers warmer weather, thriving in a moist, sandy, slightly alkaline soil. Garlic must be grown in full sun. It is easily propagated from nursery sets (bulbels), or by planting individual garlic cloves, the easiest method for the home gardener. Plant the pointed end up, about an inch deep. Space plants 6 to 12 inches apart. In regions free from ground frost, plant garlic in late fall for harvest the following summer. In regions where the ground freezes, plant as soon as the ground thaws in spring.

Fresh garlic and dried (dehydrated) garlic are treated as two separate commodities commercially. Like fresh vegetables, fresh garlic reaches consumers through produce supply chains. Dried garlic products reach grocery store shelves through the spice trade. In the U.S. the fresh and dehydrated garlic industries are centered in five counties in central California. The city of Gilroy, east of the southern Santa Cruz Mountains, is the epicenter of American garlic production.

Therapeutic Uses

+ *Diarrhea*
+ *Coughs and colds*
+ *Heart health*

Garlic is a key ingredient in many ethnic cuisines and has a cherished history in herbal medicine. It also has a stunning reputation for fighting off infections, especially in the gut and lungs. With the growing problem of antibiotic resistance (when bacteria and parasites are no longer vulnerable to antibiotics), garlic could be critical.

Louis Pasteur first documented garlic's antibacterial activity in 1858. Albert Schweitzer relied on garlic

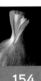
over the (kitchen) counter TIERAONA'S GARLIC

Soften garlic cloves by soaking or steeping. Then crush 2 small to medium cloves and put in a teacup. Pour 1 cup near-boiling water over the garlic and add 1 teaspoon honey and 1 teaspoon lemon juice. Drink warm at the first sign of a cold.

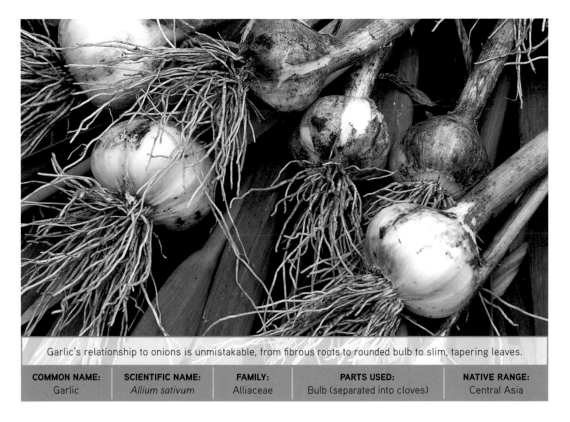

Garlic's relationship to onions is unmistakable, from fibrous roots to rounded bulb to slim, tapering leaves.

COMMON NAME:	SCIENTIFIC NAME:	FAMILY:	PARTS USED:	NATIVE RANGE:
Garlic	*Allium sativum*	Alliaceae	Bulb (separated into cloves)	Central Asia

to treat amoebic dysentery for years in Africa. Now modern research has confirmed that garlic can kill a number of diarrhea-causing organisms, including *Salmonella, Escherichia coli, Entamoeba histolytica,* and *Giardia lamblia.* Fresh garlic also impairs many organisms that cause colds and pneumonia. In fact, a preliminary study found that taking a garlic supplement helped prevent the common cold.

Not only can garlic help fight infection but it may reduce the risk of some cancers. In 2002, the *Journal of the National Cancer Institute* reported results of a population-based study showing reduced risk of prostate cancer for men with a high dietary intake of garlic and scallions. Garlic also protects the gastrointestinal tract. Seven studies evaluating garlic consumption found that those who ate the most raw and cooked garlic had the lowest risk of colorectal cancer. Multiple studies have found that aged garlic **extracts** prevent or reduce gastrointestinal toxicity resulting from methotrexate, a drug often prescribed for autoimmune conditions.

There are also good reasons to include garlic in a heart-healthy diet. It helps lower cholesterol and blood pressure, though its effects are mild. Garlic also makes **platelets** a little less sticky, thus reducing the risk of clots.

How to Use

Cooking deactivates some of garlic's activity, so one of the easiest ways to take garlic is simply to eat it! Raw garlic is probably the optimal form. Crush a couple cloves and put in olive oil, add a dash of lemon, and toss over a salad.

CAPSULES: If buying garlic in capsule form, look for products standardized to allicin, a key ingredient. Research suggests garlic products providing 4 to 8 mg allicin daily are optimal.

Precautions

Garlic is safe and well tolerated in the regular diet. There is a small risk that eating larger quantities of raw garlic (more than 4 cloves per day) can affect platelets' ability to form a clot, so it makes sense to reduce consumption 10 days before surgery and to not exceed this amount if taking anticoagulant medications. Garlic can also interfere with medications used to treat HIV infection.

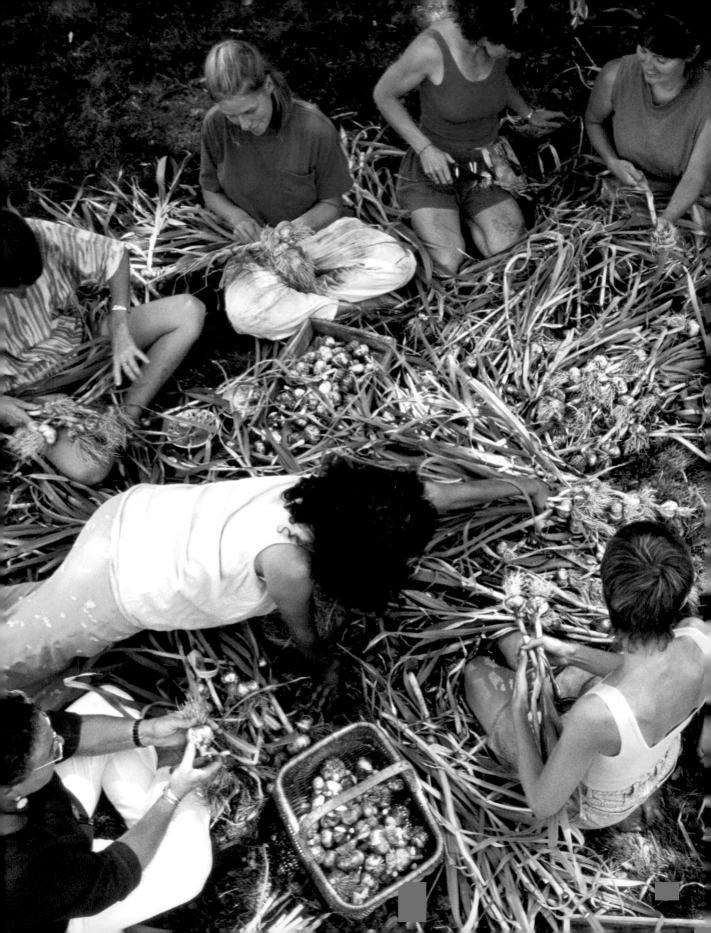

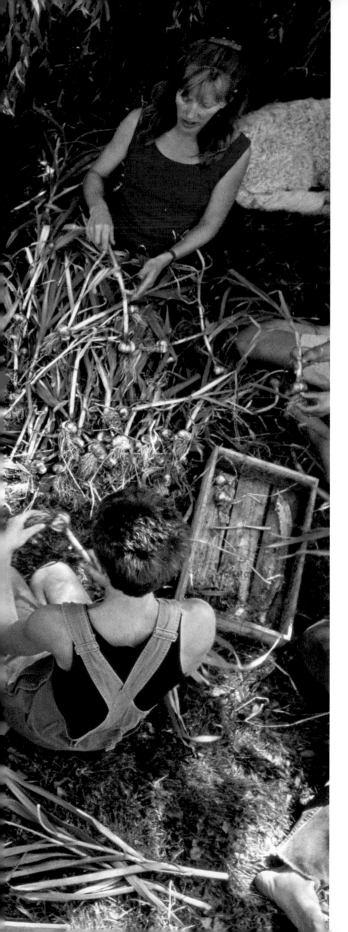

Garlic
Harvest

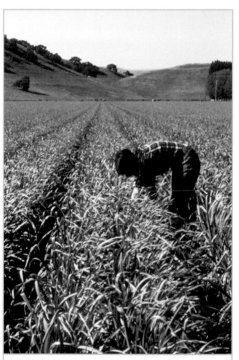

In the United States and much of Europe, garlic is harvested in mid- to late summer, usually commencing in July and continuing through August, depending on the variety and strain. Leaf condition is one key to timing a garlic harvest. A bulb is typically ready to be lifted when slightly more than half of its lower leaves have begun to brown and die off. Final determination is made after close examination of a sampling of bulbs. A worker (above) inspects bulb condition in a field near Gilroy, California, a garlic-producing hub in the central part of the state known for its annual garlic festival. Workers in Rockport, Maine (left), gather around mounds of freshly harvested garlic to remove dirt and detritus. Bulbs must be handled with care, as they are surprisingly fragile; the slightest bump can bruise the inner cloves, causing decay and loss of quality. After being allowed to dry, or cure, for about 2 weeks after harvesting, garlic bulbs are trimmed of their stalks, placed in containers, and stored or shipped. Alternatively, the stalks are left on and woven together to create simple or elaborate garlic braids.

DIGESTIVE SYSTEM

Ginger

ᚲᚷ *Zingiber officinale* ᚷᚳ

Ginger is native to Asia, where it has been used as a spice for at least 4,400 years. Over the centuries, it has become one of the world's most popular culinary flavorings. Its intensely clean, slightly sweet and zesty heat is an essential element in everything from Indian curries and Thai stir-fries to gingerbread and ginger ale. Ginger's genus name, *Zingiber*, is derived from the Greek *zingiberis*, which, in turn, came from the Sanskrit *sringabera*, meaning "horn shaped." The reference is to the knobby shape of the plant's roots, or more accurately, rhizomes.

Its tuberous, underground stems are the part of ginger used in cooking and in herbal medicine, where ginger is prized as an aid to digestion and remedy for stomach upset, diarrhea, and nausea.

Since ancient times, ginger has played a role in Arabic, Indian, and Asian herbal medicine. It has been an essential ingredient in traditional Chinese medicine since the fourth century B.C. In ancient India, ginger was known by its Sanskrit name, *vishwabhesaj,* meaning "universal medicine," and used to treat digestive upsets and intestinal gas and stimulate circulation in the body's extremities. The Greeks and Romans imported ginger from the East and ate it as a cure for intestinal parasites. During the Middle Ages, it was held in such high esteem that it was said to have come from the Garden of Eden. Ginger was used to treat a variety of

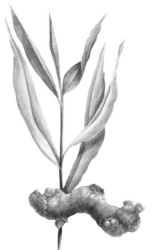

complaints, from stimulating digestion and easing nausea to treating colds, bronchitis, and flu.

Modern herbal medicine practitioners prescribe ginger to prevent or treat nausea and vomiting associated with motion sickness. Unlike many prescription and over-the-counter motion sickness medicines, ginger does not cause drowsiness or dry mouth. Ginger is also used to treat nausea associated with pregnancy and cancer chemotherapy and after surgery. Because of its **antiseptic** properties, ginger is suggested for infections of the digestive tract and the effects of food poisoning. Fresh gingerroot can be chewed to relieve sore throat. Ginger tea is used to treat colds, flu, headaches, and painful menstruation. Ginger is also used in traditional medicine to reduce pain and inflammation associated with arthritis and ulcerative colitis.

Fresh or dried, ginger's gnarled roots possess a fragrant fiery heat as well as compounds that aid digestion.

TIME LINE OF USAGE AND SPREAD

500 B.C.
Confucius notes that he is never without ginger when he eats.

A.D. 200
Ginger is listed as a taxable commodity by the Romans.

1547
Export to Europe of large quantities of West Indian and American ginger begins.

1884
Great Britain imports more than 5 million pounds of ginger root.

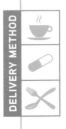

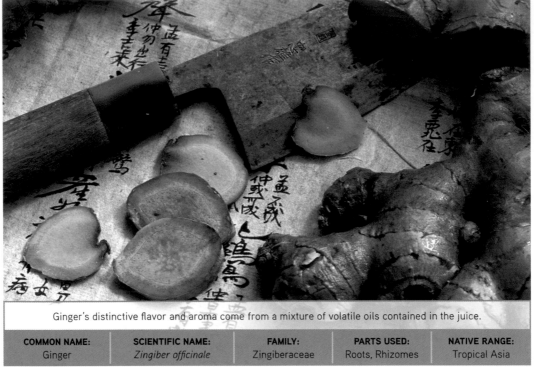

Ginger's distinctive flavor and aroma come from a mixture of volatile oils contained in the juice.

COMMON NAME:	SCIENTIFIC NAME:	FAMILY:	PARTS USED:	NATIVE RANGE:
Ginger	*Zingiber officinale*	Zingiberaceae	Roots, Rhizomes	Tropical Asia

Zingiber, a genus with a center of diversity in Southeast Asia extending throughout tropical Asia and tropical Australia to southern Japan, includes about 100 species. The best known is common ginger (*Zingiber officinale*). Ginger is a robust, herbaceous perennial that reaches a height of more than 20 inches. It has linear, lance-shaped leaves closely hugging the stem. They are about 7 inches long and an inch or so wide, narrowing to a slender tip.

Greenish yellow flowers with dark purplish lips crowd into a clublike spike on a flowering stalk. Many cultivated **varieties** rarely flower. Most flowering plants are grown for several years as tropical perennials before a bloom appears. The **rhizomes** (underground stems), the familiar plant part of commerce, are highly aromatic, with thick, branching lobes, varying in size and shape depending on the cultivated variety.

Growing Habits

Ginger has been cultivated in tropical Asia since ancient times, but its origins are obscure. No wild forms of ginger are known in tropical Asia. Perhaps originating in India, it spread throughout the Asian tropics before recorded history. Today ginger is grown around the world in humid tropical climates.

Like pepper, ginger arrived in Europe at least 2,000 years ago. Greek and Roman authors surmised that gingerroot was a product of the Arabian Peninsula, since it arrived in southern Europe via Arab trading routes. Long before potatoes, tomatoes, or red peppers arrived from the Americas, ginger was familiar to Europeans who could afford it. By the 13th century, Marco Polo had observed it growing in India and China. Tariff duties were levied on ginger in Barcelona, Paris, and Marseilles. In 14th-century England, ginger was second only to black pepper in popularity. A pound of ginger was about equal to the price of 1 sheep. In the 16th century, Portuguese traders carried ginger from East to West Africa, then to South America. The Spanish established plantations in Jamaica, still known as a producer of high-quality ginger.

Cultivation and Harvesting

Ginger is grown locally and commercially throughout the tropics. It is usually the rhizome's outer lobes—with a bud or an eye—that propagate ginger. The first shoots pop up within 2 weeks. Ginger likes a moderately rich loam and warm, humid, sunny conditions.

It is usually harvested about 9 months after planting. Products include fresh rhizomes (green ginger), dried ginger, preserved ginger, and **essential oils**. The fragrant oils that come from fresh and from dried roots are sold as 2 distinctly different products.

Therapeutic Uses

+ *Motion sickness*
+ *Morning sickness*
+ *Nausea and vomiting*
+ *Inflammation*
+ *Coughs and colds*

In herbal medicine, ginger is prized for treating indigestion and nausea. This traditional use has been strongly confirmed by science. Many human studies have shown that ginger eases nausea and reduces vomiting in pregnancy, motion sickness, and chemotherapy. A National Cancer Institute study found that if patients take 0.5 to 1.0 g of ginger for three days before and after chemotherapy along with antinausea medications, nausea is reduced by an additional 40 percent. The way ginger relieves nausea is not completely understood, but current thinking is that **compounds** in ginger bind to receptors in the gastrointestinal tract that then act to turn down the sensation of nausea and to accelerate digestion, thus reducing the time food sits in the stomach.

Ginger is being investigated for reducing the inflammation and pain of arthritis. Human studies have shown that ginger relieves osteoarthritis pain in the knees better than **placebo** but not as well as ibuprofen.

Sip a cup of hot ginger tea on a cold winter night and you will appreciate the warming properties of ginger, as it improves circulation by gently opening blood vessels in the feet and hands. Ginger tea not only warms your toes but may keep you from getting sick. Compounds in ginger have been shown to destroy many of the viruses that cause the common cold!

How to Use

FRESH GINGER TEA: Slice one inch of fresh ginger rhizome into small pieces. Simmer in 2 cups water on low heat for 15 minutes. Strain. Drink 1 to 3 cups per day for coughs and colds and to enhance circulation.

DRIED GINGER TEA: Pour 1 cup boiling water over ¼ to ½ teaspoon ginger powder and steep for 10 minutes. Pour liquid tea off and discard powder. Drink 1 cup after meals for gas/bloating or to ease nausea.

CAPSULES: Take 250 to 500 mg 2 to 3 times per day.

EXTRACTS: Concentrated **extracts** are typically used for osteoarthritis. Use as directed.

Precautions

Adding ginger to the diet is safe for young and old. Ginger may possibly cause mild heartburn in some. Pregnant women should not take more than 1 g of dried ginger per day. Do not combine high doses of ginger with anticoagulant drugs (blood thinners) without medical supervision.

over the (kitchen) counter HOMEMADE GINGER ALE

Combine in a saucepan 1 inch fresh ginger rhizome, grated, with 1 cup water and ¾ cup raw sugar. Cook over medium heat until the sugar is dissolved. Remove from heat and steep, covered, for 1 hour. Strain the syrup and refrigerate for another hour. Pour into a 2-liter container with tight-fitting lid. Add ⅛ teaspoon active dry yeast, 2 tablespoons fresh lemon juice, and 6 cups water and shake to mix. Leave container at room temperature for 48 hours and then refrigerate. Use within 10 days.

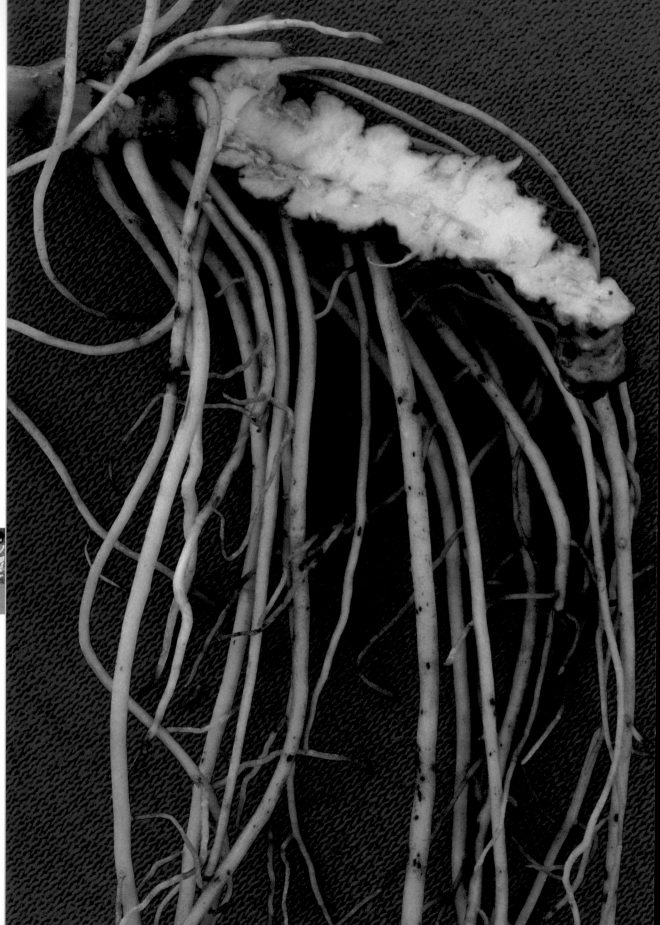

Goldenseal

An American native, goldenseal is a member of the buttercup family that once grew in great abundance in the eastern deciduous forests of the United States. The "golden" part of its common name comes from the bright yellow interior of the plant's fleshy rhizomes (underground stems). "Seal" is a reference to small, circular marks on the rhizome's twisted, wrinkled surface that were thought to resemble the decorative seals once used to stamp warm wax onto envelope flaps. Native American tribes used goldenseal to produce a beautiful golden yellow dye.

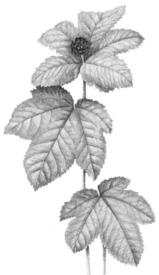

They also used the herb medicinally and introduced European settlers to its healing properties in the 1700s. A century later, goldenseal had gained such popularity that it was severely overharvested, an assault that continued into the 20th century, until wild stocks were legally protected. Now cultivated, but still scarce in the wild, goldenseal is a top-selling herbal supplement marketed to aid digestion, treat infection, and boost the immune system.

The Cherokee used the bitter-tasting **rhizomes** of goldenseal as an eyewash and for skin problems. It was also given to settle stomach upsets, stimulate appetite, as an **antiseptic** to ease inflammation, and as a general cure-all. European settlers adopted goldenseal primarily as an eyewash and a soothing remedy for sore throats, mouth sores, and digestive upsets.

Goldenseal was little more than a folk remedy until the late 1800s, when American physicians practicing **Eclectic** medicine began promoting its use in traditional ways. Soon goldenseal's popularity soared.

Some of goldenseal's traditional applications have been retained in modern herbal medicine. Today goldenseal is recommended for soothing the stomach and aiding digestion. It is used to treat inflammations of the skin, eyes, and mucous membranes, including sinusitis, conjunctivitis, urinary tract infections, vaginitis, sore throats, and canker sores. Many herbalists recommend goldenseal for colds, hay fever (allergic rhinitis), flu, and certain types of diarrhea. Goldenseal is also used topically as a disinfecting antiseptic for minor wounds.

Goldenseal's fleshy rhizomes—and Medusa-like tangle of rootlets—are the source for extracts and topical remedies.

TIME LINE OF USAGE AND SPREAD

1852
Eclectic physician John King writes about goldenseal in *The Eclectic Dispensatory.*

1860
Commercial demand for goldenseal root begins around this time.

1884
Declines in wild goldenseal due to overharvesting are documented.

1997
U.S. Fish and Wildlife Service lists goldenseal as endangered.

There is only one species of *Hydrastis*. An erect, hairy perennial, goldenseal grows to scarcely a foot tall. One forked stem, bearing 2 leaves, unfurls in early spring. One leaf is smaller than the other, bearing the flower at the base of its stalk. Leaves may be up to 1 foot wide and about 8 inches broad but are typically about half that size. The leaves have 5 to 9 distinct lobes, with irregular sharp teeth around the margins. As they unfurl in spring, and before fully expanded, a white flower emerges with the leaves. It is only about a half inch in diameter, without petals. Lasting only a week, the spray of up to 50 stamens give the flowers a soft beauty. By July to early August, a round, fleshy, bright red fruit, superficially resembling a raspberry, ripens, tempting and then disappointing with its dry, bitter flavor. The horizontal, knotty rhizome, scarcely thicker than a pencil, is brilliant yellow within. Beneath, fibrous rootlets anchor the plant.

Growing Habits

Goldenseal is found in moist, deep-shaded woods of the Appalachians and Ozarks, a range extending from Vermont to Georgia, west to Arkansas, and north to Minnesota.

For more than a century botanical writers have observed the scarcity of goldenseal, attributed to overharvesting of the root. Supply shortages in the late 1990s and a dramatic rise in the price of the dried root led the United States Fish and Wildlife Service to list goldenseal under the CITES (Convention on International Trade in Endangered Species of Wild Fauna and Flora) treaty, an agreement among nations governing international trade in plants and animals. Goldenseal is allowed as an export, but exporters must validate that it was obtained in a sustainable manner. Supply shortages, trade restrictions, and increase in price are factors that stimulated goldenseal commercial cultivation—a real success story in conservation efforts for a wild medicinal plant.

DIGESTIVE SYSTEM

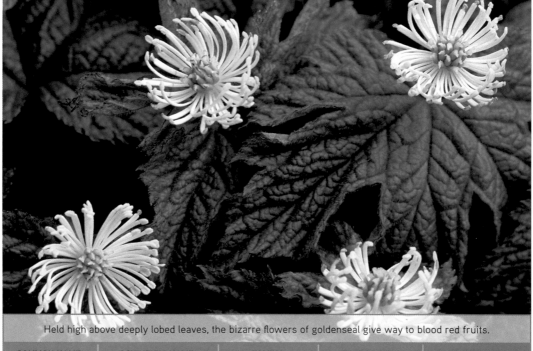

Held high above deeply lobed leaves, the bizarre flowers of goldenseal give way to blood red fruits.

COMMON NAME:	SCIENTIFIC NAME:	FAMILY:	PARTS USED:	NATIVE RANGE:
Goldenseal	*Hydrastis canadensis*	Ranunculaceae	Roots, Rhizomes	E. North America

To make a mouthwash, simmer 1 teaspoon of goldenseal in 1 cup water for 5 to 7 minutes. Strain and let cool. Swish for 10 to 15 seconds and spit out. Repeat 3 to 4 times per day. Make a fresh supply of mouthwash every 2 to 3 days.

Cultivation and Harvesting

Each rhizome is studded with rootlets and undeveloped buds. Any piece of the rhizome with a bud or "eye" and a few strands of fibrous root can be replanted. On average, about 5 plants can be divided from each mature rhizome. Plant 1 inch deep, 8 inches apart. Break roots into pieces and plant in September. A well-drained, deep, loose, friable soil, high in organic matter, is optimal. The rhizome is harvested after the third or fourth year of growth.

Therapeutic Uses

+ *Digestive aid*
+ *Diarrhea*
+ *Antimicrobial*

The woodland goldenseal is one of the best known **indigenous** North American plants. It was widely used by eastern tribes. Goldenseal was an official drug in the United States almost continuously from 1830 to 1955. During the late 19th and early 20th century, a number of pharmaceutical companies, including Parke-Davis, Eli Lilly, and Squibb, manufactured and sold goldenseal products. Today, goldenseal remains a popular herbal remedy in the United States, particularly for the treatment of gastrointestinal complaints.

Looking to the past can often prove useful when researching medicinal plants. As a clear demonstration of that, scientists at the University of Chicago recently found, in test-tube studies, that goldenseal **extracts** are highly active against multiple strains of *Helicobacter pylori*, a bacterium that is responsible for the majority of peptic ulcers and gastric cancers. While there are many **compounds** that contribute to the overall medicinal effects of goldenseal, it is berberine, a yellow **alkaloid**, that is the primary infection fighter. Berberine destroys many microorganisms that cause diarrhea,

including *Giardia lamblia* and *Entamoeba histolytica*. These organisms cause chronic diarrhea and can lead to significant dehydration and weight loss. Goldenseal and other plants containing berberine could play an important public health role given that approximately 20 percent of the world's population is chronically infected with *Giardia* and some 50 million people with the amoeba *E. histolytica*.

Goldenseal can be found in salves and ointments designed to help heal skin infections. Research has shown that berberine is effective for the treatment of psoriasis and may also be useful for minor fungal infections of the skin. While the taste of goldenseal is quite bitter, it can be very effective as a mouthwash and can also be used for treating canker sores and mouth ulcers.

How to Use

TEA: Due to its bitterness, goldenseal is quite unpalatable as a tea.
CAPSULE: Generally, 1 to 3 g per day.
TINCTURE: Take 2 to 4 ml, 2 to 3 times per day.
TOPICAL: Salves and ointments are readily available. Use as directed.

> **NOTE:** Claims for using goldenseal orally to mask illicit drug use in a urine test are not accurate. Studies show that goldenseal has no effect on urine drug assays.

Precautions

Goldenseal may stimulate uterine contractions and is therefore generally not recommended for use during pregnancy. Goldenseal can also interact with **enzymes** in the body that metabolize certain prescription medications. Those taking other medications should check with their health care professional or pharmacist before taking goldenseal.

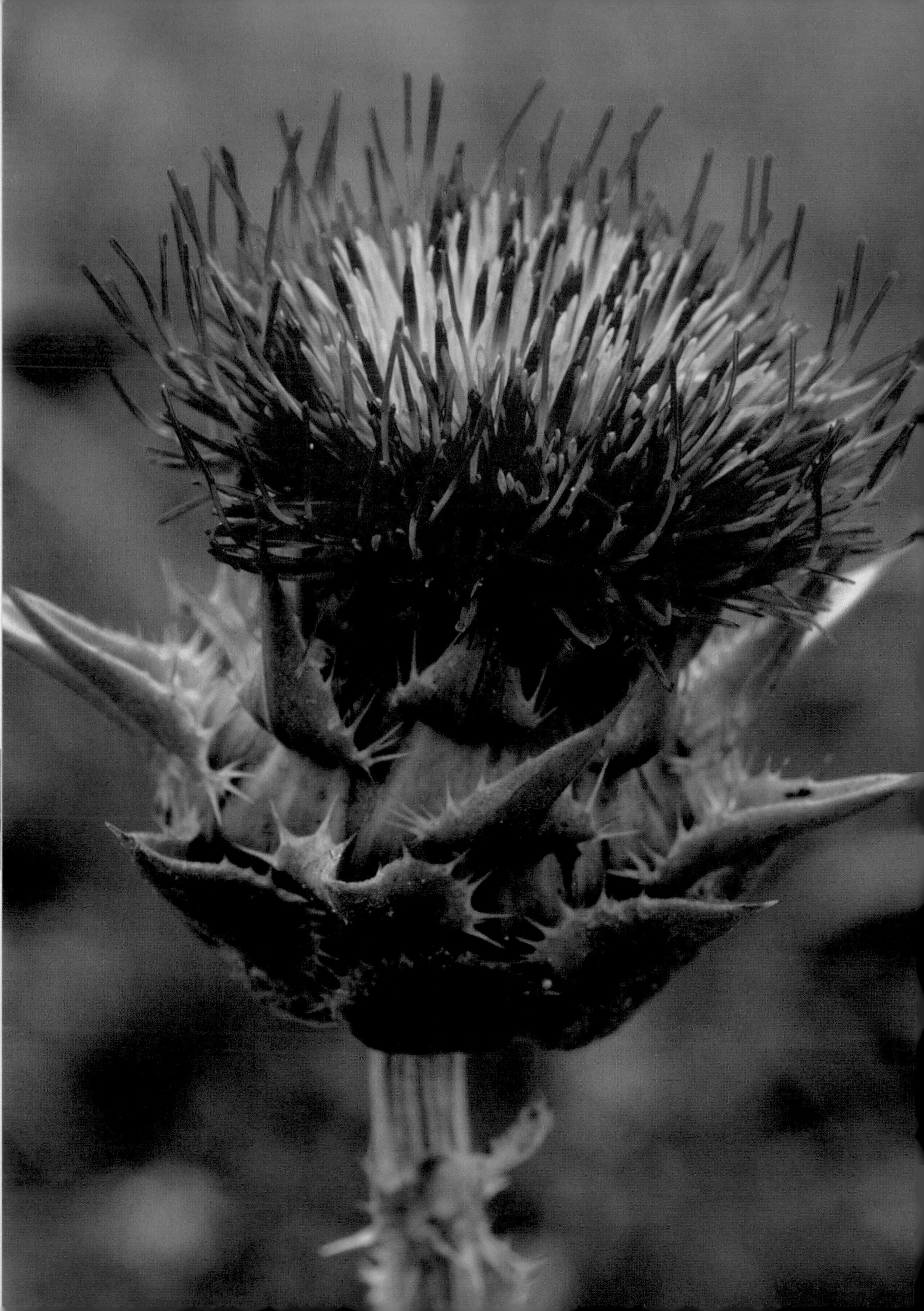

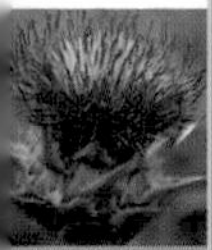

Milk Thistle

Silybum marianum

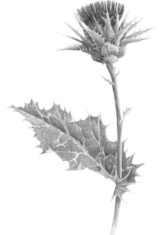

ilk thistle is a statuesque plant, with purple pincushion flowers borne on strong, furrowed stems. At first glance, milk thistle closely resembles other thistles in that its green parts are well armed with sharp prickles. But milk thistle's leaves set it apart, with distinctive white mottling along their branching veins. Other common names for this herb are St. Mary's thistle, Our Lady's thistle, and holy thistle. Along with the species name, *marianum*, they are all a reference to the Virgin Mary. According to a medieval legend, a drop of Mary's milk once spilled on the leaves of the plant. At the touch of the milk, the white markings appeared and have persisted ever since. During the Middle Ages, people believed that a plant's appearance contained clues as to how it should be used medicinally. Milk thistle was given to nursing mothers to stimulate milk flow. This use aside, milk thistle's primary role in herbal medicine has remained the same for more than 2,000 years—as a treatment for liver problems.

All parts of milk thistle are edible. The Romans cultivated it as a vegetable, and they combined milk thistle sap with honey to create a concoction thought to regulate bile. By the 12th century, the herb had become well established in the medical traditions of several European countries, particularly Germany, for treating conditions believed to be linked to a poorly functioning liver. Milk thistle is mentioned in several herbals from the Middle Ages. Over the centuries, milk thistle's popularity remained strong in Europe, and later in America, as a treatment for liver, spleen, and kidney ailments and as a remedy for jaundice. But by the early 20th century, milk thistle was considered old-fashioned, an herb whose time had passed.

In the 1960s, interest in milk thistle was rekindled when researchers isolated a complex of chemicals from the herb's seeds with pronounced liver-protecting properties. Today, milk thistle is taken to protect the liver against many toxins, including certain drugs such as **acetaminophen**, which can cause liver damage in high doses. It is recommended for viral hepatitis, chronic liver disease, and certain types of liver cirrhosis.

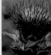

Atop stout, spiky greenery, milk thistle's tufted blooms are the source of the tiny dark seeds used in herbal medicine.

TIME LINE OF USAGE AND SPREAD

1ST CENTURY
Roman physician Pliny the Elder writes that milk thistle is good for "carrying off bile."

1150
Hildegard of Bingen touts milk thistle in *Physica*, first herbal penned by a woman.

1653
English herbalist N. Culpeper recommends milk thistle for clearing the liver and spleen.

1960
Research on the active components in milk thistle begins in Germany.

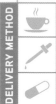
The small genus *Silybum* is represented by only 2 spine-armed thistles, originating in Europe. The other species is *Silybum ebernum*, found from Spain to eastern North Africa. Milk thistle is an annual or biennial growing to 5 feet tall. The spiky, white-mottled leaves at the base of the plant are smooth, with deeply divided lobes armed with a stout spine at the end of the toothed segments. The leaves are up to 8 inches long and 4 inches broad and generally lance shaped in outline. Stem leaves are smaller with yellowish-white spines. The flower head, crowded with violet ray flowers, sits atop the main stalk. Small, curved bracts surround the flower. The shiny, dark, ¼-inch seeds are the parts used.

Growing Habits

Native to dry soils and found along roadsides, waste places, and fields in the Mediterranean region and southwestern Europe, milk thistle has been cultivated since Roman times. It has become naturalized or is a casual escapee from gardens throughout much of Europe. Introduced to North America and temperate South America, milk thistle is particularly common in California, where the Mediterranean-like climate of the central coast provides a perfect home. Elsewhere in North America, it is occasionally established in scattered populations.

Cultivation and Harvesting

Growing milk thistle in your herb garden might make the neighbors question your sanity. The plant is propagated from seeds, which readily germinate, as one might expect from an herb sometimes regarded as a weed. It is not particular, thriving in poor, dry soils, as long as they are well drained. It likes full sun.

Milk thistle was once grown as a vegetable in English gardens, and the young leaves, with spines removed, were eaten in early spring. Young stalks with their skin peeled away were eaten like asparagus. The seeds, relished by goldfinches, also have been used in birdseed mixes. The seeds, and in particular an **extract** made from them, are used in herbal medicine. Their use for liver conditions dates to the first century.

As a commercial crop, milk thistle presents challenges as flowering stalks in a field may bloom at different times and at widely varying heights, complicating the timing of seed harvest. The seeds are harvested with a wheat combine when completely ripe. The combine separates most of the chaff from the seed; usually quite dry at the time of harvest, they are stored in a barn or shed until shipped to the customer.

Therapeutic Uses

+ *Liver protectant*

Milk thistle has been used for more than 2,000 years as a treatment for liver and gallbladder disorders, especially "when the eyes and skin turneth yellow," an early reference to jaundice and liver disease. These historical writings spurred researchers to study the usefulness of milk thistle for hepatitis, cirrhosis, and toxin- or drug-induced liver damage. Science has confirmed that **compounds** in milk thistle called flavonolignans (collectively referred to as **silymarin**) protect liver cells from damage caused by alcohol, acetaminophen (Tylenol), and the very poisonous deathcap mushroom (*Amanita phalloides*). In fact, special preparations of silymarin are available in

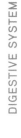

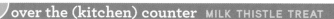

over the (kitchen) counter MILK THISTLE TREAT

It's not just for the birds. Milk thistle seeds are a good source of protein and **amino acids** and can be delicious when added to cereals or smoothies. Grind organic milk thistle seeds and cook with your oatmeal or substitute milk thistle for flax seeds in recipes.

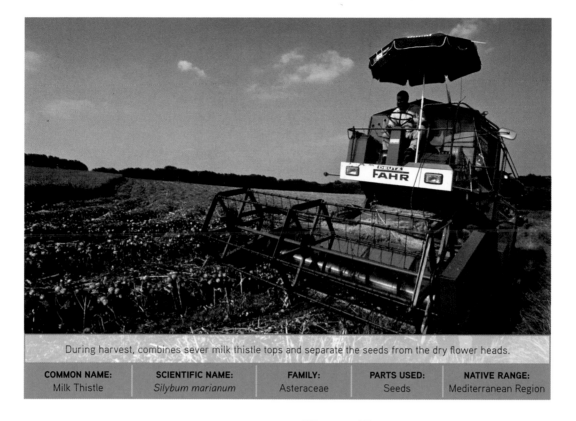

During harvest, combines sever milk thistle tops and separate the seeds from the dry flower heads.

COMMON NAME:	SCIENTIFIC NAME:	FAMILY:	PARTS USED:	NATIVE RANGE:
Milk Thistle	*Silybum marianum*	Asteraceae	Seeds	Mediterranean Region

European emergency rooms to use as an antidote for mushroom poisoning. It is not surprising then that Germany's Commission E, which studies the safety and efficacy of herbs, recommends milk thistle for liver damage caused by toxins or cirrhosis of the liver and as therapy for liver inflammation.

Milk thistle and its active compounds are undergoing research in the U.S. and abroad. According to the National Cancer Institute, silymarin protects the liver by preventing toxins from entering cells and by revving up **enzymes** that detoxify toxins in the liver. Silymarin can protect liver cells during chemotherapy and appears to boost the effect of certain chemotherapy drugs. Protective effects of milk thistle may extend even beyond the liver. Researchers have found that it shields the kidney against injury from drugs and radiation and prevents ultraviolet damage to the skin. However, despite encouraging research on the ability of milk thistle extracts to protect liver cells, studies in people with alcoholic liver disease and with type B or C viral hepatitis have yielded conflicting results.

How to Use

TEA: Simmer 1 teaspoon crushed milk thistle seeds in 1 cup water for 10 minutes. Strain. Drink 1 to 3 cups per day.

TINCTURE: Alcohol extracts are not advisable if using for liver protection.

EXTRACT: When using milk thistle for liver protection, use a product that contains a minimum 70 percent silymarin. The dose for these products is generally 210 to 420 mg per day. Research suggests absorption is enhanced when milk thistle is combined with phosphatidylcholine.

Precautions

No contraindications are associated with this herb, even in substantial dosages. Milk thistle has been extensively used in Europe, and many studies have shown it to be safe. While it was once thought that milk thistle might interact with certain medications, recent human studies have failed to demonstrate any interaction with oral dosing. Despite its safety, individuals who have liver disease or are being treated for cancer should discuss the use of any dietary supplement with their health care provider.

Peppermint

Mentha x piperita

Peppermint is the aromatic plant that gives the candy of the same name its cool, refreshing taste. It is one of more than two dozen species of mint that belong to the genus *Mentha*. The name comes from Minthe, a nymph in Greek mythology who had the misfortune to be loved by Hades, god of the underworld, and subsequently was turned into an insignificant little plant by Hades's jealous wife. According to the story, Hades tried to make it up to Minthe by sweetly scenting her small, green leaves. While several mints appear to have been cultivated since the time of the

ancient Egyptians, peppermint is a relative newcomer. It was discovered in England in 1696, a natural hybrid of two other mint **species**. Cultivation of peppermint spread rapidly across Europe, and colonists transported the herb to the New World. Today, peppermint ranks near the top of the world's favorite flavorings. It is also a respected herbal remedy for upset stomach and other digestive issues.

Mint leaves have been used in herbal medicine for several thousand years, according to writings and relics from the Greek, Roman, and ancient Egyptian periods. Spearmint *(Mentha spicata)* was likely the mint the Romans prized as a flavoring for food and a scent for bathwater and cosmetics. The Roman physician Pliny the Elder thought mint was supreme among herbs; he wrote that the very smell of it could reanimate the spirit.

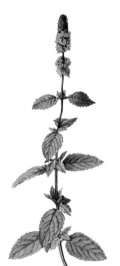

Many medieval herbals speak of mint as the best treatment for stomach ailments. Mint steeped in wine or vinegar made an effective mouthwash, and mint leaves applied to the forehead and temples were an early headache remedy. In England and the American colonies, mint was an herb of choice for treating indigestion, flatulence, colic, heartburn, nausea, headaches, fevers, and colds.

Peppermint appears to calm the muscles in the walls of the stomach and intestines. Modern herbal practitioners recommend peppermint for soothing upset stomach or improving digestion; the herb is often used to treat the pain, gas, and diarrhea associated with irritable bowel syndrome (IBS). Applied to the skin, peppermint has a cooling effect on rashes, hives, and other irritations. Peppermint is widely used to treat colds and flu, soothe sore throats, and quiet dry coughs.

Peppermint's aromatic leaves, and the flavorful oil they contain, have been used since antiquity as an aid to digestion.

TIME LINE OF USAGE AND SPREAD

1597
English herbalist J. Gerard writes mint is "wholesome for the stomacke."

1696
Peppermint is discovered growing in an English field and subsequently cultivated.

1721
Peppermint is officially included in the *London Pharmacopoeia*.

1790s
Mint is grown commercially for the first time in the U.S. in western Massachusetts.

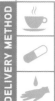

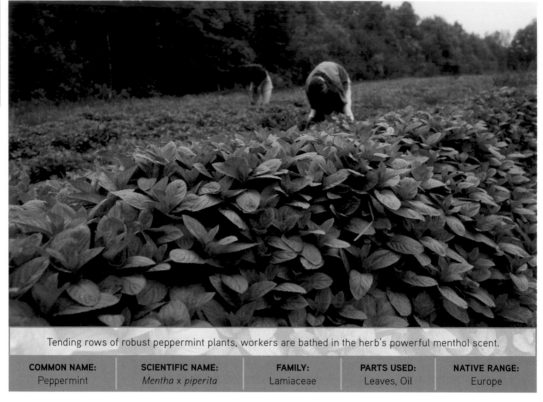

Tending rows of robust peppermint plants, workers are bathed in the herb's powerful menthol scent.

COMMON NAME:	SCIENTIFIC NAME:	FAMILY:	PARTS USED:	NATIVE RANGE:
Peppermint	*Mentha x piperita*	Lamiaceae	Leaves, Oil	Europe

DIGESTIVE SYSTEM

The genus *Mentha* defines genetic diversity. There are 25 true species of *Mentha*, but through hybridization endless variations have resulted in more than 2,300 named varieties. Peppermint is a hybrid cross of spearmint *(Mentha spicata)* and watermint *(Mentha aquatica).* A perennial growing up to 3 feet tall, peppermint spreads by runners, traveling across or just beneath the soil surface. The square stem is usually reddish purple and smooth.

Its leaves are smooth, shiny, wrinkled, egg or lance shaped, sharply toothed, and usually up to 2 inches long. Unlike spearmint, all of the leaves of peppermint are distinctly stalked. The pink or lilac flowers bloom from mid- to late summer. They are arranged in a head or oblong spike and are almost all completely sterile.

Peppermint is also defined by the high percentage of menthol in its **essential oil**, giving it the flavor and fragrance Americans associate with candy canes. The species name, *piperita*, honors its warm, peppery fragrance.

Growing Habits

Native to Europe, peppermint is widely naturalized in European gardens; it was brought to America by early European settlers. In naturalized situations, it is often found growing next to a spring or moist stream banks. Perhaps arising as a natural hybrid in nature, the first known specimens were collected in 1696 in Herefordshire County in the western English countryside, and were described by English botanist John Ray in 1704. By 1750, commercial cultivation began in England near Mitcham, a famous mint-producing region. By 1812, commercial production in the U.S. began on a small scale in Ashfield, Massachusetts.

Cultivation and Harvesting

Peppermint is a perennial of easy culture. The savvy herb gardener, however, knows not to buy peppermint seeds. Any plants resulting from a packet of seeds will not be true peppermint.

A field of peppermint may produce a few viable seeds, but according to mint expert Arthur Tucker at Delaware State University, their fertility rate is about 0.0002 percent. Propagation is by cuttings, division, or most easily by a cutting of the runners. Any piece of the runner with a node will produce a new plant. Peppermint thrives in a cool climate and rich, moist soil.

Peppermint leaves or oil is harvested just as the plant begins flowering. In the United States, production is primarily in the Pacific Northwest, and also in Michigan and Indiana. Recently imports from China, India, Canada, and Germany have increased.

Therapeutic Uses

+ *Indigestion*
+ *Irritable bowel syndrome*
+ *Colds and coughs*
+ *Muscle aches*
+ *Tension headache*

Peppermint is a long-standing digestive herbal remedy. This aromatic herb calms the muscles of the digestive tract and improves the flow of bile from the gallbladder, helping the body to digest fats. It is for these reasons that peppermint alleviates intestinal gas, reduces abdominal cramping, and can settle an upset stomach. Studies show that peppermint oil, especially when combined with caraway seed oil, is equal or superior to conventional treatments for indigestion.

Peppermint oil is the most widely studied herbal product for treating irritable bowel syndrome (IBS), characterized by recurring abdominal pain along with bouts of constipation, diarrhea, or both. IBS disproportionately affects women, and there are few effective treatments. The majority of clinical studies show that peppermint oil is superior to **placebo** and equivalent to prescription medications for improving IBS,

especially when diarrhea is the predominant symptom. Peppermint oil is very well tolerated.

Peppermint and its active constituent, menthol, are good for the respiratory system. A cup of warm peppermint tea can thin mucus, help loosen phlegm, and relieve a stuffy nose. The Food and Drug Administration approves the use of mentholated ointments, lozenges, and steam inhalants for coughs. Applied to neck and chest, the vapors quickly relieve coughing. Applied topically in products such as Ben-Gay and Tiger Balm, peppermint also soothes the skin, reducing itching from bug bites or poison ivy and relieving arthritis and headache.

NOTE: Never apply peppermint oil to the face of an infant or small child under the age of 5, as it may cause spasms that inhibit breathing.

How to Use

TEA: Pour 1 cup boiling water over 1 teaspoon dried peppermint leaves, or 6 to 8 fresh leaves. Steep for 10 minutes. Strain and cool. Enjoy 2 to 3 times per day after meals.

CAPSULES: 500 to 1,000 mg dried peppermint leaf taken after meals. Sustained release peppermint oil capsules are used for IBS. In studies 0.2 ml peppermint oil was given 2 to 3 times a day with meals.

LOZENGES: For sore throat and cough, lozenges should contain 5 to 10 mg menthol. Children under 2 should not be given menthol products.

TOPICAL: Ointments, rubs are available. Apply 2 to 3 times daily, or as directed.

Precautions

Do not use peppermint if you have gastroesophageal reflux disease (GERD) or if you have a hiatal hernia, as peppermint can make heartburn worse.

over the (kitchen) counter PEPPERMINT HEADACHE COMPRESS

Pour 3 cups hot water over 3 peppermint tea bags. Steep, covered, for 5 to 7 minutes. Remove tea bags. Add 1 cup ice cubes. Dip washcloth into cold tea and apply to forehead to relieve sinus or tension headache.

Psyllium

Native to India, Pakistan, Iran, and parts of the Mediterranean, psyllium—also called ispaghula or isphagula—is an annual with narrow, straplike leaves that grows no more than knee high. Its small, white flowers give way to tiny, glossy seeds that have a slight reddish tint. Psyllium is prolific: Each plant can produce up to 15,000 seeds. The common name for *P. ovata* in India is *isabgol,* which comes from the Persian words *isap* and *ghol,* meaning "horse ear." The name aptly describes the peculiar shape of psyllium seeds. The word "psyllium" comes from the Greek word for flea, also a reference to the tiny seeds. The husk of psyllium seed contains large amounts of soluble fiber; when wet, it becomes slippery and mucilaginous and expands to 10 times its size as it absorbs water. Completely indigestible, the husks are used as a source of dietary fiber to relieve constipation and maintain a healthy digestive tract.

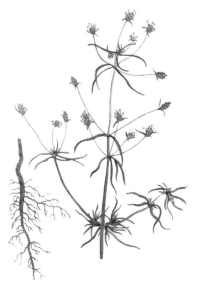

Psyllium has a long history as a medicinal herb, having been used in Indian **Ayurvedic medicine** for centuries, and as part of other healing traditions in Asia and Europe. More recently, psyllium has become a widely used laxative agent throughout Europe, Asia, and North America. The United Sates is currently the world's largest importer of psyllium husk, with much of the product going into over-the-counter bulk laxatives, such as Metamucil, and into high-fiber breakfast cereals.

Psyllium is recommended by both herbal and conventional medical practitioners to relieve constipation. Combined with water, psyllium husk produces a slippery mass that stimulates intestinal contractions and speeds waste through the digestive tract. Recently, psyllium has been found effective in treating mild to moderate cases of inflammatory bowel disease, irritable bowel syndrome, hemorrhoids, and other intestinal problems. Psyllium appears to effectively lower blood cholesterol levels, particularly **low-density lipoprotein** (LDL), or "bad," cholesterol, when added to a low-fat, low-cholesterol diet.

Herbalists and conventional physicians alike recommend psyllium seeds as a source of heart-healthy dietary fiber.

TIME LINE OF USAGE AND SPREAD

1934
G. D. Searle Co. markets Metamucil with psyllium husk as active ingredient.

1990s
Germany approves the use of psyllium to reduce blood cholesterol levels.

1997
The FDA allows cereal manufacturers to make health claims for psyllium husk.

1998
Astronaut John Glenn snacks on psyllium wafers on space shuttle *Discovery*.

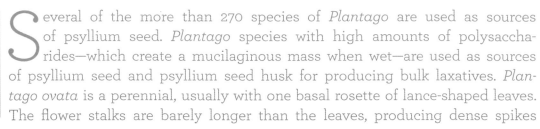
several of the more than 270 species of *Plantago* are used as sources of psyllium seed. *Plantago* species with high amounts of polysaccharides—which create a mucilaginous mass when wet—are used as sources of psyllium seed and psyllium seed husk for producing bulk laxatives. *Plantago ovata* is a perennial, usually with one basal rosette of lance-shaped leaves. The flower stalks are barely longer than the leaves, producing dense spikes about an inch long. The tiny flowers are crowded in the flower spikes, with stamens barely extending outside the flowers. *Plantago afra* and *P. arenaria* have opposite leaves up the stem (rather than all leaves at the base of the plant) and are annuals.

Growing Habits

The perennial *P. ovata* is found in southeastern Spain and is widespread in North Africa and southwestern Asia, growing in dry, semiarid poor soils. It occurs in southern California and Arizona, with scattered populations in southern Utah and Nevada and western Texas. *Plantago afra* is found in dry soils throughout much of southern Europe. *Plantago arenaria* is more widely distributed throughout southern, central, and Eastern Europe, thriving in poor, dry soils. It is often naturalized in northern Europe as well. In North America, it is established from Quebec south through New England to the Carolinas, west to Missouri, north to Minnesota. In western North America, it occurs from British Columbia south to California. Despite its widespread geographical distribution in North America, in most states it is limited to waif populations in only 1 or 2 counties.

Cultivation and Harvesting

Plantains (from the **genus** *Plantago*), abundant in many parts of the world, are often regarded merely as weeds. They are easily grown from seed and thrive in soils where other plants may not easily grow.

Plantago ovata is the most widely cultivated psyllium source, as its seeds are larger than

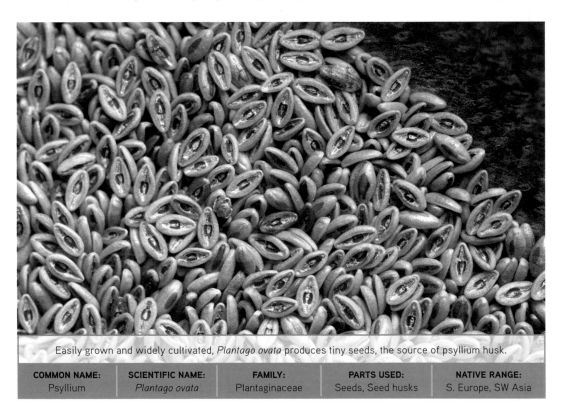

Easily grown and widely cultivated, *Plantago ovata* produces tiny seeds, the source of psyllium husk.

COMMON NAME:	SCIENTIFIC NAME:	FAMILY:	PARTS USED:	NATIVE RANGE:
Psyllium	*Plantago ovata*	Plantaginaceae	Seeds, Seed husks	S. Europe, SW Asia

In a bowl, mix ⅓ cup psyllium husk, 1 tablespoon olive oil, 1 tablespoon Parmesan cheese, and 1 tablespoon sesame seeds. Add ½ cup water, stir well, and let sit for 10 minutes. Roll out resulting "dough" to a ¼-inch thickness on parchment paper and lift onto cookie sheet. Sprinkle with salt (optional). Bake 25 to 30 minutes at 350 degrees. Cool and break into crunchy chips.

those of other psylliums, thereby increasing yield. In India it is grown as a winter annual in semiarid regions where some irrigation is available. It likes a light, well-drained sandy loam with a slightly alkaline pH and low fertility. From seeding to harvest, this short-lived crop completes its life cycle in about 120 days.

Much of the world's commercial production is in India and Pakistan. Since the plant is so small in stature, mechanical harvest is problematic, making it a labor-intensive crop. The whole plant is harvested once the seeds are mature, then dried in fields for 2 to 3 days, after which the plants are bundled and taken to a shed, where the seeds are threshed from the dried herbage.

Therapeutic Uses

+ *Fiber*
+ *Bulk laxative*
+ *Heart health*

Psyllium seed husks are an excellent source of soluble fiber. Every 100 g of psyllium provides 71 g of soluble fiber. A similar amount of oat brain contains only 5 g of soluble fiber! When psyllium combines with water, it swells up to 10 times its original volume, which explains why it has long been used as the primary ingredient in bulk laxatives such as Metamucil and Serutan. When taken over a period of weeks, psyllium can speed up the time that it takes for food to travel through the digestive tract. Interestingly, psyllium is also effective for the treatment of diarrhea and even can be particularly useful for those with irritable bowel syndrome who experience periods of constipation interspersed with periods of diarrhea.

Soluble fiber has been associated with lowering both total and low-density lipoprotein (LDL), or "bad," cholesterol; controlling weight; lowering blood pressure; and improving **insulin** resistance to reduce the risk of diabetes. The U.S. Food and Drug Administration has formally recognized the role of psyllium in lowering blood cholesterol levels by allowing health claims to be made for products containing its fiber. Several psyllium-containing cereals such as Kellogg's Heartwise and Bran Buds have appeared in the marketplace and are promoted for their potential cholesterol-lowering and heart health-promoting effects. Due to the overwhelming evidence that high-fiber diets prevent many of the risks associated with heart disease, the National Cholesterol Education Program recommends 5 to 10 g of soluble fiber daily.

How to Use

ADULTS: Generally 2 to 3 tablespoons per day, taken in divided doses before breakfast and before dinner. Mix each dose in a tall glass of water, stir well, drink, and follow with another glass of water.

CHILDREN (YOUNGER THAN 18 YEARS): Generally from 1 teaspoon to 1 to 2 tablespoons, depending upon the age and size of the child.

Precautions

Psyllium fiber can reduce the absorption of certain drugs, so drugs should be taken either 1 hour before or a few hours after psyllium is taken. Obstruction of the gastrointestinal tract has happened in people taking psyllium fiber, particularly if they had undergone previous bowel surgery or when psyllium was taken with inadequate amounts of water. Those who have difficulty swallowing should not take psyllium.

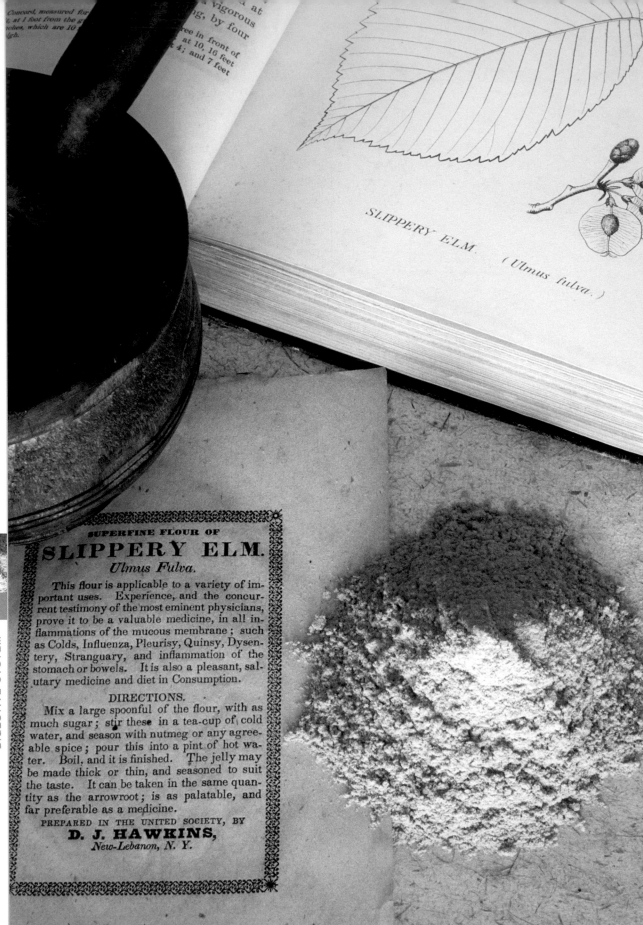

SLIPPERY ELM. (*Ulmus fulva.*)

SUPERFINE FLOUR OF

SLIPPERY ELM.

Ulmus Fulva.

This flour is applicable to a variety of important uses. Experience, and the concurrent testimony of the most eminent physicians, prove it to be a valuable medicine, in all inflammations of the mucous membrane; such as Colds, Influenza, Pleurisy, Quinsy, Dysentery, Stranguary, and inflammation of the stomach or bowels. It is also a pleasant, salutary medicine and diet in Consumption.

DIRECTIONS.

Mix a large spoonful of the flour, with as much sugar; stir these in a tea-cup of cold water, and season with nutmeg or any agreeable spice; pour this into a pint of hot water. Boil, and it is finished. The jelly may be made thick or thin, and seasoned to suit the taste. It can be taken in the same quantity as the arrowroot; is as palatable, and far preferable as a medicine.

PREPARED IN THE UNITED SOCIETY, BY

D. J. HAWKINS,

New-Lebanon, N. Y.

Slippery Elm

❦ Ulmus rubra ❦

True to its name, this plant is slippery in both taste and texture. Its source is the pleasant-smelling inner bark of *Ulmus rubra*, a medium-size tree native to North America. The species name, *rubra*, means "red" and refers to the flower buds, which are a rust red color. A number of Native American tribes used slippery elm bark as a food. American settlers later followed their example. During the American Revolution, for example, George Washington and his troops apparently survived for nearly 12 days at Valley Forge on slippery elm porridge, made by boiling

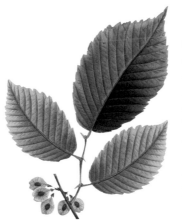

a ground-up preparation of the tree's inner bark with water or milk. Nutritionally, such a porridge is roughly on a par with oatmeal. Native Americans used slippery elm medicinally, too, a practice also adopted by the early settlers. The herb has remained a staple in American herbal medicine as a gentle and effective remedy for soothing irritations of the mouth, throat, stomach, and intestines.

For centuries, slippery elm was used medicinally by **indigenous** tribes in eastern North America. Externally, the powdered inner bark was mixed with fats or oils to make healing salves for burns, skin ulcers, boils, and minor wounds. Taken internally, it helped ease the discomfort of sore throats, quieted coughs, and relieved stomach and bowel complaints. The Cherokee also used slippery elm as an eyewash. American colonists adopted slippery elm for many of these same applications. **Poultices** made of slippery elm bark were a standard treatment for gunshot wounds in the late 1700s. By the 19th century, slippery elm was being recommended by physicians and herbal practitioners for pneumonia and other lung infections, tapeworms, rashes and boils, syphilitic eruptions, broken bones, and even leprosy.

Slippery elm remains a popular herbal medicine and is widely available. It is one of the few herbs approved by the U.S. Food and Drug Administration and sold as a nonprescription drug. Slippery elm helps soothe and heal inflamed mucosal tissues, such as the lining of the throat, stomach, and intestines. Herbal practitioners also suggest it for gastroesophageal reflux disease (GERD), Crohn's disease, ulcerative colitis, and diarrhea.

Native Americans introduced early settlers to slippery elm's inner bark, typically ground into a fine powder.

TIME LINE OF USAGE AND SPREAD

1787
J. Schoepf lists slippery elm as a "salve bark" in his *Materia Medica Americana*.

1812
U.S. Army troops in the War of 1812 feed horses slippery elm bark when hay runs out.

1875
Boston schoolmaster George Emerson notes slippery elm is being overharvested.

LATE 1800s
Thayers Slippery Elm Lozenges, still sold today, appear on U.S. market.

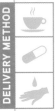
About 30 or 40 species of *Ulmus* occur in the Northern Hemisphere. Slippery elm is one of 7 species indigenous to the United States. An open crown deciduous tree, it grows from 60 to 100 feet tall. The part used is the tawny inner bark—lying beneath the brown outer bark—which is mucilaginous, giving it a slimy or slippery feel. Slippery elm has several distinct features separating it from other North American elms. Before opening in the heart of winter, the flower buds are easily distinguished by their dark rust color (hence the **species** name *rubra*, "red"). It flowers in late winter and early spring. Often its papery, waferlike, winged fruits mature before the first leaves appear in spring. There are no hairs along the edges of the fruit's margins. The 4- to 9-inch-long leaves are half as wide. Oblong to oval in shape, they contract into slender tips. The margins are double serrated (smaller sharp teeth between larger sharp-pointed teeth). The upper surface and especially the lower surface feel rough like sandpaper.

Slippery elms are often confused with the American elm. A distinguishing characteristic is the trees' leaf surfaces. The leaf surface of the American elm *(Ulmus americana)* above and below is much smoother, and if hairs are present, they are softer than in slippery elm. American elm is the much lamented victim of Dutch elm disease.

Growing Habits

Slippery elm occurs in a variety of soils, but it is most at home on lower slopes of hills, in alluvial flood plains, stream banks and riverbanks, and bottomland forests. This wide-ranging native occurs from the St. Lawrence River Valley south through New England, stretching down the continent to northern Florida, west to eastern Texas, and north through the eastern edge of the prairie states to North Dakota. *Ulmus* is the classical Latin name for elm trees, from which the name "elm" is derived, an ancient word from Anglo-Saxon, Celtic, Gothic, and Teutonic dialects, remaining unchanged in modern English.

Cultivation and Harvesting

Though not as stately as the famous American elm, the broad, flat crown produced by the straight or forked trunk of slippery elm makes it a good shade tree, particularly in soils with a good supply of moisture. Slippery elms will tolerate a wide range of soils, but the tree grows best in compact, moist, limey soil. Propagation is by seed, which generally germinates without pregermination treatments, though seed from northern sources may exhibit dormancy. Seeds can be planted in spring or fall.

Slippery elm is common in the wild throughout most of its range, so it is seldom cultivated. The inner bark is harvested in the spring. The best time for harvesting slippery elm is when the sap rises in early spring and temperatures climb above freezing during the day and plummet at night—the same time frame for collecting maple sap. When the time is right, the bark can be removed easily in long strips, almost popping off the tree. Most commercial production of slippery elm bark comes from wild populations in Appalachia.

Therapeutic Uses

+ *Occasional heartburn*
+ *Coughs*
+ *Sore throat*
+ *Itchy, inflamed skin*

over the (kitchen) counter SLIPPERY ELM GRUEL

Add 1 to 2 tablespoons water to 1 teaspoon of the powdered bark, making it into a paste. Then add 2 cups boiling water. Stir well and let steep for 10 minutes. Pour off the liquid and add a pinch of cinnamon or pumpkin pie spice, with a little maple syrup. It's great for soothing a sore throat, easing a cough, or relieving occasional heartburn.

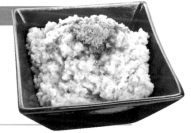

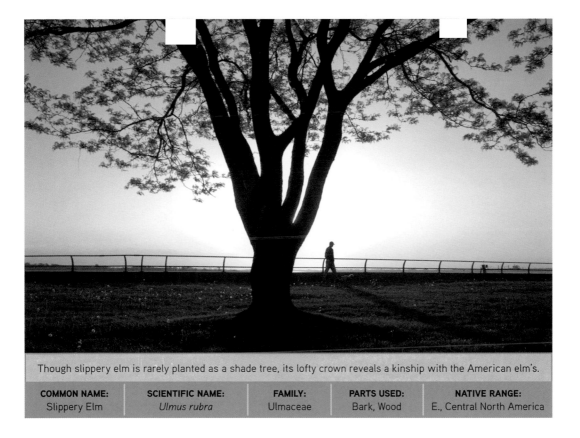

Though slippery elm is rarely planted as a shade tree, its lofty crown reveals a kinship with the American elm's.

COMMON NAME:	SCIENTIFIC NAME:	FAMILY:	PARTS USED:	NATIVE RANGE:
Slippery Elm	*Ulmus rubra*	Ulmaceae	Bark, Wood	E., Central North America

Slippery elm bark has been used as a food and medicine for centuries. Slippery elm bark was an official drug in the *United States Pharmacopeia* from 1820 to 1936. Although there are virtually no modern studies, the FDA has approved slippery elm as a safe nonprescription demulcent for soothing minor throat irritation and protecting irritated tissue. The tissue-coating activity in slippery elm results from the presence of a group of **compounds** called **mucopolysaccharides** that become mucilaginous, or slimy, in contact with water. It is this property that explains the popularity of slippery elm for relieving sore throats, dry coughs, and occasional heartburn. Indeed, the herb is still listed in the *British Herbal Compendium* as a treatment for inflammations of the esophagus and stomach and for diarrhea.

Although slippery elm is usually recommended for internal use, it can also be made into a paste or included in an ointment and applied topically to soothe itchy, inflamed skin. Examples for use include eczema, insect bites, and acne.

How to Use

TEA: Add 1 cup of boiling water to 1 to 2 teaspoons powdered bark and steep 5 minutes. Drink 2 to 3 times per day.

CAPSULES: 800 to 1,000 mg 3 times daily, taken with a full glass of water.

LOZENGES: Widely available, both flavored and unflavored. Follow the dosing instructions on the label.

TOPICAL: Mix 2 tablespoons powdered bark with ¼ cup water and make a paste. Add more water as needed to thoroughly mix. Apply to inflamed or itchy area for 20 to 30 minutes. Reapply as needed. Do not use on open wound.

 NOTE: Other drugs should be taken 1 hour prior to or several hours after consumption of slippery elm, as it may slow the absorption of oral medications.

Precautions

Slippery elm is generally well tolerated. But it is not recommended for those with bile duct obstruction or gallstones.

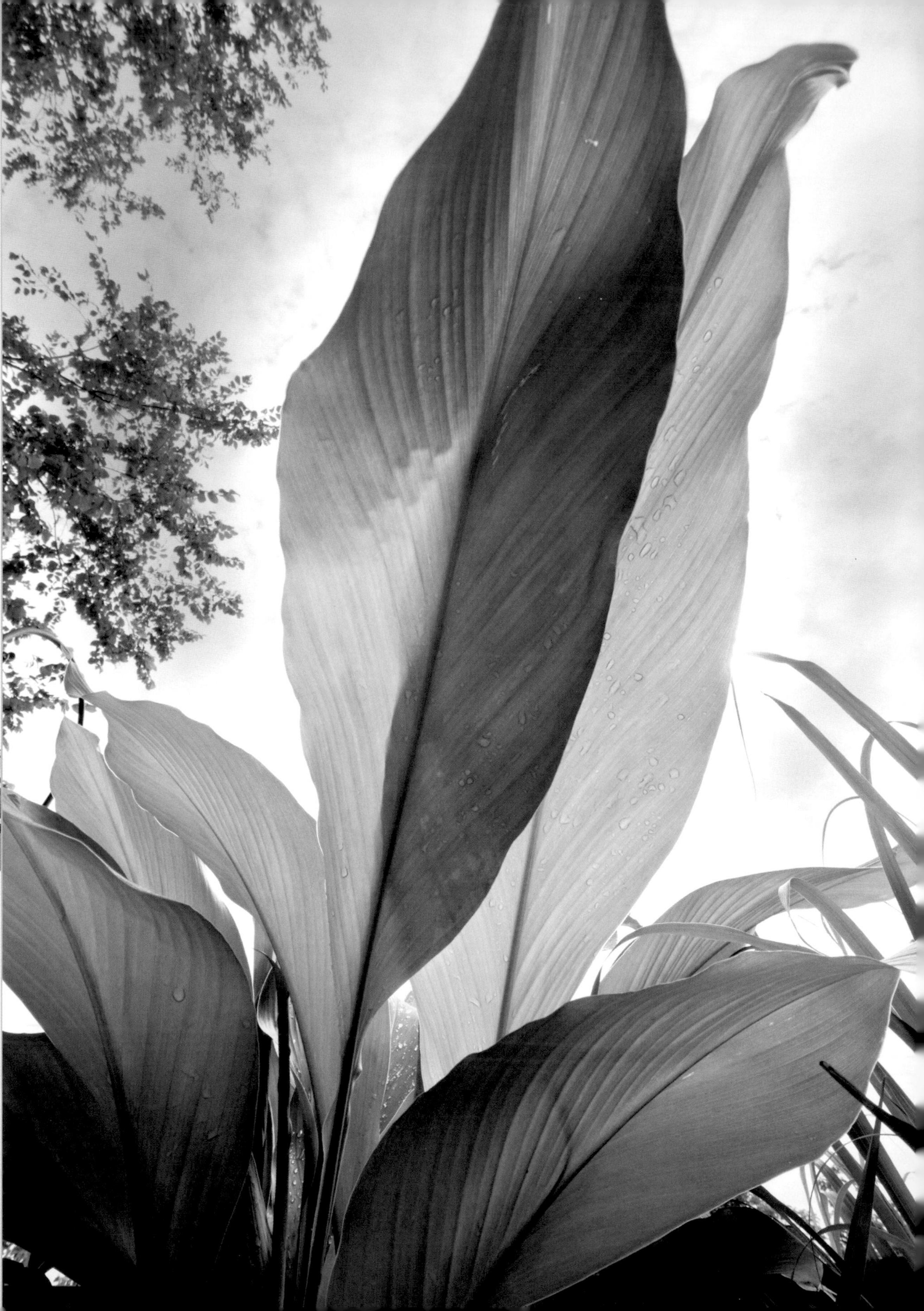

Turmeric

Curcuma longa

Turmeric is the source of the brilliant golden-orange spice that gives many curries their peppery, somewhat musky flavor and ballpark mustard its bright yellow hue. It comes from the tuberous root, or rhizome, of a stately, large-leafed perennial that belongs to the same family as ginger. The genus name of turmeric, *Curcuma*, comes from *korkum*, a word used in ancient Rome for saffron, a much costlier, more subtly flavored spice. Turmeric is mentioned in the Vedas, the oldest sacred texts of Hinduism, as being associated with purity and cleansing. Even today, orthodox Hindu brides and bridegrooms take part in a ceremony called *haldi*—the Hindi word for turmeric—in which their faces and hands are coated with turmeric paste before they take their vows. As a healing herb, turmeric has its roots deep in the medicinal traditions of India, China, and several Southeast Asian cultures. In Western herbal medicine, it has recently gained popularity as a potent, but safe **anti-inflammatory** treatment for a host of digestive ailments and other conditions.

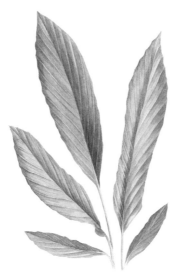

Native to India and Indonesia, turmeric has been used in Indian **Ayurvedic** and Unani traditional medicine for at least 2,500 years, primarily to treat digestive and liver disorders, skin infections and irritations, and arthritis. In China, turmeric was prescribed by traditional medical practitioners for abdominal pain, jaundice, and menstrual conditions. The ancient Greeks knew of the herb, but it never became part of Greek or Roman medicinal culture. In Western herbal medicine, serious interest in turmeric began in the mid-20th century, when German scientists began to investigate the herb's therapeutic properties.

Today turmeric is used in herbal medicine to treat digestive and liver problems, joint pain, and skin conditions. Herbalists recommend turmeric for indigestion and diarrhea, as well as inflammatory bowel diseases such as Crohn's and ulcerative colitis. Other uses include clearing up skin conditions such as eczema and psoriasis, preventing cardiovascular disease and cancer, and reducing blood cholesterol levels.

Turmeric's large, elegant leaves arise from fleshy roots, the source of both cooking spice and medicinal powder.

TIME LINE OF USAGE AND SPREAD

650 B.C.
Clay tablets describe turmeric as a brewing spice, stomach tonic, and dye plant.

A.D. 1280
Marco Polo mentions turmeric in notes of his travels to China.

1815
French chemists Vogel and Pelletier isolate curcumin from turmeric.

1971
Studies of turmeric's anti-inflammatory properties initiated.

Distinctively hued turmeric root has been included in East Asian herbal pharmacopeias for millennia.

COMMON NAME:	SCIENTIFIC NAME:	FAMILY:	PARTS USED:	NATIVE RANGE:
Turmeric	*Curcuma longa*	Zingiberaceae	Roots, Rhizomes	Southern Asia

Some 50 species of *Curcuma* are native to Southeast Asia. Turmeric is most easily identified from its knotty, fingerlike rhizome segments, which when fresh are brilliant orange within; when dried and powdered they are the familiar yellow-orange turmeric of commerce. A perennial, often grown as an annual, the plant reaches 3 to 6 feet in height. The leafy shoots have up to 10 alternate leaves, surrounded by conspicuous folding sheaths. The oblong, lance-shaped leaf blades are dark green above, with a thick green midrib. The underside of the leaf, if held to the light, is covered with dots containing **essential oil**. Leaves are up to 27 inches long and 7 inches wide. The flowers are borne on a terminal cylindrical flower spike, with spirally arranged, white, yellow-streaked flowers opening 1 at a time. The sterile flowers never produce seeds.

Growing Habits

Turmeric, like ginger, defies a specific origin. Probably originating in southern Asia, most likely India, it is not known from the wild, except for naturalized plants in areas where it may have been cultivated, such as teak forests of East Java in Indonesia. A sterile plant that does not produce viable seed, it is believed to have developed as a result of selection and vegetative propagation over many centuries. Today India is thought to be the center of domestication. It was introduced to China before the seventh century, and reached East Africa by the eighth century. By the 13th century it was grown in West Africa. The Spanish introduced it to Jamaica by the 18th century.

Cultivation and Harvesting

Turmeric is always propagated from dividing the **rhizomes** with a bud or eye. These so-called daughter rhizomes, separated from the primary mother rhizome, are usually used for propagation. Turmeric likes hot weather and humid conditions. It likes a loose, friable loam, with good amounts of organic matter, and does best in a slight acidic soil, struggling if the soil is waterlogged or too alkaline. Turmeric also makes an excellent container plant for a patio. Plants can be bought from nurseries specializing in herbs. Turmeric is cultivated throughout the tropics, with India and China growing most of the world's supply.

Simmer 1 teaspoon turmeric powder in 2 cups water for 10 minutes, stirring until the turmeric is thoroughly dissolved. Turn the heat to low and add 2 cups milk (dairy or soy), 1 tablespoon almond oil, and 1 to 2 tablespoons honey or maple syrup. Remove from heat, drink, and enjoy. This tea may be refrigerated and consumed warm or cold.

Therapeutic Uses

+ *Inflammatory bowel disease*
+ *Rheumatoid arthritis (joint pain)*

This ancient spice is one of the most intensely researched herbs in the marketplace. Interestingly, studies in animals suggest turmeric may offer protection from Alzheimer's disease. Scientists have discovered that **curcumin**, a group of highly active yellow-colored **compounds** in turmeric, stops the accumulation of plaque in the brain. Destructive protein fragments known as **beta amyloid** plaques build up in the brains of people with Alzheimer's, leading to memory loss. Studies in humans are currently under way to confirm this preliminary finding.

Turmeric seems to have a special affinity for reducing **inflammation** in the body, particularly in the gastrointestinal tract. Curcumin has been shown to be beneficial for reducing symptoms in patients with Crohn's disease and ulcerative colitis. These conditions are collectively referred to as inflammatory bowel disease. Patients given doses of 1 to 2 g per day of curcumin experienced fewer symptoms and less systemic inflammation.

Curcumin may protect against colon cancer. A small pilot study in patients with familial adenomatous polyposis (FAP) disorder—characterized by the development of hundreds of benign tumors in the colon, eventually leading to colorectal cancer—garnered positive results. A combination of 480 mg of curcumin and 20 mg of quercetin taken orally 3 times a day reduced the number and size of tumors in patients by roughly 60 percent over a 6-month period. A larger study is currently under way at Johns Hopkins University.

Researchers around the world are showing a tremendous interest in turmeric. In the United States alone, the National Institutes of Health is currently funding studies on turmeric and curcumin for a variety of conditions, including colorectal cancer, pancreatic cancer, Alzheimer's disease, psoriasis, inflammatory bowel disease (IBD), irritable bowel syndrome (IBS), and rheumatoid arthritis.

How to Use

TEA: Pour 2 cups boiling water over 1 teaspoon turmeric and steep for 10 minutes. Strain. Add honey and/or lemon if desired.

CAPSULES: 2 to 3 g turmeric per day provides 60 to 100 mg curcumin, the daily amount typically consumed in the diet in India.

STANDARDIZED EXTRACT: To replicate the levels of curcumin used in the clinical trials on turmeric, purchase an **extract** that guarantees a specific level of curcumin (sometimes written as curcuminoid on the label). Most studies used turmeric extracts providing 1 to 2 g per day of curcumin, taken in 2 to 3 divided doses.

> **NOTE:** The best way to absorb turmeric/curcumin is with piperine, an **alkaloid** found in black pepper. Try adding pepper to your curry dishes.

Precautions

Eating turmeric is very safe. Scientists have shown that taking curcumin at doses of up to 12 g per day was also very well tolerated, though there is little reason to take that much. Some people may get indigestion when taking high amounts of turmeric/curcumin.

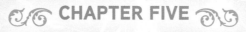

CHAPTER FIVE

Joints, Muscles, and Skin

Plants & Joints, Muscles & Skin

✦

T he last of the great English herbalists and one of the first great English botanists, John Parkinson (1567-1650) was both an eminent gardener and an expert on medicinal plants. Early in his career he was appointed apothecary—the medieval equivalent of a pharmacist—to James I of England, and in 1618, helped create the first London *Pharmacopeia*, the official listing of medicinal herbs and other substances approved for use in English medicine, including instructions on their preparation. Many botanists and medical historians consider Parkinson's greatest work to be the monumental *Theatrum Botanicum: The Theater of Plants*. It is by far the largest classic herbal in the English language and describes some 3,800 plants. One of them is comfrey *(Symphytum officinale)*.

"The rootes of Comfrey," Parkinson wrote, "taken fresh, beaten small, spread upon leather, and laid upon any place troubled with the gout, doe presently give ease of the paines and . . . giveth ease to pained joynts, and profiteth very much for running and moist ulcers, gangrenes, mortifications and the like." Parkinson was likely familiar with comfrey's effect on painful joints, for when he published *Theatrum Botanicum* in 1640, he was 73.

Age is rarely kind to joints, the places in the skeleton where bones come together. Ligaments are strong, tough tissues that hold the bones of a joint in proper orientation. Joints give our bodies the flexibility to move in many ways. The shoulder and hip are two of the body's most freely movable joints. Wrist, ankle, knee, thumb, and neck joints are a bit less mobile but still exhibit a remarkable range of motion.

Of course, no joint could move without muscles. Those that move joints are formed from skeletal muscle tissue and are under conscious control. Skeletal muscles are anchored to bones by tendons. Like the smooth muscles in many organs and the cardiac muscles of the heart, skeletal muscles are made of specialized muscle cells that can contract, or shorten. When muscles contract, body parts move, whether to reposition bones by skeletal muscles, squeeze a meal through the digestive tract by smooth muscles, or pump the heart's four chambers by cardiac muscles.

The contours of many muscles and joints are somewhat visible, and easily felt, under the skin. The skin, the body's largest organ, accounts for nearly 16 percent of the average person's weight. Thin, stretchy, and relatively tough, skin is far more than just a veneer. With minute receptors for touch, pressure, and pain, skin is a sensor, monitoring the body's surroundings and everything it contacts. With tiny blood vessels, sweat glands, and hairs, skin is also a thermostat, ready to release heat or conserve it to regulate body temperature. Skin is also a watertight barrier and shield, the first line of defense against the outside world.

For all its toughness, however, skin is easily bruised, burned, and abraded in everyday life. It can erupt with welts, rashes, hives, and sores as a result of allergies, disease, exposure, and stress. For all their strength, muscles can be overstretched, bruised, or torn. And for all their versatility, joints can be strained, sprained, or dislocated. They are also targets for inflammatory, degenerative, and autoimmune diseases, such as osteoarthritis and rheumatoid arthritis.

Ancient healers invariably turned to plants for solutions to these problems. Skin conditions were often treated with oils pressed from plant leaves or fruits, salves made from mixing plant parts with fats, and infusions brewed by steeping herbs in hot water. In many cases, applying herbal preparations to the skin was also the most effective way to treat problems associated with muscles and joints. Many herbs, such as comfrey, common in Parkinson's day, are still employed by modern practitioners of herbal medicine to treat skin, muscle, and joint complaints. Herbalists also recommend several herbs native to Australia, South America, and Africa that have entered the modern pharmacopoeia. This chapter includes 11 herbs commonly used to treat problems relating to the skin, joints, and muscles.

Popular as a home remedy and an ingredient in many over-the-counter skin products, aloe *(Aloe vera)* is widely recommended for soothing and healing burned or irritated skin. Arnica *(Arnica montana)*, another skin soother, also penetrates the skin to bring about healing in muscles and joints. Popular in Europe, arnica is effective for bruises, muscle soreness, and joint pain. Herbalists suggest preparations of edible calendula *(Calendula officinalis)* flowers to treat skin irritations, from simple chapping to fungal infections. Internally, calendula soothes inflamed mucosal tissues forming the lining of the mouth, throat, and other parts of the digestive tract.

Prior to the 1970s, cat's claw *(Uncaria tomentosa)* was largely unknown outside South America. In less than four decades it has become a popular remedy for inflammatory joint, nerve, and muscle complaints, as well as viral skin infections such as shingles *(Herpes zoster)*. Native to the Americas, cayenne *(Capsicum annuum)* is another effective herbal painkiller. Applied to the skin, it desensitizes nerve endings and dulls pain. Cayenne is popular for relieving pain associated with many joint and muscle conditions, including arthritis, fibromyalgia, and lower back pain, as well as skin inflammation. Used carefully—and never taken internally—comfrey works much as Parkinson described it, to ease joint pain, sprains, sore or stiff muscles and to heal certain types of skin conditions.

Devil's claw *(Harpagophytum procumbens)* is another fairly recent introduction into Western herbal medicine. Native to southern Africa, it is an effective remedy for eruptive skin problems, but its primary use in herbal medicine is for relieving the pain and inflammation of degenerative joint diseases. Rosemary *(Rosmarinus officinalis)* is familiar to most people as a culinary herb, but rosemary oil is commonly prescribed to improve circulation and ease muscle and joint pain. Tea tree *(Melaleuca alternifolia)* hails from Australia; the pungent oil extracted from its leaves has powerful antibacterial and antifungal properties. An ingredient in many over-the-counter skin and hair products, tea tree helps prevent, control, and heal a host of skin infections and irritations.

The last two herbs profiled in this chapter were used extensively by Native Americans. Willow bark *(Salix alba, S. purpurea, S. fragilis)* was the abundant source of the compounds later used to create aspirin. Its pain-relieving properties are effective for joint and muscle pain. Witch hazel *(Hamamelis virginiana)* is a traditional remedy for clearing skin problems, relieving muscle and joint soreness, and soothing irritations of the digestive tract lining.

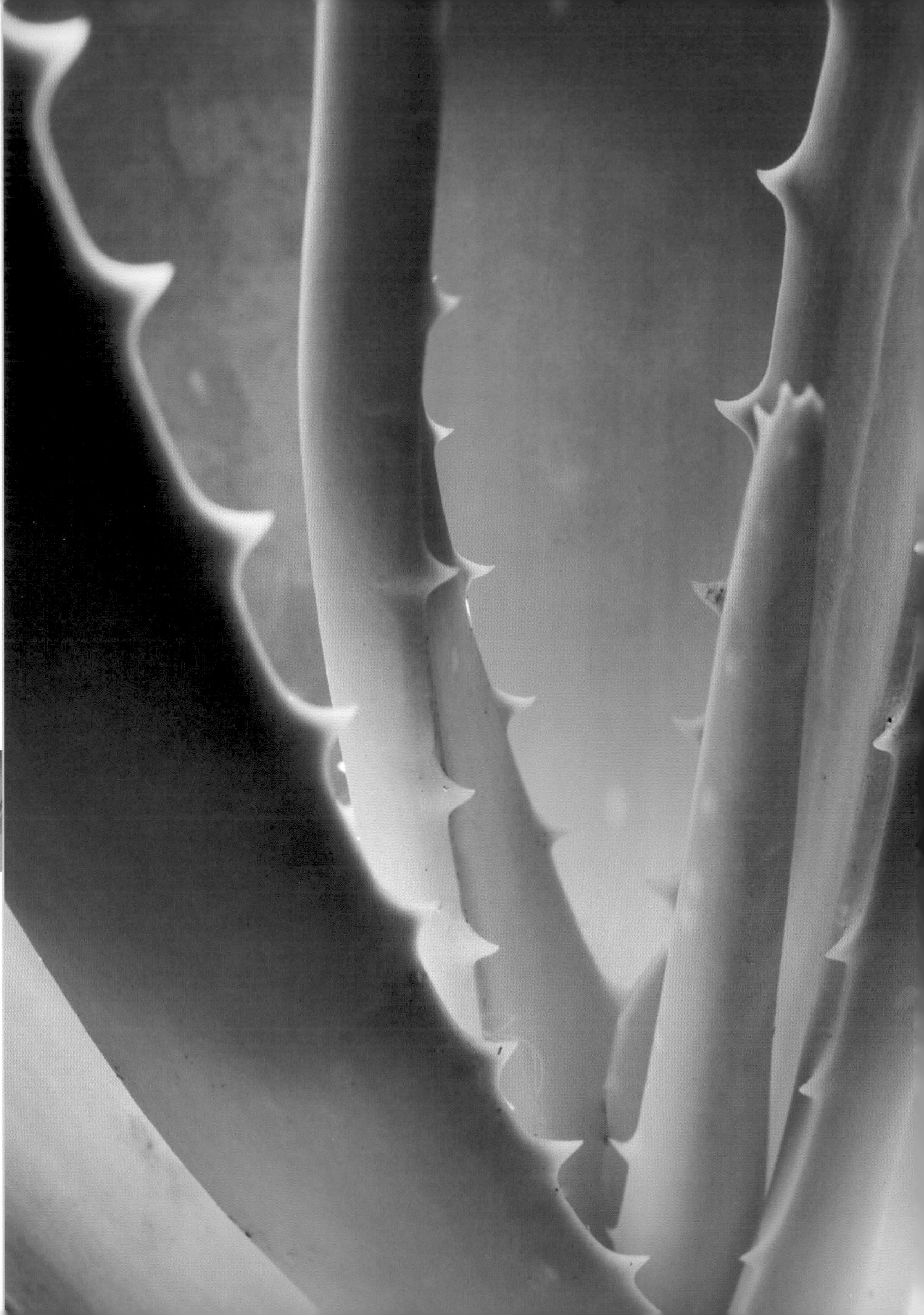

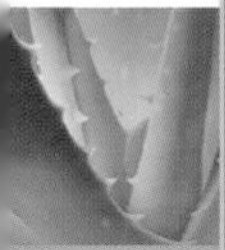

Aloe

Aloe vera

Native to North Africa and coastal areas surrounding the Mediterranean Sea, aloe is one of the most familiar of all herbal remedies. Pots of aloe grace many sunny kitchen windowsills, where the thick, fleshy leaves stand ready to become a quick and easy treatment for scalds and burns. A leaf plucked from the plant and sliced open shelters at its core a clear mucilaginous gel remarkably effective for soothing wounds and burns, speeding healing, and reducing risk of infection. The bitter, yellowish sap that oozes from the leaf's skin—not to be confused with the gel—is dried to form aloe latex, a crystalline substance.

In ancient Egypt, aloe was known as the plant of immortality. Legend has it that Cleopatra massaged aloe gel into her skin as part of her daily beauty routine. Greek philosopher Aristotle is said to have urged his student Alexander the Great to claim a group of islands off the Horn of Africa to acquire the aloes that grew there for his army's medicinal arsenal. Aloe found its way into European herbal medicine by the tenth century. The gel was applied externally to soothe and heal wounds and maintain healthy skin. Internally, herbalists prescribed it for stomach disorders, insomnia, hemorrhoids, headaches, gum diseases, and kidney ailments. Aloe latex was prescribed for constipation.

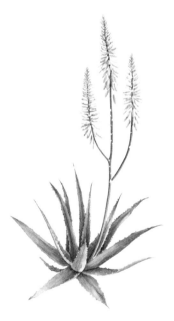

Today, aloe is one of the most commonly used herbs in the U.S. Applied externally, it provides immediate relief for burns, sunburn, skin irritations, scrapes, and minor wounds. It is useful in treating genital herpes and psoriasis. Aloe gel contains active **compounds** that decrease pain and inflammation and stimulate skin repair. Preparations of aloe gel are widely available, but many consider it most effective when taken directly from fresh-cut leaves. It is a common ingredient in over-the-counter skin care products. Internally, aloe gel and aloe juice (from aloe gel) are taken for osteoarthritis, stomach ulcers, irritable bowel syndrome, and asthma. Studies suggest that aloe juice may help lower blood sugar levels in type 2 diabetes and speed wound healing in diabetics.

Inside aloe's succulent leaves is a cooling astringent gel, prized for its power to soothe irritated skin.

TIME LINE OF USAGE AND SPREAD

1552 B.C.
Aloe vera mentioned in the *Codex Ebers*, a medical document of ancient Egypt.

A.D. 50-70
Aloe's use is described by Dioscorides in *De Materia Medica*.

1590s
English herbalist J. Gerard notes two aloes used for their healing powers.

1930s
Aloe gains popularity in West for treating skin ailments and reactions to radiation burns.

The genus *Aloe* includes some 450 species of tropical herbs, shrubs, and trees native to South Africa and Madagascar, as well as the southern Arabian Peninsula and Canary Islands. The common *Aloe vera* is familiar to many as a houseplant, often kept handy for the fresh leaf gel so good for minor burns, bites, or sunburn. Aloes in cultivation are notoriously difficult to identify, as they change in size and appearance when grown under different conditions.

Hybridization further confuses identification. In some books aloe is listed as *Aloe barbadensis*. Under the rules of botanical nomenclature, which botanists follow in naming plants, the earliest validly published name has priority. N. L. Burman published the name *Aloe vera* on April 6, 1768. Philip Miller published the name *Aloe barbadensis* on April 16, 1768. Hence, Burman's name, *Aloe vera,* bestowed 240 years ago, has priority over Miller's *A. barbadensis* by 10 days. The name *Aloe* is derived from a Greek name for this or a similar plant.

Aloe vera grows to 36 inches or so. The thick, fleshy, lance-shaped leaves, with soft-spiny margins, grow from 6 to 20 inches long, usually in a rosette of up to 16 leaves. Outdoors in tropical climates, or in greenhouse-grown potted plants, aloe produces a single flowering stalk with pendant, inch-long drooping yellowish flowers, slightly swollen at the base.

Growing Habits

Aloe vera has been cultivated for thousands of years, obscuring with certainty its geographical origin. A commonly accepted theory is that *Aloe vera* originated in the Canary Islands and was brought to the Mediterranean region by early seafaring traders. The plant was found throughout the Mediterranean region some 2,000 years ago. Dioscorides, a physician in the Roman army of Nero, mentioned it in his medical compendium, *De Materia Medica*. A recent study theorizes that *A. vera* may have originated in the southern Arabian Peninsula,

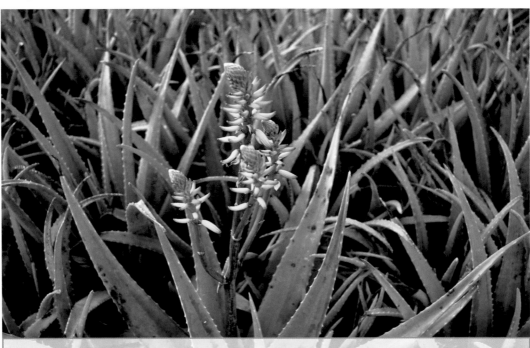

At home in arid places, aloe has been cultivated for its medicinal effects since the time of the ancient Egyptians.

COMMON NAME:	SCIENTIFIC NAME:	FAMILY:	PARTS USED:	NATIVE RANGE:
Aloe	*Aloe vera*	Asphodelaceae	Leaves	Tropics, Mediterranean

Grow an aloe (purchased from any good garden center) on a kitchen windowsill so it's within easy reach. To use fresh aloe gel as topical first aid for minor burns and scrapes, first rinse injury with cool water. Cut off 1 of the plant's outer leaves at its base. Slice the leaf down the middle and carefully scrape out the gel inside. Gently apply to injured skin.

once a key trading point for medicinal plants in the ancient world, and subsequently spread through the Egyptian empire. Today it is the most widely grown medicinal plant in American households.

Cultivation and Harvesting

Aloe prefers a gravelly, well-drained, infertile soil; it likes full sun but is tolerant of shady windowsills. A plant of dry climates (think desert), it requires little water. Offsets at the base of the plant can easily be separated and repotted. Large-scale commercial cultivation occurs in south Texas and Mexico, supplying cosmetic and dietary supplement markets worldwide.

Therapeutic Uses

+ *Burns (first- and second-degree)*
+ *Psoriasis*
+ *Colitis*
+ *Diabetes*

Aloe is famous for soothing sunburn. Perhaps less well known is how broadly its healing properties extend—from soothing minor cuts and skin conditions to possibly lowering blood sugar levels in diabetics.

Aloe gel is the inner mucilaginous—or gooey—part and is used topically for many skin conditions. Recent research shows that ingesting this gel confers benefits in lowering blood glucose in people with diabetes and easing symptoms in people with ulcerative colitis. Aloe gel contains **polysaccharides**, compounds that have a soothing effect on mucous membranes, and **enzymes** that coat irritated skin and ease pain. Aloe may also be antibacterial. For these reasons, aloe has been used in some skin conditions, such as first- and second-degree burns and psoriasis, sometimes showing better effects than more conventional

therapies. In a study of 30 people with second-degree burns, aloe cream, containing 0.5 percent of the gel in powdered form, helped to heal the burns faster than sulfadiazine, a commonly used antibacterial cream. In addition, a study of 80 people with psoriasis showed that a 70 percent aloe cream worked as well as 0.1 percent triamcinolone cream, often prescribed for psoriasis.

So-called aloe juice is made from aloe gel. The gel—either fresh or powdered dried aloe gel—is just one ingredient in aloe juice products. Marketed as aloe juice, these products may also contain water, citric acid, fruit juices, preservatives, and more. Aloe gel is also an ingredient in many cosmetic products, including topical creams, lotions, and shampoos.

How to Use

ALOE GEL: Apply to the skin several times daily for burns and other skin conditions. For colitis, take 25 to 30 ml (about 2 tablespoons) twice daily; for diabetes, 10 to 20 ml (about 1 tablespoon) daily. Follow manufacturer's guidelines.

Precautions

Topically applied, aloe is safe. However, aloe may delay healing in deep, open wounds, as from surgery. Aloe gel should be free of **anthraquinones** and soothing to the gastrointestinal tract, but leaf **extracts** can contain all parts of the leaf, and thus both gel and latex. It is important to buy aloe gel that says it is made from the inner fillet and/or that is free of aloin. Aloe juice containing aloin can act as a laxative and can irritate the intestines. Prolonged use can lead to electrolyte loss and dependence on juice for normal bowel function. Those with acute or severe gastrointestinal symptoms should not take the juice. Children and pregnant or nursing women should not take aloe internally.

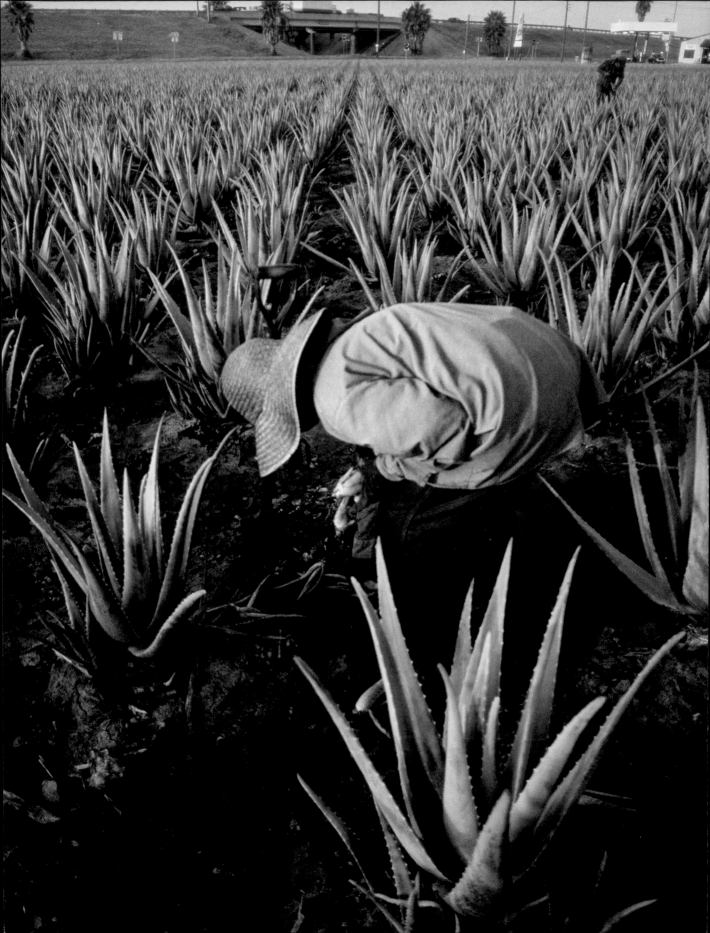

Aloe Harvest

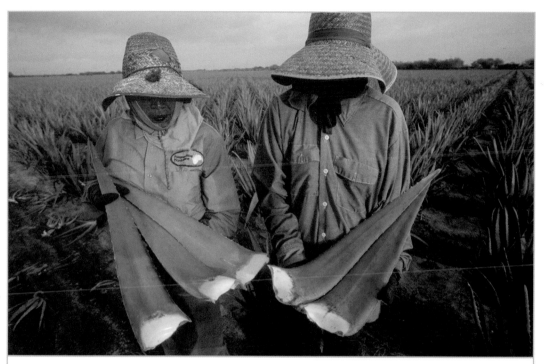

On an aloe plantation in south Texas, a worker (opposite) thins a field of aloe plants. Commercially raised plants grow in long rows—some 5,000 plants per acre. Aloe harvesting (below) takes place 4 times a year, with 2 to 3 of a plant's outer leaves removed each time. Workers display freshly cut leaves (above), each weighing roughly 2 pounds. Machine processing of freshly harvested leaves has largely replaced traditional methods.

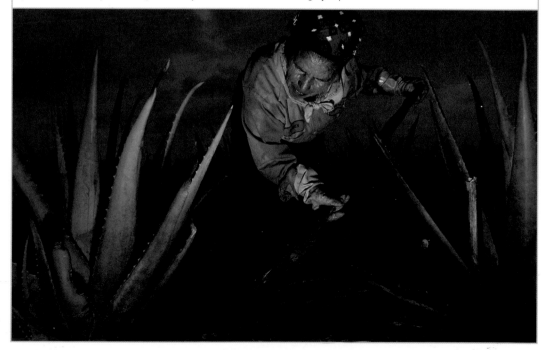

JOINTS, MUSCLES & SKIN

Arnica

Arnica montana

As the second half of its scientific name suggests, *Arnica montana* is a mountain dweller, native to sunny alpine meadows of Europe, Central Asia, and Siberia. Sporting deep yellow, daisylike flowers, arnica has been prized for centuries in these regions for its ability to ease the pain and inflammation of sore muscles, bruises, and sprains. Across the Atlantic, Native Americans used related species, such as *Arnica fulgens*, in a similar way for bruising, muscle soreness, and back pain. Long before the healing properties of arnica were recognized in Europe, though, the herb

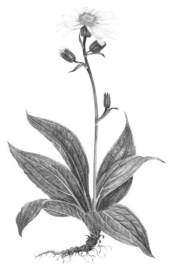

was used in pagan rituals designed to ensure a good harvest. Arnica blossoms, brilliant as tiny suns, were thought to be especially potent on the summer solstice. Bunches of the flowers were gathered on Midsummer Day and placed in fields to enhance the fertility of crops.

By the 1500s, interest in arnica had shifted from the magical to the medicinal. Italian physician and herbalist Pietro Andrea Mattioli wrote favorably about the herb's healing properties in his botanical masterpiece, *Commentarii in Sex Libros Pedacii Dioscoridis*, which was first published in 1544. Arnica found a place in the folk medicine of many other European countries, especially Germany and Austria, where it remains an important medicinal herb to this day. *Arnica montana* is currently an ingredient in more than a hundred German herbal preparations. Originally, the entire plant, including the roots, was used in preparing herbal remedies, but now typically only the flower heads are used.

In the U.S., arnica has never enjoyed the popularity it does in Europe. Nevertheless, preparations of this herb are readily available—as gels, ointments, creams, and sprays—for external use in treating bruises, muscle strains, sprains and dislocations, arthritis and rheumatic pain, phlebitis, and swelling due to fractures. Arnica salves can be an effective remedy for chapped lips and acne. **Tinctures** of arnica are also common for use as a base in making compresses and **poultices**. Arnica in its herbal form is primarily restricted to these types of topical applications because it can cause serious side effects if taken internally.

Herbalists employ remedies made from the dazzling blossoms of arnica to treat bruises, sprains, and swellings.

TIME LINE OF USAGE AND SPREAD

1820	1830s	1880	1981
Arnica is officially added to the *U.S. Pharmacopeia* (and removed in 1960).	German writer Goethe (1749-1832) drinks arnica tea in old age for angina.	Homeopathy founder S. Hahnemann notes arnica's use for bruises and sprains.	*A. montana* compounds with anti-inflammatory and antibiotic activity identified.

A rnica—from a Greek word meaning "lambskin," referring to the leaf texture—serves as both the scientific genus name and the plant's common name. It is an herbal medicine primarily associated with European species, especially the well-known *Arnica montana*. However, of the 29 species in the genus, only 2 occur in Europe—*A. angustifolia* and *A. montana*. One species is found in Japan, but the vast majority of arnicas, 26 in all,

grow in western North America, ranging from Canada to Mexico. Several American **species**, including *A. chamissonis, A. cordifolia, A. latifolia,* and *A. sororia,* are used as substitutes for *A. montana*. Arnica (*A. montana*) grows from 10 to 22 inches tall. Its basal rosette of leaves and stem leaves is egg shaped to lance shaped, densely hairy, about 3 to 7 inches long, and an inch wide. The daisylike flowers are yellow to yellow-orange. All of the aboveground parts, harvested in flower, are used in herbal medicine.

Growing Habits

The **genus** ranges around the colder regions of the Northern Hemisphere. The narrow-leaved *A. angustifolia,* found in Arctic Europe, also

occurs in Greenland and throughout Canada, south to Montana. European *A. montana,* as its name implies, is usually found in the mountains, growing in poor, often acidic soils from southern Norway and Latvia to southern Portugal in the Carpathian Mountains to the northern Apennines. Half of the North American species (13) are rare or **endemic** to very narrow areas or found only in Canada and Alaska. Of the 17 California species, 4 are relatively common in mountain meadows and are used locally by herbalists. North American meadow arnica (*A. chamissonis*) is cultivated on a small scale in other parts of the U.S. and used in arnica products. One of the most widespread western North American species is an alpine to subalpine plant found in moist meadows and

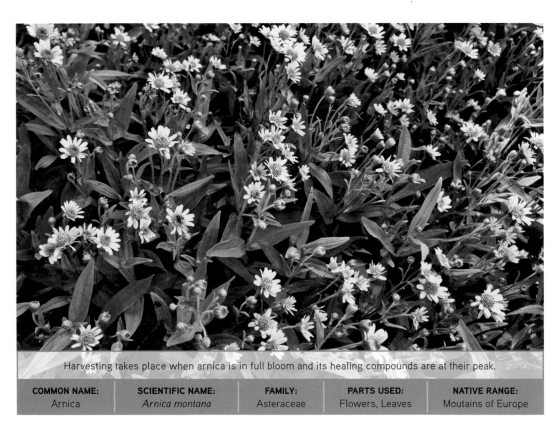

Harvesting takes place when arnica is in full bloom and its healing compounds are at their peak.

COMMON NAME:	SCIENTIFIC NAME:	FAMILY:	PARTS USED:	NATIVE RANGE:
Arnica	*Arnica montana*	Asteraceae	Flowers, Leaves	Moutains of Europe

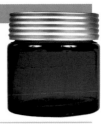

Pack a widemouthed jar with arnica leaf and fill it with almond oil. Screw on the lid. Let the mixture steep for 2 to 3 weeks, stirring daily. Strain the oil into a clean container and refrigerate. To make the salve, heat ½ cup of the arnica oil in a saucepan to 100°F. Add ¾ ounce of grated beeswax. Stir until the wax is melted. Let mixture cool slightly. Pour into sterile half-ounce jars with secure lids and store in the fridge.

late snowmelt belts at the edge of coniferous forests. Another species, common leopardbane (*A. caulis*), is found in moist soils, mostly along the coastal plain from Delaware to Florida.

Cultivation and Harvesting

Arnicas are locally protected in the wild, and the harvest of wild plants is discouraged. As a predominantly subalpine to alpine plant group, arnicas succeed in cool climates and poor, acidic soils. They do best in a well-drained, humus-rich soil, with drainage improved by pea gravel added to the soil. Propagation is by root division early in the season or by seeds. The aboveground portions of the plant are harvested in full bloom and used fresh or dried.

Therapeutic Uses

+ *Bruises*
+ *Contusions and other musculoskeletal injuries*
+ *Swelling (from injuries)*
+ *Joint pain (from injuries or osteoarthritis)*

Arnica is the herb to go to immediately after an injury. Whether for the pain and swelling after bumps and sprains or the resulting bruising, arnica salves, ointments, gels, and creams are a common externally applied herbal remedy. (**Homeopathic** formulations of arnica, in dilute formulations given as capsules or pellets taken under the tongue, are also prescribed for the purpose of treating the symptoms immediately after an injury.) Arnica has a long history of use for these conditions in Europe and has been endorsed by the German health authority's Commission E, responsible for evaluating the safety and efficacy of medicinal herbs in Germany. Currently it is becoming a common addition to first-aid kits in the United States.

This popular herbal treatment is supported by research. Many studies have been done after patients had surgery—plastic surgery, tonsil removal, hand operations—to manage the pain, swelling, and bruising. In a study involving 204 people with osteoarthritis in their hands, arnica gel was compared with a similar-appearing gel containing 5 percent ibuprofen; after 3 weeks, each group had similar improvements in both pain relief and hand function. This research result needs further investigation, but arnica could be an interesting option for osteoarthritis. Many beneficial effects of arnica are thought to come from **sesquiterpene lactones**, a group of **compounds** that fight inflammation and relieve pain.

How to Use

CREAMS, GELS, OINTMENTS, AND SALVES: Arnica topicals can be applied to an injury several times daily; or follow product instructions. Commercial arnica topical preparations are widely available.

POULTICE: Steep 3 tablespoons of arnica flowers in a cup of hot water. Let stand for 10 minutes. Cool and apply saturated plant material to injury for 10 to 15 minutes. Repeat 3 to 4 times daily for an acute injury.

 NOTE: To prevent the absorption of dangerous compounds, topical preparations of arnica should not be applied to broken skin or near the mouth or eyes.

Precautions

Arnica should not be taken internally. It can cause heart arrhythmias and possible respiratory collapse; this concern is avoided with homeopathic preparations, because the arnica has been significantly diluted. Applied externally, arnica is generally safe and is usually well tolerated; if a rash should appear, discontinue use.

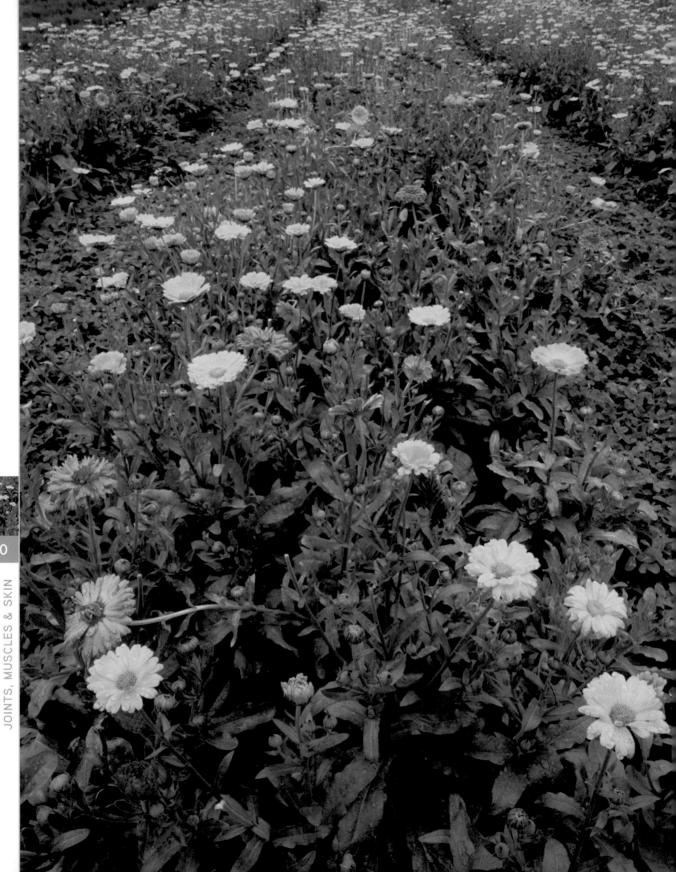

Calendula

⚬⁄ᵒ Calendula officinalis ᵒᵥ⚬

Nicknamed pot marigold, poet's marigold, or simply "gold," calendula is not to be confused with the rather unpleasantly scented common garden marigold of the genus *Tagetes*. Calendula flowers have little scent, and unlike any *Tagetes*, are edible. Decked out with single or multiple rows of petals in sunny yellow or bright orange, the flowers seem to hover above the plant's grayish green, slightly sticky stems and leaves. Calendula is a profuse bloomer. Its name is likely derived from the Latin *calendae*, meaning "little calendar" or "little clock." The reference could be to calendula's propensity for being in bloom during the new moon of summer months (in some climates, nearly every month) or to its habit of partially closing its petals along with the setting sun.

For centuries, calendula has been prized for its ornamental, culinary, and cosmetic properties. The flowers have been used to decorate Hindu temples; color food, cosmetics, and fabric in ancient Greece; and garnish dishes in ancient Rome. In medieval England, the petals were dried by the barrelful, then churned into syrups and conserves, added to winter stews, and baked into breads. Medicinally, calendula's colorful petals have been used since at least the 12th century. Traditionally, preparations were administered internally for fevers, stomach upsets, ulcers, and more. Its

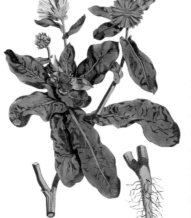

chief use, however, was external, as a remedy for skin conditions and for infection in minor wounds.

Calendula is used to treat many of the same conditions today. Whether applied to the skin or taken internally, calendula preparations appear to speed healing. Modern herbalists recommend calendula lotions, creams, and ointments for chapped skin, eczema, minor cuts and burns, diaper rash, insect bites, hemorrhoids, athlete's foot, and varicose veins. Calendula-containing eardrops are used to treat ear infections in children. Taken internally, calendula may relieve throat infections, improve digestion, and heal gastric and duodenal ulcers. Recently, calendula has been shown to help prevent dermatitis in breast cancer patients during radiation.

The cheery blooms of calendula brightened medieval herb gardens just as they do their modern counterparts.

TIME LINE OF USAGE AND SPREAD

1100s	**1477**	**1699**	**1860s**
Calendula is cultivated in European gardens.	*Macer's Herbal* claims herb improves eyesight, draws out "wicked humours."	The *Countrie Farme* notes calendula helps "headache, jaundice, red eyes and ague."	Calendula is used by field doctors during the American Civil War to staunch bleeding.

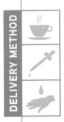
Of the dozen species of *Calendula,* the best known is *Calendula officinalis.* Calendula is both the scientific name and the common name for this widely grown herb. It is annual or perennial in warmer regions, with erect, branched, leaf stems from 8 to 20 inches. The alternate leaves are oblong lance shaped, usually wider at the top than toward the base. Leaves are somewhat hairy and 3 to 6 inches long, and up to 1½ inches broad. The flower heads have the typical disk and ray flower arrangement of a daisy, ranging from light yellow to vivid orange in color. Dozens of cultivars (cultivated **varieties**) are found in American, European, and Japanese horticulture, where calendula is highly developed as a cut flower for the floral trade.

Growing Habits

Probably native to southern Europe and North Africa, calendula has been widespread in cultivation for centuries, its exact origins lost in time. It is found throughout Europe, mostly near gardens, where it escaped from cultivation.

In North America, calendula has escaped and naturalized, mostly as scattered localized plants. It is found in eastern Canada, south through New England, west through Pennsylvania and Ohio, north to Michigan and Wisconsin. In the West it has escaped from cultivation in California; there it is also an ornamental, as it is in Washington and southern British Columbia.

Cultivation and Harvesting

Calendula is cultivated in gardens worldwide from subarctic regions to the tropics. It is a plant that is adaptable to various growing conditions. It is easily grown from seed. Once it begins flowering after about 6 weeks of growth, it will continue to bloom even after the first frost. It succeeds well in any average garden soil with good drainage, thriving in full sun, though in the South dappled shade will improve its chances of flourishing during summer heat and humidity. Flowers can be picked continuously throughout the growing season. The flowers and the whole plant are used in herbal medicine. The dried ray flowers or whole flower heads are used for coloring and, given their somewhat sweet-salty flavor, for flavoring as well. The whole plant is harvested fresh for **tinctures** and **extracts**. Usually the dried flower heads are used in teas.

Therapeutic Uses

+ *Dermatitis*
+ *Wounds*

The warm gold blossoms of calendula have long been a signature remedy for skin ailments, from eczema and abscesses to acne and abrasions. The German health authority has

over the (kitchen) counter CALENDULA COMPRESS

Steep 2 teaspoons of calendula flowers in a cup of hot water. Strain, cool, and then use the liquid to saturate a cloth to make a compress. Alternatively, the moistened flower material itself can be used as a poultice. Wrapped in gauze to contain the moisture, the poultice can be placed on the skin for 15 minutes. Either a poultice or a compress can be used several times daily, giving caledula's anti-inflammatory and antibacterial effects a chance to take effect.

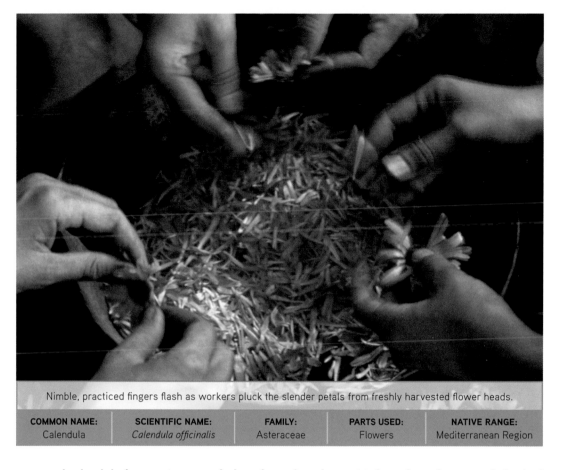

Nimble, practiced fingers flash as workers pluck the slender petals from freshly harvested flower heads.

COMMON NAME:	SCIENTIFIC NAME:	FAMILY:	PARTS USED:	NATIVE RANGE:
Calendula	*Calendula officinalis*	Asteraceae	Flowers	Mediterranean Region

approved calendula for treating wounds, based on research showing its **anti-inflammatory** effects and effectiveness in helping wounds seal over with new tissue. Calendula is thought to have 2 main medicinal actions on skin. The **triterpenoid compounds** such as oleanolic acid appear to inhibit a variety of bacteria. Its anti-inflammatory effects may be the result of a triterpenoid compound acting as an **antioxidant**, to reduce damage from oxygen **radicals** in the healing process.

Calendula products have been developed and studied for a host of human ailments. For example, a calendula extract combined with green tea, tea tree oil, and manuka oil was developed into a mouth rinse—a spinoff of research showing calendula rinses fight gum inflammation, or gingivitis. Another study randomized 254 breast cancer patients about to undergo radiation treatment to apply either a calendula ointment or a commonly used medicine, trolamine, twice daily. The calendula group exhibited less dermatitis from the radiation and also had fewer interruptions to their treatment.

One method for making a calendula ointment is to heat the plant in petroleum jelly, strain, and cool for use on the skin. Calendula's anti-inflammatory effects and its effectiveness for various skin ailments may be more pronounced when the flowers are first extracted with high-dose alcohol, before being incorporated into creams or ointments.

How to Use

TOPICAL PREPARATIONS: Extracts are incorporated into many skin products: soaps, creams, ointments, salves, and lotions with various concentrations of calendula. Apply preparations 3 to 4 times daily to heal minor skin conditions.

Precautions

Those allergic to plants in the Asteraceae **family** can develop a sensitivity to topical use. Should a rash develop, discontinue use.

Cat's Claw

✦ *Uncaria tomentosa* ✦

Armed with inch-long hooked thorns that closely resemble sharp feline claws, cat's claw, or *uña de gato* in Spanish, is a large, woody vine native to the Amazon rain forest and other tropical regions of South and Central America. The thorns may deter animal predators, but their primary function is to help the plant anchor itself to tree trunks and branches as it climbs more than a hundred feet up into the rain forest canopy. For centuries, two species of cat's claw—*Uncaria tomentosa* and the closely related *U. guaianenesis*—have been used by indigenous

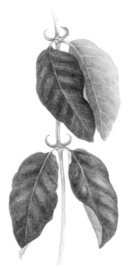

peoples, particularly in Peru, to treat a wide variety of health problems and conditions.

Since the rise of the Incas, a number of Peruvian tribes have used cat's claw bark and root preparations for treating asthma, arthritis, rheumatism, urinary tract infections, kidney problems, inflammation, and cancer. The herb has also been used as a remedy for fevers, intestinal ailments, gonorrhea, and as a form of birth control. Traditional use of cat's claw continues today in many **indigenous** rain forest communities.

Before the 1970s, cat's claw was essentially unknown to the rest of the world. Since its introduction first in Europe and then worldwide, it has become one of the most popular Amazonian herbal remedies available. So popular that overcollection of cat's claw has become a serious concern.

In modern herbal medicine, cat's claw is thought to be a powerful stimulator of the immune system. It is recommended for many chronic illnesses, such as fibromyalgia, chronic fatigue, mononucleosis, and shingles. Because of its potent **anti-inflammatory** properties, cat's claw is used to treat joint problems such as those occurring in osteoarthritis and rheumatoid arthritis; for the same reason it is recommended for gastritis, ulcers, and neuralgia. The herb may protect against gastrointestinal damage associated with nonsteroidal anti-inflammatory drugs (NSAIDs) such as ibuprofen. Because it possesses tumor-fighting properties, cat's claw may be a complement to cancer treatments. Since the early 1990s, it has also been used for treatment of HIV and other diseases or disorders of the immune system.

Amazonian tribes were the first to discover that the bark of cat's claw vine can ease pain in arthritic joints.

TIME LINE OF USAGE AND SPREAD

1400s	**1970s–1980s**	**1980s**	**EARLY 1990s**
Use of cat's claw predates the time of the Inca's dominance in Peru.	Austrian Klaus Keplinger does the first comprehensive research on cat's claw.	International trade in cat's claw begins, following significant research.	Cat's claw used in Peru and Europe as adjunct treatment for cancer and AIDS.

An herbalist in Puerto Maldonado, Peru, displays rain forest products, including cat's claw bark (bottom shelf).

COMMON NAME:	SCIENTIFIC NAME:	FAMILY:	PARTS USED:	NATIVE RANGE:
Cat's Claw	*Uncaria tomentosa*	Rubiaceae	Bark, Roots	Amazon, Tropical S. America

Cat's claw bark can be seen in virtually every local market in western Amazonia. Two of the 40 tropical species of *Uncaria*—*U. tomentosa* and *U. guianensis*—occur in South America. High-climbing lianas (woody vines), they stretch toward the top canopy in the Amazon rain forest. The stems of *U. tomentosa* can be densely or sparsely hairy but become nearly hairless with age. The 3½- to 6-inch leaves are opposite, broadly rounded or heart shaped at the base, oval in outline, mostly bright green and shiny above, and white hairy beneath. Just beneath the leaf node are prominent clawlike thorns—modified tendrils that allow branches to hook on to trees and climb into the rain forest canopy. It is this feature that makes the plant most recognizable. *U. guianensis* is very similar in appearance, but is mostly smooth stemmed, with smooth, shiny, hairless leaves. Its thorns are usually more strongly curved than those of *U. tomentosa*.

Growing Habits

Native to the American tropics from Belize south to Paraguay, *U. tomentosa* is a rain forest **species**. It thrives in forest openings where sunlight allows it to reproduce, and it does so vigorously in disturbed clearings; to mature, however, it needs to climb. Cat's claw matures in about 10 years, when the central vine reaches a diameter of about 4 inches. *U. guianensis* has a similar range and grows in the same rain forest habitat; however, it also thrives along roadsides and forest trails and in disturbed areas around rivers, sites that make it much more accessible for harvesting.

The two species contain different **alkaloids**, and some of the important medicinal components of *U. tomentosa* are not present in *U. guianensis*, making *U. tomentosa* the preferred species in herbal medicine. However, because of the greater accessibility of *U. guianensis*, the bark of both species is collected and sold in the herb trade. Visual inspection of the bark or wood defies identification as one species or the other.

Cultivation and Harvesting

Both South American sources of cat's claw are wild-harvested. Peruvian government institutions and private companies are studying cat's claw commercial cultivation. The findings suggest that it must be grown with trees to facilitate climbing and vertical growth. Outside its rain forest habitat, if grown in low light and shade, the plants do not do well. In some South American villages, farmers have encouraged cat's claw cultivation near their homes as a ready source of income. Despite attempts at cultivation, the supply is primarily harvested from rain forests in tropical South America. The majority of dried bark in the herb trade comes from Peru.

Therapeutic Uses

+ *Osteoarthritis*
+ *Rheumatoid arthritis*
+ *Immune system booster*

This woody climber of the Amazon rain forest holds promise for people suffering from the painful, stiff joints of both osteoarthritis and rheumatoid arthritis. Many of the medicinal benefits of cat's claw come from one group of chemicals called pentacyclic oxindole alkaloids, which act as boosters to the immune system. The concentration of these alkaloids varies depending on when and how the plant is harvested. Other **compounds** in cat's claw may be responsible for its **antioxidant** and anti-inflammatory properties.

When 40 people with rheumatoid arthritis were given 20-mg capsules of cat's claw *(U. tomentosa)* 3 times daily for 6 months, joint pain decreased. The formulation used in this study was the brand Krallendorn containing 14.7 mg per g of alkaloid compounds. Subjects in another study, using 100 mg of an **extract** of *U. guianensis* for osteoarthritis of the knee, reported less pain with activities.

In a study exploring the immune system effects of cat's claw, either **placebo** or 300 mg of a cat's claw extract was given twice a day for a month to 23 men; subsequently, they received a vaccine immunizing them against pneumonia. After 6 months, the group receiving cat's claw maintained their immunity, whereas the placebo group showed some waning of immunity, as measured by **antibody** levels. This particular extract contained fewer alkaloids and more of other compounds, demonstrating that the alkaloids are not the only important ingredients in cat's claw.

 NOTE: Those with autoimmune diseases or those taking immunosuppressive medications or blood pressure medicines should not use cat's claw.

How to Use

Dosages depend on which of the 2 species are used and how the product is prepared. The herb can be taken as tea (**decoction**), **tincture**, powdered, or in capsule form. Follow manufacturer's dosage guidelines. The following preparations apply to *U. tomentosa:*

TEA: Boil 1 g of root bark for 15 minutes in 250 ml water (about a cup). The decoction is strained, cooled, and taken 1 to 3 times a day.

TINCTURE: Take 1 to 2 ml, 2 to 3 times daily.

EXTRACT: Dried, powdered extracts are mixed into water; follow product label instructions.

CAPSULE: Capsules of cat's claw contain standardized amounts of alkaloids or other compounds. Extraction techniques are designed to favor the presence of particular medicinally active compounds. A range of techniques is used to make extracts, including freeze-drying or ultrafiltration of water extracts.

Precautions

Some people experience mild side effects from cat's claw. Symptoms can include stomach upset, headache, and dizziness. Do not take if pregnant or nursing. Not recommended for children under age 3.

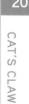

---

over the (kitchen) counter CAT'S CLAW TEA

To make cat's claw tea, simply add 1 teaspoon of cat's claw root bark to 4 cups of boiling water. Stir well and pour into a saucepan with a tight-fitting lid. Simmer this mixture for 10 to 15 minutes. Cool, strain, and drink 1 cup approximately 3 times per day.

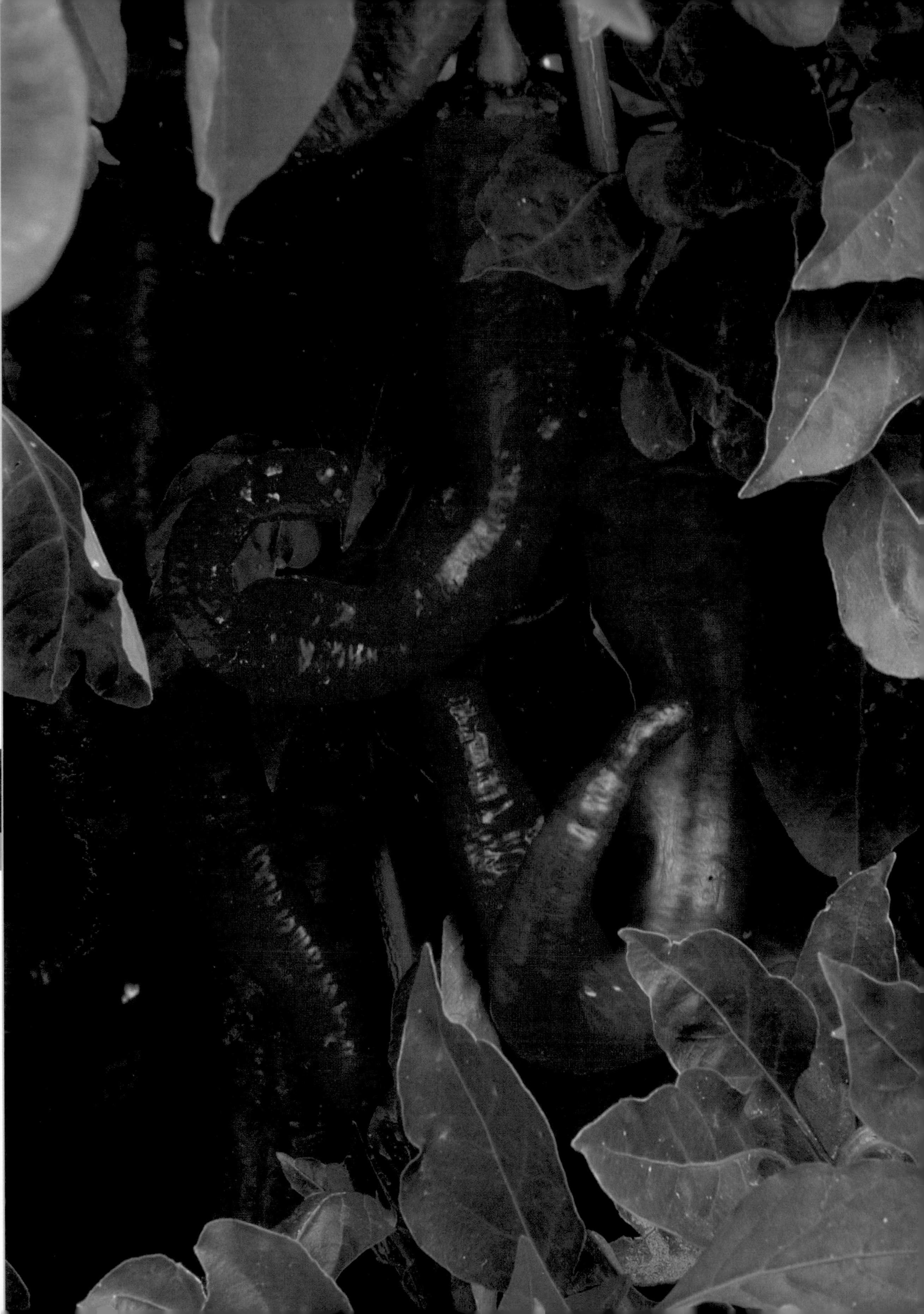

Cayenne

✦ *Capsicum annuum* ✦

The spicy cuisines of Mexico, Southeast Asia, China, southern Italy, many Caribbean islands, and North America's Cajun cultures share an ingredient: hot pepper. Not the tiny black peppercorns ground in pepper mills, but the fleshy fruits borne by plants belonging to the genus *Capsicum*. More than a thousand different varieties of *Capsicum* are grown worldwide. They produce colorful fruits that vary considerably, not only in color, size, and shape, but in the intensity of their heat. That heat comes from a plant chemical called capsaicin, which, in addition to adding zest to food, has pain-relieving properties.

Cayenne peppers, native to Central and South America, were being cultivated in these regions more than 9,000 years ago. Not until the 15th century was cayenne introduced to the rest of the world. Cayenne seeds were first brought to Europe following Columbus's voyage of 1492. Vasco de Gama is credited with introducing *Capsicum* into Africa and India.

Cayenne has been used for millennia to dull pain and increase circulation. The Maya used it to treat infections; the Aztec to quiet throbbing toothaches. Cayenne has also been used in traditional **Ayurvedic**, Chinese, Japanese, and Korean medicines as a topical for arthritis and muscle pain and as an oral remedy for circulatory and digestive problems.

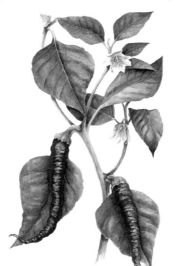

Applied to the skin, cayenne is thought to desensitize nerve endings. In modern herbal medicine, cayenne is added to lotions and salves to relieve the pain of osteoarthritis and rheumatoid arthritis, shingles, and fibromyalgia-related joint or muscle pain and to reduce itching and inflammation associated with psoriasis. Concentrated capsaicin creams (often available only with prescription) are sometimes used for post-surgical pain and certain types of neuropathy. Taken internally, cayenne may reduce blood cholesterol and triglyceride levels, relieve cluster headaches, improve circulation, relieve heartburn, stimulate stomach-lining cells to secrete substances that prevent ulcers, and help regulate blood sugar levels by affecting the breakdown of carbohydrates after a meal.

The flaming hues of cayenne peppers hint at their heat, exploited by herbalists for centuries to ease pain.

TIME LINE OF USAGE AND SPREAD

CA 5000 B.C.
Peppers are cultivated by indigenous tribes in Central and South America.

A.D. 1493
Cayenne's arrival in Italy is documented after Columbus's voyage to the New World.

MID-1700s
Botanist Carolus Linnaeus names the genus *Capsicum*, identifying two species.

1912
Scoville scale developed for measuring the hotness of cayenne and other peppers.

When Christopher Columbus arrived on the Caribbean Island of Hispaniola in 1492, he was in search of the Far East Spice Islands and, in particular, black pepper. Instead, he found red peppers. Though *Capsicum* has been grown in the Americas for some 9,500 years, scientists are only beginning to understand its astounding genetic diversity. The genus is represented by at least 10 tropical American species, 5 of which are cultivated today.

Some 1,700 **varieties** of *Capsicum* are known, most derived from *Capsicum annuum,* the source not only of cayenne but also of bell peppers, pimento, paprika, and chili, to name just a few. A perennial, cayenne is smooth stemmed, with shiny, alternate, oval to lance-shaped leaves. The familiar seedpods range from inch-long globes to banana-shaped fruits more than a foot long. The delicate, star-shaped flowers are milky white.

from which they spread to various parts of South and Central America. In Latin America, centuries before the arrival of Columbus, 5 species had been domesticated. In addition to *Capsicum annuum* and *C. frutescens,* other domesticated species include *C. chinense* (originating in the Amazon region, not China), *C. pubescens,* and *C. baccatum,* the preferred chili in the Andean region from Ecuador, Peru, and Bolivia to Chile.

Growing Habits

Cayenne is usually grown as an annual, reaching 3 feet in height, though in frost-free tropical regions it is a perennial of 6 feet or more.

Capsicum **species** are believed to have originated in an area of southern Brazil and Bolivia,

Cultivation and Harvesting

Peppers are sown from seed indoors 6 to 8 weeks before spring's last frost. In southern states, cayenne can be sown directly in the garden after danger of frost has passed. Seedlings should be spaced 8 to 12 inches apart. A rich,

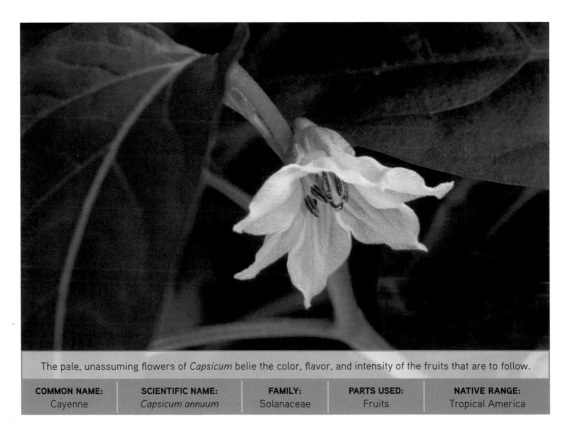

The pale, unassuming flowers of *Capsicum* belie the color, flavor, and intensity of the fruits that are to follow.

COMMON NAME:	SCIENTIFIC NAME:	FAMILY:	PARTS USED:	NATIVE RANGE:
Cayenne	*Capsicum annuum*	Solanaceae	Fruits	Tropical America

At the first sign of stuffiness or of a head cold, or if you're simply feeling the chills or aches on a bitter winter day, try this peppery treat. Combine 1 cup of boiling water, the juice of 1 lemon, and 2 to 3 dashes of dried ground cayenne. Stir well, sweeten to taste with honey or stevia—and let this zingy drink perk you up.

sandy loam is preferred for pepper culture. Peppers like full sun but will tolerate some shade. Gardeners should remember that the plant's irritating **compounds** are easily transferred to the hands. When harvesting peppers, keep hands away from the eyes.

China and India have become the largest suppliers of cayenne to world markets. Red peppers in their myriad forms are grown throughout the world. They are the most widely consumed spice in the world, representing about 25 percent of world spice consumption.

Therapeutic Uses

+ *Arthritis*
+ *Nerve pain*

Despite its bite in spicy cuisines, purified cayenne pepper, yielding the essential compound capsaicin, is an effective topical pain reliever. Capsaicin is absorbed through the skin and binds to specific receptors that act to deplete a compound responsible for conveying pain sensations to the brain.

One category of conditions that cause pain originates from nerve damage resulting from diabetes or other nervous system problems. For this discomfort, creams containing at least 0.075 percent capsaicin applied to a painful area over 6 to 8 weeks have been shown to provide relief. In some cases, just one high-dose patch containing 8 percent capsaicin can be beneficial. A common pattern in the treatment is that the pain gets worse for a few days before it gradually gets better; benefits are often sustained even after treatment stops. Some studies have shown that preparations with a lower percentage capsaicin, some of which are available over the counter, are less effective, either because of the lower dose or because of poorer absorption. These creams are also used by those experiencing the lingering pain of shingles.

Osteoarthritis may also benefit from capsaicin creams. Creams containing 0.025 percent capsaicin have shown to help ease joint pain of adults suffering from osteoarthritis over a 6-week period; one study, in which subjects used the 0.075 percent cream for 4 weeks, decreased arthritis pain and tenderness in the hands.

How to Use

CREAM: For nerve-related pain, apply cream containing 0.075 percent capsaicin 3 to 4 times daily. Lower dose creams containing only 0.025 percent capsaicin applied 4 times daily may be effective for arthritis. For optimal benefit, treatment is usually recommended for 6 to 8 weeks; benefits for arthritis may occur before 8 weeks. Researchers also are developing other higher dose forms of cayenne, including a patch and injections, which look promising for pain relief.

 NOTE: Use gloves to apply creams, and wash hands after application to prevent spreading to eyes, nose, mouth, or other mucous membranes.

Precautions

Application of cayenne preparations to the skin can cause a rash as well as burning, stinging, and redness. The rash, often an irritation rather than an allergic reaction, is usually worse on first applications of the preparation and then gets better with repeated use. However, if the rash gets worse with time, treatment should be discontinued and improvement should occur quickly. Do not apply to broken skin. Occasionally, people will develop a cough after using higher strength preparations, presumably from the spicy substance that gets inhaled.

Comfrey

Symphytum officinale

The leaves and stems of comfrey bristle with rough hairs, a characteristic it shares with other members of the borage family. Both this herb's scientific and common names speak to its use in traditional herbal medicine. Comfrey may be a corruption of the Latin *confirma*, meaning "to make firm," or *confervere*, meaning "to boil or grow together." The genus name, *Symphytum*, comes from the Greek *sympho*, which has a similar meaning. Colloquial names such as knitbone, boneset, and bruisewort reflect comfrey's use through many centuries to promote healing of bruises, sprains, fractures, and bones.

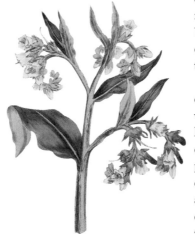

Comfrey has been used since at least the time of the ancient Greeks, perhaps as early as 400 B.C. The Roman naturalist Pliny the Elder (A.D. 23-79) discovered that when comfrey roots were boiled in water, a sticky paste was produced that could bind pieces of meat together. This finding seemed to underscore comfrey's value in mending broken bones and torn flesh. Comfrey enjoyed great popularity during the Middle Ages. Widely cultivated, it was a mainstay in monastery gardens. The herb was applied externally, often as a **poultice** of leaves or roots, to help clear bruises, heal sprains and minor wounds, and mend broken bones. Comfrey tea and other preparations of the plant were also taken internally for bronchial problems, stomach disorders, ulcers, diarrhea, and more. In both Europe and the U.S., comfrey was an herb garden staple and herbal remedy through the 1700s and 1800s.

Comfrey was held in high esteem until the late 1970s, when research revealed that its leaves, and especially its roots, contain **compounds** called pyrrolizidine **alkaloids** that can cause severe liver damage when ingested. In light of these findings, many countries banned the internal consumption of comfrey products. Topical preparations of the herb, however, are considered safe. Comfrey ointments, creams, poultices, and **liniments** are applied to heal bruises, ease sore muscles, and speed the healing of fractures, sprains, and strains. Recently, comfrey has shown promise as a topical treatment for relieving acute upper or lower back pain.

The rough leaves and fleshy roots of comfrey have long been mainstays to promote healing of joints and skin.

TIME LINE OF USAGE AND SPREAD

484–425 B.C.
Greek historian Herodotus notes use of comfrey to staunch severe bleeding.

A.D. 1672
English writer J. Josselyn catalogs comfrey as plant in colonial herb garden.

1978
Researchers report lab rats get liver tumors after diet of comfrey leaves and roots.

2001
Oral comfrey-containing products are banned in the United States.

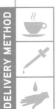

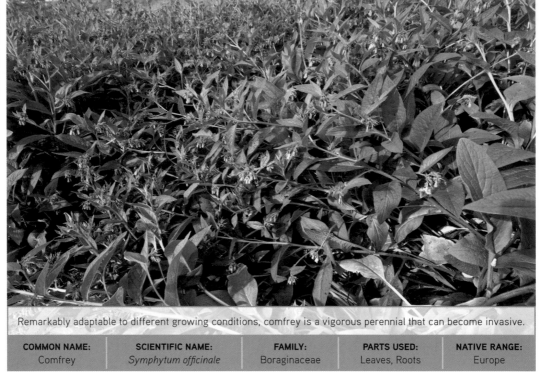

Remarkably adaptable to different growing conditions, comfrey is a vigorous perennial that can become invasive.

COMMON NAME:	SCIENTIFIC NAME:	FAMILY:	PARTS USED:	NATIVE RANGE:
Comfrey	*Symphytum officinale*	Boraginaceae	Leaves, Roots	Europe

Of the 35 species of *Symphytum*, 2 are commonly used in herbal traditions, common comfrey (*S. officinale*) and Russian comfrey (*S. x uplandicum*). Common comfrey is a perennial growing from 2 to 4 feet in height. The broad lance-shaped leaves at the plant's base grow to more than a foot in length and up to 4 inches wide, becoming progressively smaller on the upper stem. The rough, hairy, sandpaper-textured leaves are distinctly winged, and the leaf base cleaves the stem. Flowers unfurl in a spiraled flower head. Tubular white, pink, or bluish half-inch flowers have short lobes at the end.

Russian comfrey is a coarse perennial that may reach 6 feet, a hybrid of common comfrey and prickly comfrey (*S. asperum*). Russian comfrey's leaves are rounded or heart shaped at the base. Flowers, about ¾ inch long, are dark purple, changing to shades of blue and pink. Comfrey has a large, fleshy, black **taproot**, which is cream colored within. Leaves and roots for Russian and common comfrey are traditionally used in herbal medicine.

Growing Habits

Common comfrey is native to most of Europe, growing in damp grasslands and along rivers and streams. It is most common in central Europe, rare in southern Europe. Comfrey has become established in eastern North America and the southern tier of the Canadian provinces and is scattered in a few western states.

Russian comfrey is naturalized in much of central and northern Europe. Its exact origins are unclear. It was once widely cultivated in Europe as a fodder crop for livestock, producing more tonnage per acre than almost any other temperate climate **species**. The deep taproot spreads by lateral offshoots, making it difficult to eradicate once it is established. If comfrey once grew at a site, it is most likely still growing there.

Cultivation and Harvesting

Comfrey is easily propagated from root cuttings. A new plant will sprout from a piece of root an inch long. Plant comfrey in a permanent location, because if you plan to move it later, you will have to remove every scrap of root, or a new plant will soon emerge. Comfrey is adaptable to most soil types. It grows in full sun.

Comfrey root is harvested when the plant is dormant. Today comfrey is primarily imported from the fields of Eastern Europe. The first leaf growth of the spring is usually cut and discarded, as the first growth is potentially higher in toxic compounds.

Therapeutic Uses

✛ *Joint pain*

Comfrey's common names, boneset and knitbone, reflect its traditional use and historic reputation as a soother of painful joints and broken bones and a healer of damaged tissue. Comfrey contains allantoin, a chemical that helps tissues to regenerate and heal, and rosmarinic acid, an **anti-inflammatory** and pain-relieving compound. These benefits are counterbalanced by the fact that comfrey is a well-documented source of a group of dangerous chemicals called pyrrolizidine alkaloids toxic to the liver and perhaps even cancer causing. Governmental and scientific groups have set limits on the amount of these alkaloids that is safe to ingest. Some herbal medicine companies have developed techniques to remove the alkaloids from comfrey, offering formulations presumed safer to use.

In a recent study, alcohol-based comfrey root **extract** with 99 percent of the dangerous alkaloids removed was incorporated into an ointment and used, over a 3-week period, on 220 people with osteoarthritis in their knees. When these subjects were compared with a **placebo** group, pain relief was noted—categorized as total, at rest, and with movement. Also noted was improvement in knee mobility and overall quality of life. This same extract was used in people with ankle sprains; findings also supported this use, showing it at least as effective as a commonly prescribed pharmaceutical gel used to control pain and swelling. Other topical preparations using extracts of species related to *S. officinale* were tested in people with back pain; improvements in mobility and pain relief supported comfrey's anti-inflammatory and **analgesic** effects.

 NOTE: Use only topical preparations of comfrey that have been purified of their toxic pyrrolizidine alkaloids.

How to Use

CREAM, GEL, OR OINTMENT: Germany's Commission E authorities recommend no more than 1 mg of comfrey daily in order to limit toxicity to the liver and other organs. Concerns over comfrey's toxicity are addressed by using specialized formulations where the dangerous alkaloids have been removed and the anti-inflammatory and pain-relieving substances retained. Extracts (Kytta Salbe f, for example, and other brands guaranteed to be free of pyrrolizidine alkaloids) are the safest way to take advantage of the benefits of comfrey. These preparations can be massaged into affected joints 3 to 4 times daily.

Precautions

Comfrey leaf and root contain liver toxins and cancer-causing compounds potentially dangerous when ingested or applied to the skin. Preparations free of these compounds are presumed safer, though most sources still warn against applying comfrey products on open wounds.

🥣 **over the (kitchen) counter** SOOTHING SALVE

Mix 1 cup olive oil with 1 tablespoon each of dried comfrey leaves, lavender flowers, and calendula petals. Stir in top of a double boiler for 40 minutes. Cool, strain, and reserve oil. Melt ¼ cup beeswax in double boiler. Stir in strained oil. Pour into salve tins.

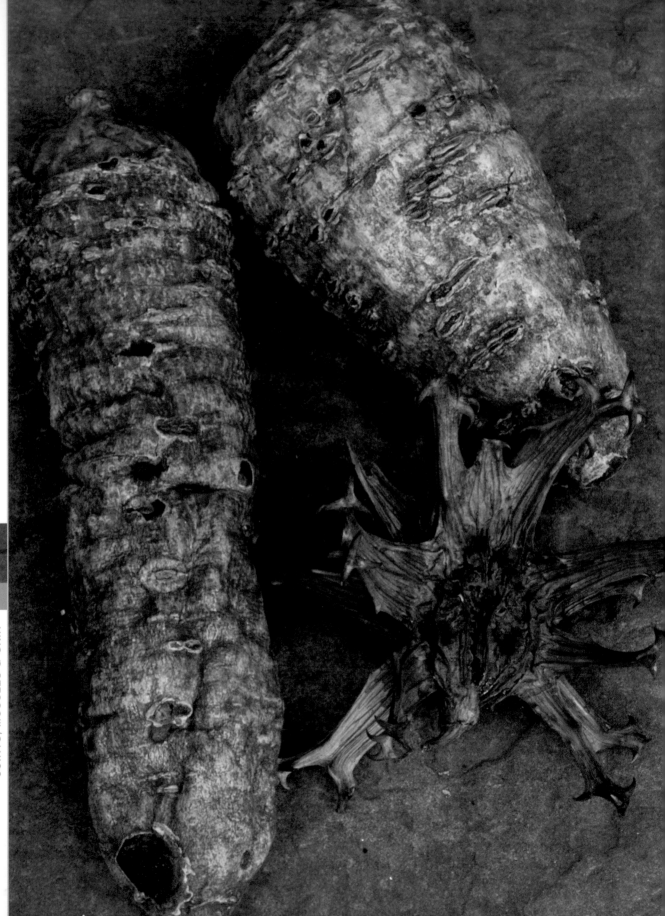

Devil's Claw

✤ *Harpagophytum procumbens* ✤

D uring the rainy season, profusions of trumpet-shaped, violet-red flowers cover the stems of *Harpagophytum procumbens*, a trailing perennial native to desert landscapes of southern Africa. Each flower lasts only a day, and is soon transformed into a formidable fruit armed with long spines. The spines, in turn, are tipped with hooked thorns sharp enough to slice through clothing. These fruits are the source of the plant's common name: devil's claw. Yet it is the roots of devil's claw, rather than its peculiar fruits, that are used in herbal medicine.

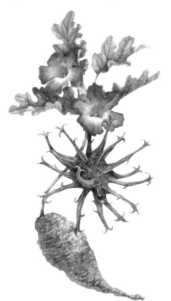

Indigenous tribes in southern Africa, such as the Khoikhoi of the Kalahari Desert, have used devil's claw as a healing herb for perhaps thousands of years. Among these tribes, devil's claw preparations have been taken internally to treat gastrointestinal problems, reduce fever, calm allergic reactions, and ease migraines. Externally, the herb has been used to treat sores, ulcers, and boils. Up until the early 1900s, devil's claw was unknown in Western medicine. In the early 1900s, a South African farmer interested in the region's native plants noted local tribes using preparations of the dried roots of devil's claw to treat various ailments. Impressed by the results, the farmer began promoting a tea made from the plant's roots. Word reached Europe of this healing plant, and soon devil's claw was being used there to reduce pain and inflammation, ease heartburn, and restore appetite.

In modern herbal medicine, devil's claw is a respected treatment for relieving the pain and inflammation of degenerative joint diseases such as osteoarthritis. Use of devil's claw to relieve arthritis-related pain is widespread in Europe and growing in the U.S. Short-term treatment may be as effective as some nonsteroidal **anti-inflammatory** medications such as ibuprofen and may allow reduced use of these medications. There is some indication that devil's claw may slow arthritis-related symptoms. The herb is also used to treat fibromyalgia and back pain; to relieve headaches, stomach upsets, allergies, and fever; and to stimulate appetite.

The fruits of devil's claw are its namesake, but its fleshy roots are the source of compounds to ease arthritis pain.

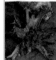

TIME LINE OF USAGE AND SPREAD

CA 1907	1970s	1997	2001
South African G. H. Mehnert witnesses use of devil's claw by indigenous tribes.	Trade in devil's claw for the herbal market begins in South Africa.	German drug firm propagates the *H. procumbens* high-quality variety in Namibia.	Devil's claw sales in Germany hit 74 percent of rheumatism prescriptions.

If you wish to see devil's claw, your best opportunity is a safari to the Kalahari Desert in southwestern Africa. There are only 2 species of *Harpagophytum*—*H. procumbens* and *H. zeyheri*. Devil's claw's life force is concentrated in a large, carrotlike central taproot and secondary tuberous roots. Each year as the scant rainy season begins, creeping stems sprout from the perennial roots. The plant's leaves are irregularly lobed and grayish green in color. The flowers are tubular, deep violet to yellow, with lighter throats. The plant part that receives greatest attention is the dry, woody fruit capsules. Some 6 inches long, with protruding arms protected by back-curved hooked spines that look like grappling hooks, this part is responsible for the names "devil's claw" and "grapple plant." These parts, which hold the seeds, also serve as a seed dispersal mechanism—reaching out to hitch a ride on passing animals.

Growing Habits

The two **species** of devil's claw are restricted to Angola, Botswana, Mozambique, Namibia, South Africa, Zambia, and Zimbabwe. Namibia is the largest supplier, followed by Botswana and South Africa. *H. zeyheri* is found in areas that receive higher rainfall.

Devil's claw seems to do best in deep, free-draining soils. Typically it will grow in clumped populations, but the distribution is spotty even within the plant's predictable habitat. Commercial export of the root began in Namibia and Botswana in 1962. Only *H. procumbens* was used in herbal medicine until 2003 when *H. zeyheri* was registered for use in Europe.

Cultivation and Harvesting

You are unlikely to see devil's claw coming to an herb garden near you. Virtually the entire world's supply is wild-harvested. Namibia is the largest producer, exporting some 1,000 metric tons of the dried roots. The secondary tubers are usually harvested, while the primary **taproot** is left in the ground.

Concern has arisen over the plant's future. Provincial governments in South Africa, as well as regional working groups, are surveying the plant's distribution and determining guidelines for sustainable harvest. In the province of North West in South Africa, the North West Department of Agriculture, Conservation, and Environment recently instituted the Devil's Claw Harvesting Project. It serves as a model for a sustainable harvest, allowing Africans in rural villages to earn income from harvesting devil's claw root, while at the same time developing management controls to ensure sustainable supplies into the future.

Therapeutic Uses

+ *Arthritis*
+ *Back pain*

Less known than other herbal **analgesics**, devil's claw has been used in the southern part of the African continent for centuries to ease pain, as well as to lower fevers and stimulate digestion. The root and secondary tubers are bitter to the taste, and these bitter **compounds** stimulate the body to secrete more saliva and digestive juices, enhancing digestion and easing gas and bloating. Research has focused primarily on the use of devil's claw for relieving pain and has confirmed the herb's potent anti-inflammatory activity. One

over the (kitchen) counter DEVIL'S CLAW TEA

Combine ½ to 1 teaspoon dried, crushed devil's claw rhizome with 1 teaspoon celery seed (not celery salt). Add 1 cup boiling water and let steep 15 minutes. Strain into a cup. Drink 1 to 2 cups a day for 1 month. Keep a daily journal during this time, and if you suffer from osteoarthritis, record any changes in arthritis pain. Avoid if pregnant or if you suffer from heartburn or gastroesophageal reflux disease (GERD) or gastrointestinal ulcers.

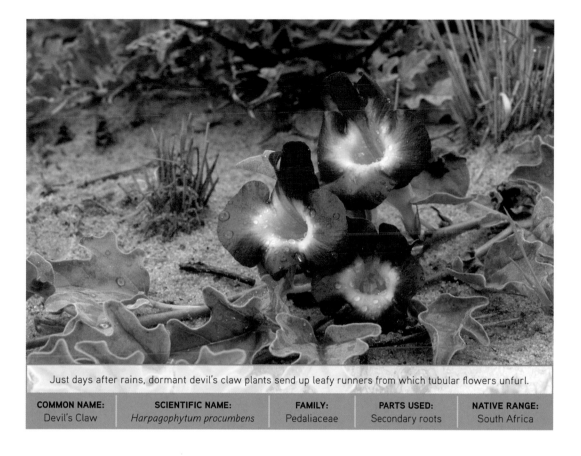

Just days after rains, dormant devil's claw plants send up leafy runners from which tubular flowers unfurl.

COMMON NAME:	SCIENTIFIC NAME:	FAMILY:	PARTS USED:	NATIVE RANGE:
Devil's Claw	*Harpagophytum procumbens*	Pedaliaceae	Secondary roots	South Africa

of the key compounds in devil's claw is harpagoside, a **glycoside** that inhibits chemicals in the body involved in generating **inflammation** and pain.

Many human clinical studies have examined the effectiveness of devil's claw for alleviating arthritis and back pain. Three high-quality clinical trials found strong evidence that devil's claw relieves back pain, with one trial finding it as effective as the prescription drug rofecoxib (Vioxx) with no significant side effects. Research studies have also confirmed that devil's claw is effective for relieving the pain of osteoarthritis of the hips and knees, averaging a 35 percent improvement after 8 weeks of treatment.

How to Use

TEA: Simmer 1 teaspoon in 1 cup water for 10 minutes. Strain and drink 2 to 3 times per day.
CAPSULES OR TABLETS: 1,200 to 2,400 mg of devil's claw per day providing 50 to 100 mg harpagoside per day, taken in 2 to 3 divided doses. (It is best to purchase devil's claw as a standardized **extract**. Most studies have found that for optimal pain relief a product should provide 50 to 100 mg of harpagoside per day.)
TINCTURE: Generally, 3 to 5 ml, 2 to 3 times a day; or follow instructions on product.

 NOTE: Devil's claw stimulates the production of stomach acid. Those who suffer from heartburn or from peptic ulcers should avoid using it.

Precautions

While safety reviews have shown that devil's claw appears to be very well tolerated when taken alone, it can nevertheless interact with some medications. Those taking the anticoagulant coumadin should not use devil's claw. Those using antidepressants or relying on proton-pump inhibitors to suppress heartburn should check with a health care professional before using devil's claw. Devil's claw should not be taken during pregnancy, as it may possibly stimulate uterine contractions.

JOINTS, MUSCLES & SKIN

Rosemary

Rosmarinus officinalis

Native to sunny Mediterranean shores, rosemary is an evergreen member of the mint family. Its genus name, *Rosmarinus*, means "dew of the sea" in Latin, a reference to the plant's coastal habitat and its delicate, droplet-size flowers of pale ocean blue. Rosemary's piney aroma and bittersweet flavor work well in both sweet and savory foods, and it has been a staple in herb and kitchen gardens for many centuries. The herb also has a long history of use as a fragrance in soaps, lotions, and cosmetics. Since ancient times, rosemary has been a symbol of love, loyalty, and remembrance, often included in rituals and ceremonies associated with both marriage and death. Sprigs of the herb were entwined into bridal wreaths or tucked into bridal bouquets. In some European countries, it is still customary for mourners to carry rosemary in funeral processions and to cast the herb into the grave during the burial.

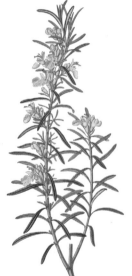

As a medicinal herb, rosemary gained an early reputation for improving memory and uplifting the spirits. In ancient Greece, students wore garlands of rosemary in the belief it would improve their recall. To this day, students in Greece burn rosemary in their homes the night before exams. Pliny the Elder (A.D. 23-79) wrote of rosemary's value in sharpening eyesight. Banckes's *Herbal*, from 1525, suggested boiling rosemary in wine as a cosmetic face wash, binding it around the legs to prevent gout, and drinking it in wine for a cough and to restore lost appetite. Other traditional uses for rosemary include remedies for skin complaints, poor circulation, jaundice, menstrual pain, fainting, nervousness, anxiety, exhaustion, and headaches.

Rosemary has several applications in herbal medicine today. Rosemary oil is used topically to treat muscle pain and arthritis and to improve circulation; Germany's Commission E, which examines the safety and efficacy of herbs, has approved rosemary's use for these conditions. The **essential oil** has been shown to exhibit antibacterial, antifungal, antiparasitic, and mild **analgesic** properties. Rosemary essential oil is also employed in aromatherapy to relieve stress and anxiety. Internally, rosemary is used for indigestion, nervous tension, and headache.

Rosemary's thick, narrow leaves—and their fragrant oil—have held an honored place in herbal medicine for centuries.

TIME LINE OF USAGE AND SPREAD

1300s
The Countess of Hainault compiles an accounting of the virtues of rosemary.

1597
In *Herball*, J. Gerard suggests a garland of rosemary for "stuffing of the head."

1665
Rosemary is burned indoors in plague-infested London to ward off the disease.

1987
Researchers patent rosmaridiphenol (from rosemary) as natural food preservative.

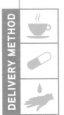

If you are familiar with the distinctive fragrance of fresh rosemary, you can identify the plant with your eyes closed, simply by stroking the leaves and inhaling the scent. Variable in habit, rosemary grows from 2 to 6 feet in height. Depending on its genetic makeup, rosemary can be a creeping or prostrate shrub, or a rigid, upright evergreen. The opposite, narrowly lance-shaped, stalk-less leaves are grayish fuzzy and hairy beneath, and leave a resinous stickiness when touched. The leaves are about an inch long, with margins that roll under. The flowers, scattered in whorls on short groups arising from upper leaf **axils**, are usually blue but may be white, pink, lavender, or sky blue. Common rosemary is one of just three **species** in the **genus** *Rosmarinus*.

Growing Habits

Native to the western Mediterranean region, especially Spain, Portugal, southern France, Tunisia, and Morocco, rosemary is often found on rocky coastal cliffs. It is not surprising that rosemary—from ground cover to hedge—is one of the most widely planted herbs in California. With its mild Mediterranean climate, buffered by morning fog, the California coast makes a perfect home for rosemary.

Cultivation and Harvesting

Cultivated **varieties** (or cultivars, denoted by names in single quotes) abound in American horticulture. The planting range for rosemary—often considered a plant for southern gardens—has been extended by the introduction of hardier cultivars.

R. officinalis 'Arp' is one of the cultivars that has proliferated in recent years, with light blue flowers and thick, widely spaced leaves. It is famous for being one of the hardiest of rosemary cultivars, managing to survive temperatures as low as –10°F. Under an arctic blast in the northeast Texas town of Arp, the late herbarist Madalene Hill discovered this hardy cultivar in 1972. Later, the National Arboretum in Washington, D.C., introduced it into commercial horticulture.

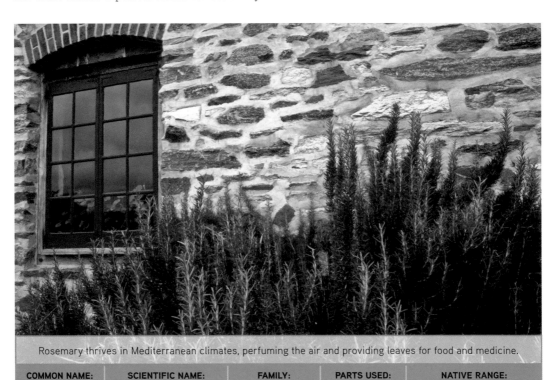

Rosemary thrives in Mediterranean climates, perfuming the air and providing leaves for food and medicine.

COMMON NAME:	SCIENTIFIC NAME:	FAMILY:	PARTS USED:	NATIVE RANGE:
Rosemary	*Rosmarinus officinalis*	Lamiaceae	Leaves, Twigs	Southern Europe

In a small bowl, blend 2 drops rosemary oil, 1 drop lavender oil, and 1 drop eucalyptus oil. Add 4 teaspoons of a carrier oil, such as sweet almond, apricot kernel, olive, or sesame. Blend well. Apply to body, especially joints, before going to the gym, running, or engaging in vigorous exercise.

The best way to obtain a rosemary plant is simply to buy one at any gardening center, where rosemary is easily found. It is difficult to grow from seed. Rosemary likes a light, well-drained, sandy loam. An excellent container plant, it should not be overwatered. Unglazed clay pots are best, as they help the soil to dry, reducing the chance of root rot. Rosemary needs a sunny, airy situation.

Rosemary is produced commercially in Spain, Portugal, and France, all countries of its natural range. Some commercial production also occurs in California.

Therapeutic Uses

+ *Topical antioxidant*
+ *Antibacterial*
+ *Muscle and joint pain*
+ *Bronchitis*
+ *Circulation*
+ *Memory/cognition*

One of those herbs that the nose knows, rosemary leaf produces **extracts** that are a common ingredient in many hair and skin care products. They can combat dandruff and greasy hair and promote general hair health. Their most convincing use, however, is as an **antiseptic** and **antioxidant**. Preliminary research indicates that rosemary extracts can kill bacteria, fight skin **inflammation** relevant to many skin conditions, even inhibit cancer in laboratory animals. They may also block the detrimental effect of sunlight on skin cells.

Applied topically, rosemary packs an antioxidant punch. One potential application is the topical use in antiaging skin care products.

To make the essential oil, rosemary leaves are distilled to yield a fragrant, concentrated oil containing **compounds** responsible for rosemary's medicinal effects. Rosemary essential oil is antimicrobial. One test-tube study found that rosemary essential oil had a synergistic action with the antibiotic **ciprofloxacin** against a bacterium that can cause pneumonia.

Ingested or inhaled, rosemary oil has been used for other conditions, such as muscle or joint pains, indigestion, bronchitis, and sinusitis or to improve circulation. There is also some data supporting the use of rosemary aromatherapy for memory and mental function. When 40 people underwent rosemary aromatherapy for 3 minutes, changes in their brain tests indicated increased alertness, reduced anxiety, and improved ability to do mathematics.

How to Use

ESSENTIAL OIL: The essential oil is used in aromatherapy to enhance mental focus. To apply the oil topically, mix 10 drops in 1 ounce of carrier oil (olive, jojoba, almond, apricot).

CREAM/OINTMENT/SALVE: Topical products use various concentrations of rosemary's essential oil for skin conditions, such as minor bacterial or fungal infections. Apply daily to skin, joints, or muscles, as per manufacturer's directions.

TEA: Add 1 to 2 teaspoons dried rosemary leaves to 1 cup of hot water. Cover for 10 minutes. Strain. Drink 1 to 3 cups a day.

CAPSULES: Generally, 500 to 1,000 mg, once or twice daily; follow product instructions.

NOTE: Ingested rosemary essential oil can cause seizures and can be toxic to the liver and heart. Use only under the guidance of a health care professional.

Precautions

Rosemary extracts with concentrated essential oils can cause a rash with sun exposure. If that happens, discontinue use. Using rosemary as a seasoning during pregnancy is fine, but medicinal doses are not recommended.

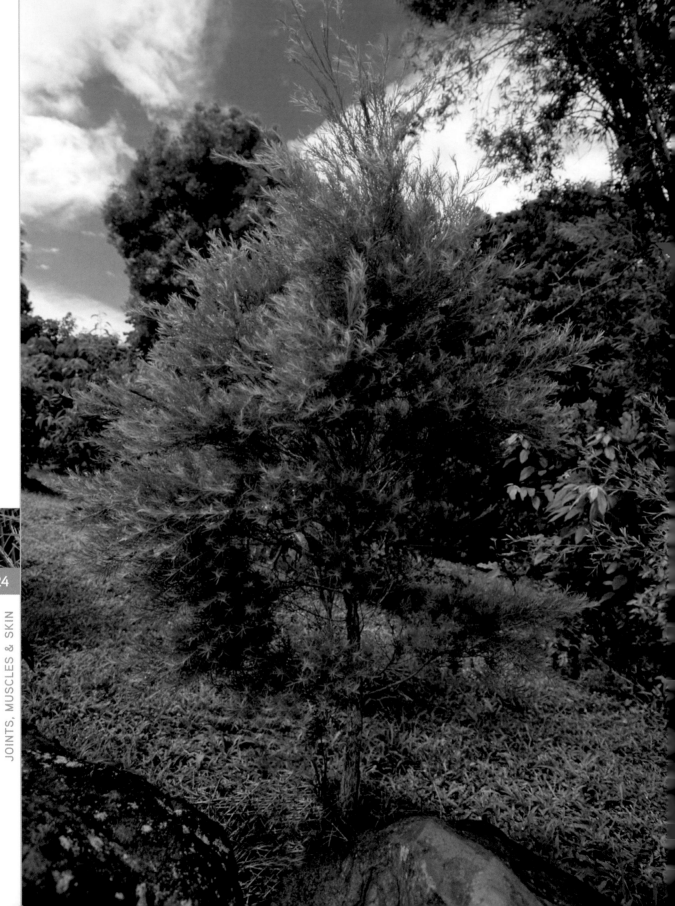

Tea Tree

🌿 *Melaleuca alternifolia* 🌿

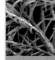

When Capt. James Cook and the crew of the *Endeavour* arrived in southeastern Australia in 1770, they were surrounded by plants and animals completely foreign to them. The sailors noticed how local Aborigines crushed and boiled the narrow, lance-shaped leaves of a small, shrubby tree to brew a hot drink resembling tea. The tree from which the leaves came was dubbed tea tree by Cook and his crew. Tea tree belongs to the genus *Melaleuca*, which includes some 200 species of evergreen trees and shrubs, most of which are native to Australia. Tea tree oil, distilled from the leaves of *Melaleuca alternifolia*, is a fairly recent addition to Western herbal medicine.

Long before Europeans arrived there, Aborigines in eastern Australia chewed tea tree leaves to ease coughs and sore throats and inhaled the oils from crushed leaves to treat respiratory ills. Crushed leaves were applied to cuts, sores, infected wounds, and burns. Tea brewed from the leaves was drunk for a host of health problems. Tea tree oil, however, was not widely used until the 1920s, when research showed it to be a powerful **antiseptic**. Australian physicians began using tea tree oil to cleanse wounds and surgical incisions. The oil found a place in home medicine cabinets for skin problems and fungal infections. During WWII, small bottles of the oil nestled inside standard-issue first-aid

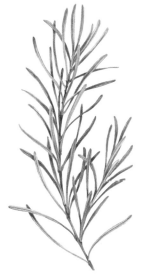

kits of Australian soldiers and sailors alike.

With the advent of antibiotics in the 1940s, interest in tea tree oil waned, only to be rekindled as antibiotic resistance grew. Tea tree oil has strong antibacterial and antifungal properties. It is used in modern herbal medicine primarily to prevent and treat skin infections. Practitioners recommend it for acne, boils, warts, athlete's foot, ringworm, toenail fungus, dandruff, head lice, vaginal yeast infections, periodontal disease, eczema, psoriasis, and more. Tea tree oil may be effective against antibiotic-resistant strains of bacteria, including methicillin-resistant *Staphylococcus aureus* (MRSA), and the herpes virus, though more research is needed to confirm this. Tea tree oil is a common ingredient in many creams, ointments, soaps, shampoos—and even toothpastes.

The slender leaves of *Melaleuca alternifolia* are the source of tea tree oil, recommended for a host of skin infections.

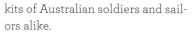

TIME LINE OF USAGE AND SPREAD

1770
Capt. James Cook arrives in Australia and notes use of tea tree leaves by Aborigines.

1929
A. Penfold and F. R. Morrison publish book that starts flurry of research into tea tree oil.

LATE 1990s
MRSA rises from 3 percent in the 1980s to 40 percent in U.S. and European hospitals.

2007
Researchers in Northern Ireland investigate tea tree oil's uses against MRSA.

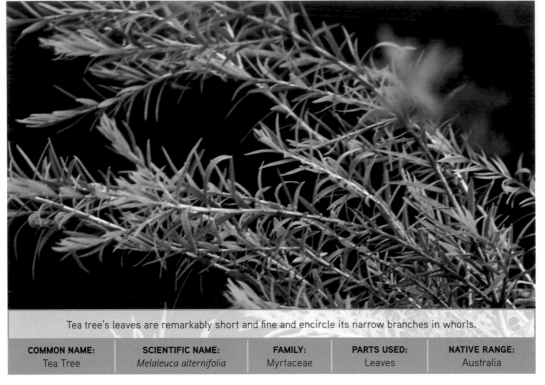

Tea tree's leaves are remarkably short and fine and encircle its narrow branches in whorls.

COMMON NAME:	SCIENTIFIC NAME:	FAMILY:	PARTS USED:	NATIVE RANGE:
Tea Tree	*Melaleuca alternifolia*	Myrtaceae	Leaves	Australia

JOINTS, MUSCLES & SKIN

Tea tree is a member of the genus *Melaleuca*, with about 250 species, more than 200 of them endemic to Australia. The genus name *Melaleuca* comes from *melas,* black, and *leukos,* white, because the main trunk is dark and the branches are much lighter, nearly white. In Australia, the common name tea tree doesn't necessarily refer to a single species, but rather is used in a generic sense for aromatic trees of the myrtle family (Myrtaceae) whose leaves have a reputation for use in beverage teas. So-called tea trees historically include members of the **genus** *Melaleuca*, as well as the genus *Leptospermum*. In international commerce, however, tea tree has come to refer to *M. alternifolia*—the only **species** of *Melaleuca* important in modern herbal medicine. *Melaleuca alternifolia* is a shrub or small tree growing up to 18 feet in height. Like many members of the genus it has a papery bark. The leaves, as the species name implies, are alternate, narrow, and about ¾ inch long. The cream-colored flowers are in loose spikes. The tree comes into bloom in Australia's summer.

Growing Habits

Tea tree is found in swampy or wet ground on the northern coast of New South Wales and in southern Queensland. The tree's swampy habitat limits efficient harvest.

Wild tea trees were first harvested for commercial use in the 1920s and 1930s, following research showing their antiseptic effects. Wild harvest virtually discontinued in the 1970s, when interest waned, and harvesting was hampered by an inhospitable habitat. In the 1980s an enterprising Australian farmer established a small plantation in northern New South Wales, where the tree grows wild. Establishment of plantations allowed for efficient harvest of the leaves, greatly increased the supply, and set the stage for the worldwide demand that followed.

Cultivation and Harvesting

Tea tree is available from some nurseries specializing in unusual herbs. It is not tolerant of cold temperatures, so in most of the United States, tea tree must be grown as a container plant. It likes a relatively rich, well-drained soil, with plenty of moisture.

Its introduction to American horticulture is a cautionary tale. A relative of the tea tree, the broadleaf paper bark tree, or cajeput *M. quinquenervia (M. leucadendron)* is a noxious weed, introduced to Florida in 1909. Like kudzu, the broadleaf paper bark tree serves as an example of a plant introduced for economic benefit that soon runs amok.

Therapeutic Uses

+ *Skin infections (fungal and bacterial)*
+ *Gingivitis*
+ *Dandruff*
+ *Acne*

Sometimes called the wonder from down under, the oil of Australia's tea tree is unrivaled as an antiseptic. Two of tea tree oil's **compounds** have been shown to inhibit the growth of many bacteria and fungi that cause human infections. They act to kill bacteria and fungi by disrupting cell membrane permeability and hampering cell metabolism.

Tea tree oil also may act against viruses, such as herpes and yeast infections, but it hasn't been as well studied for these indications. It is being investigated for treating gingivitis (gum disease), for fighting halitosis (bad breath), and for reducing plaque in the mouth, presumably by altering the presence of certain bacteria. With the growth of virulent drug-resistant staphylococcus infections, such as methicillin-resistant *Staphylococcus aureus*, or MRSA, researchers are turning to potent antibacterials such as tea tree oil for innovative treatments.

Tea tree oil has been studied extensively for its use in treating fungal infections. The formulation and concentration of the oil are important variables to consider when choosing the right product for a given use. For example, 25 percent tea tree oil in ethanol seems to work almost as well as pharmaceutical treatments for athlete's foot infections, and this formulation also seems to limit the occurrence of adverse reactions, such as dermatitis, which often occur with higher concentrations of tea tree oil. It is difficult to treat toenail fungus with creams, but the use of tea tree oil added to antifungal creams may increase the cure rate.

How to Use

ESSENTIAL OIL: Steam distillation of the leaves and small branches yields a potent **essential oil** containing germ-killing chemicals. Various concentrations of the oil are mixed with a base of desired consistency to create products for various conditions.

CREAM OR GEL: Preparations of 5 percent tea tree oil control acne as well as a commonly used medication, benzoyl peroxide, and possibly with fewer side effects.

> **NOTE:** Tea tree oil is a concentrate and should never be used undiluted or near sensitive areas such as eyes, nose, mouth, or genitals without guidance.

Precautions

Tea tree oil should never be taken internally; it can be toxic if ingested. Allergic reactions and contact dermatitis have also been documented. If redness, itching, or oozing develops after the topical application of tea tree oil, use should be discontinued and a health care provider consulted.

---

over the (kitchen) counter ATHLETE'S FOOT OINTMENT

In a small bowl, combine 1 drop lavender oil, 2 drops tea tree oil, and 1 teaspoon lightly scented oil (sweet almond, olive, or sesame oils are all good) and stir gently. Using a cotton swab, apply to infected areas of foot several times daily. To prevent staining carpets or slipping on smooth floors, you might want to slip on clean cotton socks. This fungicide can be used for infections under the nails as well.

Willow Bark

Salix alba, S. purpurea, S. fragilis

Willows and water seem to go together. Of the 400 or so willow species, most thrive in moist soils found around lakes and along rivers and streams. The affinity of willows for water is reflected in their genus name, *Salix,* a derivative of the Celtic phrase *sal lis,* meaning "near water." The inner bark of white willow *(Salix alba),* along with the closely related basket willow *(S. purpurea)* and crack willow *(S. fragilis),* is a rich source of salicin, a chemical converted in the body to salicylic acid. Salicylic acid is closely related to one of the most widely used drugs in the world: aspirin.

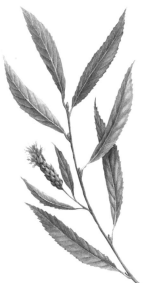

Using willow bark to relieve pain is an ancient practice. The Egyptians and Assyrians used it, as did the Chinese as far back as 500 B.C. The Greek physician Hippocrates praised willow bark's therapeutic powers a century later, advising his patients to chew it to reduce fever and inflammation. In the Middle Ages, willow bark was a common remedy for relieving pain associated with arthritis and rheumatism and for reducing fever. In North America, a number of Native American tribes used local willow **species** to treat headaches, ease joint and muscle pain, and reduce fever and chills. **Salicin** was isolated by several European scientists in the 1820s. Subsequently, an Italian chemist made a synthetic form of salicin—salicylic acid—that was an effective pain reliever but a serious stomach irritant. Around the turn of the century, the German pharmaceutical firm Bayer began marketing a "buffered," less harsh form of salicylic acid that it called aspirin. The drug quickly became number one worldwide.

Despite aspirin's effectiveness, many people experience stomach upsets and even intestinal bleeding when taking it. This is one reason willow bark, which has fewer gastrointestinal side effects, has once again become a popular treatment for alleviating pain. Recent studies confirm that willow bark contains not only salicin but other **compounds** with **antioxidant, antiseptic**, and immune-boosting properties. In modern herbal medicine, willow bark is recommended for back pain, osteoarthritis and rheumatism pain, sprains, toothache, headache, fever, colds, and flu.

The bark of several willow species is the source of remarkable aspirin-like compounds for pain relief.

TIME LINE OF USAGE AND SPREAD

4TH CENTURY B.C.
Hippocrates notes using willow bark and leaves for headaches, pain, and fever.

A.D. 1838
Italian chemist R. Piria, at the Sorbonne in Paris, converts salicin into salicylic acid.

1853
French chemist C. Gerhardt creates acetylsalicylic acid but abandons his discovery.

1899
German chemist F. Hoffmann unearths Gerhardt's formula, and aspirin is born.

The genus *Salix* is a complex plant group with more than 500 species. China is the center of diversity with some 250 species. Since willows readily hybridize, their identification confounds even the botanical specialist. About 80 *Salix* species are found in North America, but only a third are trees; the rest are shrubs. Most willows are easily recognized by their narrow, lance-shaped leaves, and dense flowering catkins,

appearing before, with, or after the leaves emerge. Male and female flowers are in separate groups. The branches have circular transverse joints and are easily broken at the base. The minute seeds are distributed by wind via silk hairs.

White willow (*S. alba*), purple willow (*S. purpurea*), and brittle willow (*S. fragilis*) are among the commercial sources of willow bark. White willow is the classic species, used medicinally since the time of the ancient Greeks. In practical terms, as long as the bark of a willow reaches a level of 1.5 percent salicins, it is considered suitable for medicinal use. For those not equipped with a chemistry lab, physician and

herb expert John King offered timeless practical advise in 1876: "There are numerous species of *Salix*, many of which, undoubtedly, possess analogous medicinal virtues. The best rule to follow is to select those whose barks possess great bitterness, combined with astringency."

Growing Habits

Willows tend to be associated with moist or wet soils, often growing next to ponds or along streams. The tenacious roots, sometimes larger and tougher than the branches, hold fast to the banks of flowing streams. When most people envision a willow tree, the weeping willow (*S. babylonica*) may come to mind, a tree from

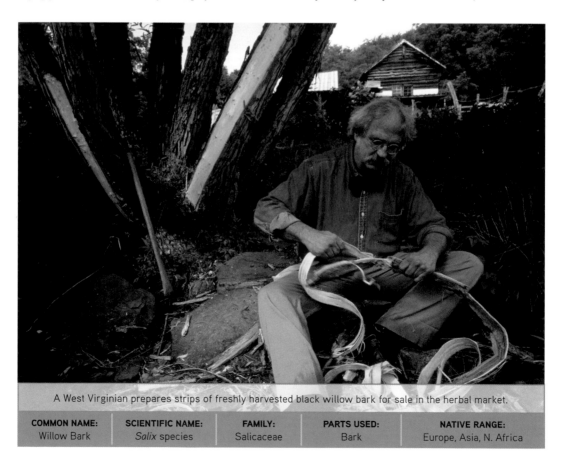

A West Virginian prepares strips of freshly harvested black willow bark for sale in the herbal market.

COMMON NAME:	SCIENTIFIC NAME:	FAMILY:	PARTS USED:	NATIVE RANGE:
Willow Bark	*Salix* species	Salicaceae	Bark	Europe, Asia, N. Africa

Grind 2 ounces of willow bark in a coffee grinder and put into a large jar with a tight-fitting lid. Cover the ground herb with 16 ounces apple cider vinegar and stir gently. Secure the lid and let mixture sit for 14 days. Strain through a cheesecloth or muslin and put strained liquid into a dark bottle. Label. This liniment can be applied topically 2 to 3 times per day to ease sunburn, muscle aches, and joint pain.

the alluvial plains of the lower Yangtze River in China. Long associated with funerary ritual in China, it has become a favorite tree for cemetery plantings in Western traditions.

Almost all of the weeping willows of Europe arrived at an unknown date, probably via Central Asia caravan routes. They are all female and may even have originated from a single tree. Willows are not confined to moist soils of temperate climates. The woody plant that grows nearest the North Pole is *Salix arctica*.

Cultivation and Harvesting

Willows prefer a rich, moist soil, though they are tolerant of poor soils. If one tree is considered the easiest to propagate, it is the willow. Passing travelers in colonial America who stuck a willow switch into the ground soon saw a tree take hold, a monument to the traveler who established it.

Therapeutic Uses

+ *Headache*
+ *Back pain*
+ *Osteoarthritis*

While most people know that aspirin was developed from a plant, many are unaware that it was the humble and graceful willow that inspired scientists to search for its pain-relieving compounds. All *Salix* species contain salicin, the precursor of salicylate, along with other compounds such as **tannins** and **flavonoids**, which contribute to the overall effect.

There is no question that willow bark can relieve mild pain, though clinical trials in humans have not always been positive. Studies in people with acute back pain and osteoarthritis generally have favored willow over **placebo**, though for those with rheumatoid arthritis, willow offered little benefit. A study

published in the *American Journal of Medicine* examined 191 patients with chronic low back pain randomly assigned to receive either a willow bark **extract** containing 120 mg or 240 mg of salicin or placebo. By the fourth week of treatment, 39 percent of those receiving the high-dose extract were pain free, 21 percent receiving the low dose were pain free, and 6 percent in the placebo group were pain free. A significant number in the placebo group required pain medication.

How to Use

The level of salicin varies considerably from one species of willow to another, so the level of pain relief may vary between teas and products.

TEA: Simmer 1 teaspoon of willow bark in 1 cup water for 10 minutes. Strain. Add honey to taste, if desired. Drink 1 cup 2 to 3 times per day.

STANDARDIZED EXTRACTS: Buy a willow bark product standardized to salicin; take daily dose equivalent to 120 to 240 mg of salicin, in 2 or 3 doses. It may take 1 week to see benefits.

Precautions

In clinical trials, 3 percent of participants experienced allergic skin reactions that disappeared soon after ending treatment. Other than this adverse effect in a small group, willow bark is well tolerated. The risks of willow bark may be similar to aspirin; thus, its use is contraindicated in children with fever to avoid the risk of Reye's syndrome. Use is also contraindicated for women who are pregnant or breast-feeding and for people with allergies. Like aspirin, willow bark affects **platelets**, cells that play a role in blood clotting, though the full dose of 240 mg per day of willow bark was shown to have less effect on platelet aggregation than a dose of 100 mg of aspirin.

Witch Hazel

Hamamelis virginiana, H. vernalis

F or most of the year, witch hazel might easily be missed amid the pines, oaks, hickories, and maples of its native eastern North American woodlands. But come November, when these larger trees have lost their leaves and gone to seed, smaller, shrubbier witch hazel bursts into bloom. Explosions of pale yellow flowers, each composed of four streamerlike petals, crowd its slender branches and often last well into December. Despite its common name, the plant has little to do with witches. The "witch" of witch hazel is likely derived from the Anglo-Saxon *wych*,

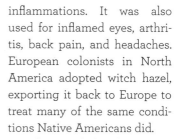

meaning "pliant" or "bendable." It refers to *H. virginiana*'s traditional use as a source of forked branches used as divining rods, or witching sticks, to locate underground sources of water or precious minerals. Witch hazel's real magic, however, lies in its mild **astringent** and **antiseptic** properties, useful primarily for treating inflamed or irritated skin.

For many centuries, Native Americans used the bark, twigs, and leaves. Teas brewed from witch hazel were used to relieve inflammation and irritation of the mouth and throat, reduce fever, and relieve menstrual pain. For feverish colds and coughs, witch hazel steam baths were common. Washes or compresses of leaves or bark were used to treat swellings, strained muscles, and bruises and to ease skin

inflammations. It was also used for inflamed eyes, arthritis, back pain, and headaches. European colonists in North America adopted witch hazel, exporting it back to Europe to treat many of the same conditions Native Americans did.

Today witch hazel water—a distilled, alcohol-based **extract** of twigs—can be found in any drugstore. But it typically contains little of the natural herb; its effects may be largely caused by the alcohol it contains. In modern herbal medicine, stronger preparations of witch hazel made directly from the bark or leaves are used to treat irritations of the skin and mucous membranes, sore throat, bleeding gums, sprains, muscle pain, eye inflammation, varicose veins, internal bleeding, hemorrhoids, and diarrhea.

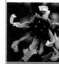

Witch hazel's peculiar blossoms adorn its branches, the source of the bark used in herbal preparations.

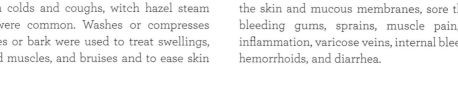

TIME LINE OF USAGE AND SPREAD

1744
American doctor C. Colden writes of "blindness" cured with witch hazel decoction.

1846
T. Pond markets witch hazel patent medicine, Pond's Golden Treasure.

1882
Fluid extract of witch hazel is added to the *United States Pharmacopeia* (deleted 1914).

1915
Poet Robert Frost laments the withering of witch hazel blossoms in "Reluctance."

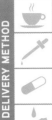
The genus *Hamamelis* includes only four species—Japanese witch hazel (*H. japonica*), Chinese witch hazel (*H. mollis*), and two North American species, Ozark vernal witch hazel (*H. vernalis*) and common witch hazel (*H. virginiana*). Witch hazel is a shrub or small tree, growing 10 to 20 feet tall, suckering at the base, and usually growing in clumps. The alternate leaves are rounded to oval in shape with scalloped margins, and up to 6 inches long and 4½ inches wide. The faintly fragrant flowers expand in leaf **axils** in autumn after the leaves have dropped. Several flowers crowd a single node. Each flower has 4 straplike, inch-long, crinkled, yellow petals. At the same time, the fuzzy, brown seed capsule (formed the previous year) matures. Within are 2 ebony black, bone-hard seeds. As the capsules dry and contract, the seeds explode from within, shooting the projectile seeds up to 30 feet from the plant.

Growing Habits

Witch hazel is found in a variety of habitats, such as dry woodlands, along the edges of bluffs, and near streams, though almost always on a slope. It is widespread in eastern North America ranging from Nova Scotia south to northern Florida, west to eastern Texas, and northward to Minnesota.

Vernal witch hazel is worth mentioning as the leaves and bark are harvested and enter the witch hazel trade, though it probably represents a small percentage of biomass sold. It begins blooming in winter, often around the first of January. Unlike the flowers of common witch hazel, those of vernal witch hazel are strongly fragrant with a reddish tint. This woody plant is confined to the Ozark Mountains of Arkansas, to Missouri, and to eastern Oklahoma.

Cultivation and Harvesting

Ironically, much of what is available in cultivated witch hazels in American horticulture is not the native *H. virginiana* and *H. vernalis*, but *H. x intermedia*—a hybrid of Japanese and Chinese witch hazels. Nevertheless, native plant nurseries do offer the **indigenous** witch hazel.

Witch hazel is easy to grow. The small trees like a humus-rich, well-drained light soil with a slightly acid pH and full sun or dappled shade. The branches are distilled to make witch hazel water, found in any drugstore.

The center of witch hazel production is in Connecticut. Woodcutters in the region cut witch hazel from their own land or parcels under contract and sell directly to the manufacturer. Witch hazel leaves and bark are also wild-harvested elsewhere in the plant's range and sold to the botanical supply trade.

Therapeutic Uses

+ *Minor cuts*
+ *Hemorrhoids*
+ *Varicose veins*
+ *Eczema*

Household first-aid kits have long held distilled witch hazel water, one of the few widely available commercial medicines made from a wild native plant. The reason for its wide distribution? Witch hazel is one of the classic astringents, the **tannins** in its leaves, bark, and twigs helping to heal a variety of skin conditions. Various preparations of witch hazel are used topically to stop bleeding from minor cuts and abrasions; calm inflamed mucous membranes and skin, such as with eczema; and decrease the size and symptoms associated with varicose veins and hemorrhoids.

over the (kitchen) counter MINTY MOUTHWASH

Mix ¼ cup aloe vera juice (not gel), ¼ cup witch hazel distillate, and 2 tablespoons distilled water in a dark bottle. Add 1 drop each of tea tree, peppermint, and spearmint oils. Mix 1 tablespoon in a glass of warm water. Swish and spit.

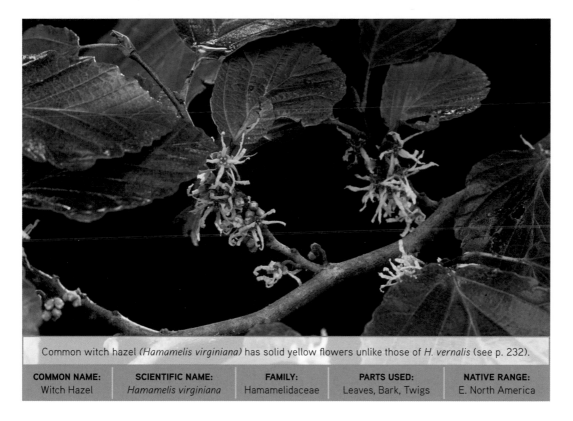

Common witch hazel (*Hamamelis virginiana*) has solid yellow flowers unlike those of *H. vernalis* (see p. 232).

COMMON NAME:	SCIENTIFIC NAME:	FAMILY:	PARTS USED:	NATIVE RANGE:
Witch Hazel	*Hamamelis virginiana*	Hamamelidaceae	Leaves, Bark, Twigs	E. North America

There are many different types of tannins in witch hazel, including **catechins** (also present in green tea and chocolate), which have **antioxidant** properties. These **compound**s may be antivirals, **anti-inflammatories**, and cancer preventives. Witch hazel also might counteract the harmful effects of **enzymes** that damage connective tissue in skin or blood vessels.

In a clinical study, researchers used a witch hazel ointment on 231 children with diaper rash, skin inflammation, and minor skin injuries and a pharmaceutical ointment on 78 children with similar conditions. The dose and duration of treatment were left to the discretion of the primary care physician for each child, and symptoms were rated over the course of 7 to 10 days. Witch hazel and the pharmaceutical ointment improved both skin appearance and symptoms over the treatment period.

Another study of 72 people with moderate to severe eczema compared the use of a cream containing witch hazel distillate with a 0.5 percent hydrocortisone cream. Findings showed that both treatments helped eczema symptoms, but the hydrocortisone worked much better.

How to Use

EXTRACT: Many different forms of witch hazel begin with a distillation of the leaves, bark, and/or twigs. This liquid is added to ointment or creams and then applied to the skin.

LIQUID: Witch hazel water is made by soaking plant parts in water and distilling the mixture. Alcohol is added to keep the distillate from spoiling (for example, 86 percent witch hazel distillate and 14 percent alcohol). The **tinctures** and other preparations commonly used by herbal medicine practitioners are usually stronger than distilled witch hazel water.

Precautions

Although witch hazel preparations can be consumed orally, there is some concern about ingesting the tannin compounds in any appreciable quantity; they can cause stomach troubles and kidney or liver damage or interfere with the absorption of vitamins and minerals. There are very rare reports of allergic reactions to topical witch hazel products, and some people develop redness and a burning sensation when witch hazel is applied to the skin.

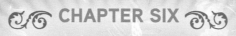

CHAPTER SIX

Urinary *and* Male Health

Plants *and* Men's Health

❦

During the late 15th and early 16th centuries, European explorers cast covetous eyes across the cobalt blue waters of the Atlantic. It was largely the fulfillment of desire that drew them west: desire to locate new routes to access the spices of Asia; expand empires in the names of kings and queens; and quench a seemingly unquenchable thirst for gold and silver. Finding botanical novelties was far down on the list, if it was there at all. Yet many of the real treasures these and later explorers "discovered" in the New World were plants. Maize, tomatoes, chili peppers, potatoes, pineapples, beans, pumpkins, and chocolate are all native to the Americas. The introduction of these foods to the rest of the world transformed not only culinary dishes but entire diets. New World plants were also the source of powerful new medicines. From the Andes, quinine-containing bark from trees belonging to the genus *Cinchona,* which the Inca used to cure cramps, chills, and other ailments, became the first truly effective treatment for malaria. From Amazonian tribes, extracts of curare from *Strychnos toxifera*, which tribal hunters used to create poison-tipped arrows, became the first treatment for tetanus; curare remains one of the most effective muscle relaxants in modern medicine even today.

Native North Americans possessed equally vast knowledge about the plants in their lands above the Equator. Of the roughly 32,000 indigenous plant species in North America, native tribes used nearly 2,900 medicinally. Over time, many of these medicinal plants were first adopted by European settlers, then transported to other countries and continents, and ultimately added to numerous pharmacopeias worldwide. For example, the bark of willow trees (*Salix* spp.), used by the Cherokee and other tribes as a pain reliever, was the source of the abundant compound modified to make aspirin. The Cascara buckthorn (*Rhamnus purshiana*), valued by Native Americans in northern California and Oregon as a cure for constipation, is now among the most commonly used herbal laxatives worldwide. And saw palmetto (*Serenoa repens)*, both food and medicine for Florida's Miccosukee and Seminole tribes, has become a staple in alternative and complementary medicine for treating one of the most universal health complaints of older men: benign prostatic hyperplasia (BPH), otherwise known as enlargement of the prostate gland.

The prostate is one of several organs integral to the male reproductive system. The largest of these is the penis, the organ used in sexual intercourse that is rich in blood vessels and composed largely of erectile tissue. Suspended below it and contained in saclike enclosures of skin are the paired testes; these organs are the production sites for male sex cells, or sperm. The testes are also responsible for making testosterone, the primary male sex hormone. A collection of tubes and ducts provide a pathway for sperm to travel from the testes to the urethra, which runs through the center of the penis. The role of the prostate, along with several other secreting and glandular structures, is to produce semen, the fluid in which sperm can be transported out of the body via the urethra.

The urinary system in both men and women is essentially the same in that it consists of the kidneys, ureters, bladder, and urethra. Kidneys filter wastes from the blood, while the ureters carry the liquid waste (urine) from the kidneys down to the bladder. Primarily a temporary storage organ, the bladder collects urine until it is excreted via the urethra. What is very different between male and female urinary tracts, however, is that in women, there are no structures that constrict the urethra. In men, the prostate gland encircles the neck of the bladder like a doughnut precisely at the point where it joins the urethra. And therein lies a problem.

As men age, the prostate typically enlarges, gradually constricting the urethra and restricting the flow of urine from the bladder. This enlargement is the culprit in BPH affecting nearly 50 percent of all men, usually after age 40. The larger the gland grows, the harder it is to urinate. BPH can lead to serious bladder and kidney problems, sometimes even requiring surgery. Other aging changes that occur in the male reproductive system include decreases in sperm production and testosterone levels, changes in the tissues that form the testes and the tubes and ducts, and erectile dysfunction.

The 8 herbs highlighted in this chapter have been selected among many as having a long history of use in treating male health-related problems or those that commonly affect the urinary tract, both in men and women.

For thousands of years, juniper *(Juniperus communis)* has been valued for its ability to warm painful joints and relieve soreness in bruised or strained muscles. Native Americans appear to have been the first to discover that preparations of juniper taken internally can help treat infections of the urinary tract. Modern herbalists continue to use juniper in this way. They also recommend parsley *(Petroselinum crispum)* for urinary tract infections and for clearing kidney stones, one of the most common—and painful—urinary tract disorders.

As men age, the chance of developing prostate cancer increases. Pomegranate *(Punica granatum)*, with its abundant seeds filled with ruby-red juice, has recently gained attention as an herb to help prevent or slow the progression of prostate cancer; it may retard the growth of other types of cancer cells as well. Native to Africa, pygeum *(Prunus africana)* is currently the most widely used herbal remedy in many parts of Europe for relieving symptoms of BPH, and use is growing in the U.S. However, it has yet to eclipse the popularity of saw palmetto in America. Yet research so far has returned mixed results on this herb's efficacy. Some studies indicate that saw palmetto can relieve many of BPH's symptoms; others have shown its effect to be minimal. More research is needed.

Stinging nettle *(Urtica dioica)* is another herb used widely in Europe for moderating the symptoms of BPH as well as clearing urinary tract infections. Most people think of tomato *(Lycopersicon esculentum)* as a food high in health-promoting nutrients. Consumption of tomato products appears to be associated with a lower risk of prostate cancer, although again, more research is needed. The chapter concludes with uva ursi *(Arctostaphylos uva-ursi)*, an herb native to Arctic regions that has a long history as a remedy for a variety of urinary tract complaints.

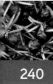

Juniper

✐ *Juniperus communis* ✐

It takes two years for the small, fleshy fruits on a female juniper to ripen, turning as they do from green to blue-black. Almost everyone calls them berries, but botanists know they are actually cones. Juniper is an evergreen conifer, a relative of cedar and cypress. Both its branches and berries exude a resinous but refreshing, cedarlike scent. Juniper was a favorite strewing herb in medieval times, scattered on floors to freshen the air and cleanse the indoor environment of infection and disease. It was also thought to possess great power to overcome evil. Burning juniper wood was a

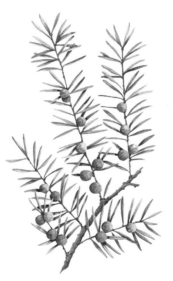

way to banish evil spirits and ward off the plague. Planting a juniper bush near a home's front entrance prevented witches from coming inside. For centuries, juniper berries have been used to flavor foods, both savory and sweet. Probably best known as the ingredient that gives gin its unique taste, juniper berries also have a long history as a medicinal herb used to treat joint pain and disorders of the urinary tract.

The ancient Greeks and Romans took juniper to ease the aches and pains associated with rheumatism. Medieval herbalists used it as a remedy for all sorts of ailments, from intestinal upsets to mental disorders. Among the **indigenous** tribes of North America, juniper was used to treat kidney problems, urinary tract infections, muscle and joint pain, stomach upset, ulcers, wounds, high fevers,

and respiratory infections. In the 1800s and 1900s, American folk medicine practitioners suggested patients chew juniper berries to relieve indigestion and stimulate appetite.

Recognized for its warming, stimulating, and disinfecting properties, juniper is still used to treat many of these same conditions. Modern herbal practitioners often suggest juniper to treat urinary tract infections and to stimulate urine production by the kidneys (but not to treat kidney infection). Juniper is also recommended, externally and internally, for relieving swelling, the pain of rheumatoid arthritis and other joint pain, muscle pain, and tendonitis. Topically, the herb's **essential oil** has been used in treating respiratory infections, congestion, and coughs and for stubborn skin conditions, including psoriasis.

Juniper berries, used in herbal medicine, are harvested from low-growing or upright forms of *Juniperus communis*.

TIME LINE OF USAGE AND SPREAD

2750 B.C.	**A.D. 77–79**	**1660**	**1653**
A coffin from Egypt's Saqqara Pyramid is made of juniper and other woods.	Pliny the Elder notes black pepper is adulterated with juniper berries.	English diarist S. Pepys touts curing colic with spirits laced with juniper berries, aka gin.	English herbalist N. Culpeper suggests juniper for countering poison.

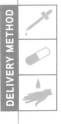
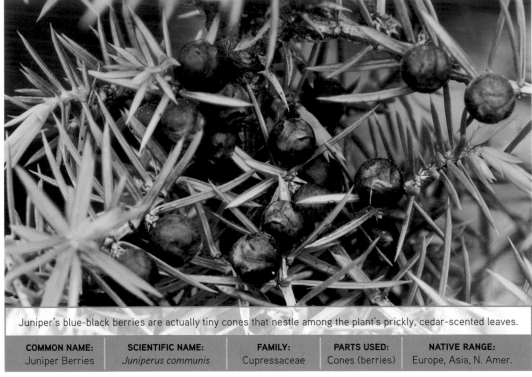

Juniper's blue-black berries are actually tiny cones that nestle among the plant's prickly, cedar-scented leaves.

COMMON NAME:	SCIENTIFIC NAME:	FAMILY:	PARTS USED:	NATIVE RANGE:
Juniper Berries	*Juniperus communis*	Cupressaceae	Cones (berries)	Europe, Asia, N. Amer.

Junipers, members of the genus *Juniperus,* are trees and shrubs native to the Northern Hemisphere, with a range extending into the mountains of tropical Africa. Of the 50 species, most of which are aromatic, essential oil-producing woody plants, common juniper *(J. communis)* is the most widespread, used in herbal medicine throughout its range. Common juniper can be a low shrub or a tree up to 30 feet tall with brown bark exfoliating into paper-thin strips.

The wide variation in growing habit segregates juniper into 5 distinct varieties, 3 of which are North American. The leaves, in whorls of 3, are evergreen, though sometimes silver and covered with a whitish film. The needlelike leaves are about an inch long, with a single white band on the upper surface, and blunt tipped to sharp pointed at the apex. The bluish black, resinous, globular berries, the part used in herbal traditions, is actually not a berry at all, but technically a seed cone.

Growing Habits

Common juniper ranges throughout cooler regions of the Northern Hemisphere, especially in the northern U.S., Canada, Greenland, Iceland, and northern Europe, circling the globe through northern Asia, south to Japan.

In North America, the most common and widespread **variety** is *J. communis* var. *depressa.* The variety name depressa suggests that this is a prostrate, or low-growing, shrub. A single plant is usually much broader than tall, spreading to about 10 feet wide, or it may be a small tree up to 30 feet tall. In much of Europe, the most common variety is typical *J. communis* var. *communis,* which was the original plant that Swedish botanist and taxonomist Carolus Linnaeus described. Herbalists from New England traveling to Europe may be surprised to learn that the dominant juniper in much of the European countryside is the same as the **species** growing in the New England countryside even though the plants appear quite different in size and shape. Typically in Europe, the variety *communis* is more like a small tree than a broad shrub. Juniper is common in fields, farmlands, fencerows, slopes, and mountain summits throughout its very wide range.

Cultivation and Harvesting

Common juniper is often grown as an ornamental evergreen, particularly *J. communis* var. *depressa*, the typical North American variety. If propagated, it strikes easily from cuttings, but it is difficult to grow from seed. Juniper prefers a well-drained, poor, slightly acidic, gravelly or rocky soil. The berries do not ripen on the plant until their second year.

Interestingly, this second-year maturation cycle of the so-called berries has presented an unusual conservation problem in the Balkans. Juniper is commonly harvested for the herb trade by workers in small rural villages. However, some pickers do not want others to come after them, so they harvest in the same area the following year. To undermine their competitors, the pickers break off the branchlets with the immature first-year fruits to prevent their harvest the following year. Much of the world's supply of juniper berries is harvested in Eastern Europe.

Therapeutic Uses

+ *Urinary tract infections*
+ *Bronchitis*

Take any part of juniper, crush it between your fingers, and the characteristic resin smell will pour forth. While the aroma may inspire thoughts of Christmas wreaths or maybe a gin and tonic (juniper berries are the flavoring source of gin), juniper has also been an effective medicine for centuries. It is the berry that contains most of the medicinal **compounds** and is the part used to make preparations. Juniper berries contain approximately 1 percent of an essential oil that has been shown to be an effective **antiseptic**, a useful topical applied to some skin infections, and a dependable inhalant for respiratory conditions.

Juniper berries have other medicinal effects as well. One of its compounds, pinene (also found in pine trees), can be mildly stimulating to respiratory tissue and act as an **expectorant.** The berries contain **terpene** alcohols that may serve as **diuretics**. The German health commission notes that juniper can combat indigestion. In Europe it is commonly used for urinary tract infections, possibly because of its antiseptic and diuretic properties.

How to Use

EXTRACT: Juniper berry **extract**, an alcohol-based liquid, is extracted from the ripe fruits; dosage is typically 1 to 4 ml, 3 times daily.

ESSENTIAL OIL: Juniper berry oil is obtained by steam-distilling juniper berries and is used in a mister for aromatherapy. Do not take the **essential oil** orally. To apply to the skin, mix 10 drops of essential oil in 1 ounce carrier oil.

CAPSULE: 425 to 850 mg, 3 times a day; often combined with other herbs for urinary health.

Precautions

Juniper berries can be strong medicine and should not be used without checking with a health care provider. When juniper oil or extracts are applied topically, skin irritations can develop. Do not apply undiluted to the skin. Some concerns also have been reported with the ingestion of juniper extracts acting as an **abortifacient** in animals; oral use of these oils should be avoided during pregnancy. Juniper oils or extracts should not be used by anyone with a kidney infection or kidney disease.

over the (kitchen) counter JUNIPER JUICE

A decoction of juniper is used to treat urinary tract infections. A typical mixture is made by boiling 1 teaspoon of dried, crushed juniper berries (they turn red when dried) in ⅔ cup of water for 5 to 10 minutes, straining, and drinking 1 to 3 times daily. To be safe, juniper should not be used for more than 1 to 2 weeks.

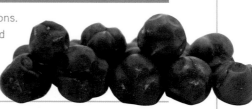

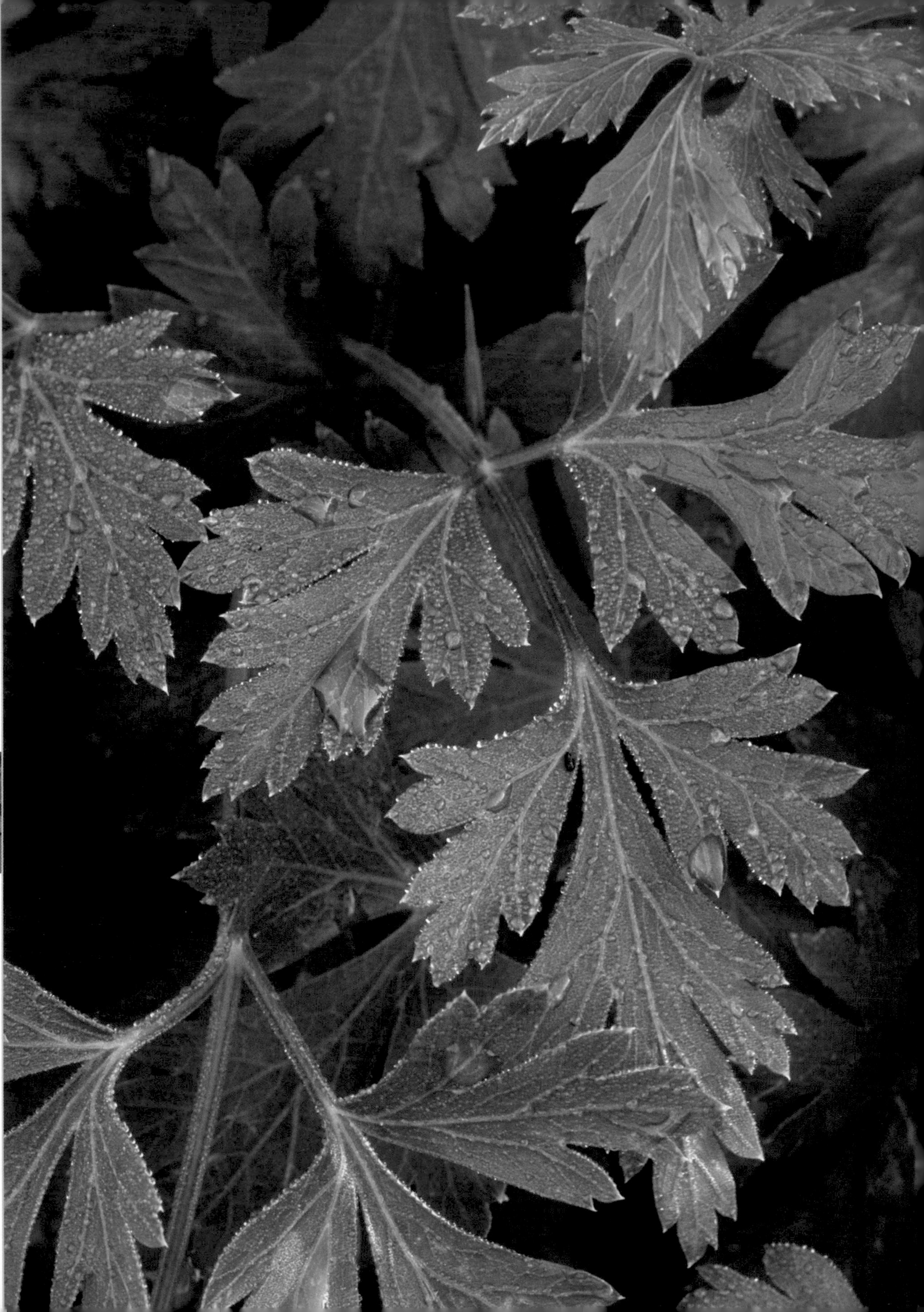

Parsley

✌ *Petroselinum crispum* ✍

With leaves either curly or flat, parsley is one of the world's most widely used herbs. It is an essential ingredient in many Middle Eastern, European, and American dishes. Parsley also has become a nearly ubiquitous garnish, typically ignored, on plates of restaurant food. The ancient Greeks treated parsley with far more respect. They associated the herb with death and oblivion, believing it to be sacred to the dead. Over the centuries, parsley attracted other superstitions. Pluck a sprig of parsley while chanting the name of an enemy,

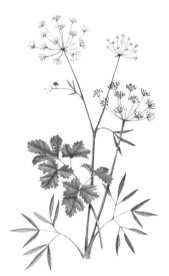

and you could bring about his or her demise. Transplant it, give it away, or pick it when in love, and disaster of some sort would inevitably follow. The Romans appear to have been the first to use parsley as a culinary herb, and its cultivation spread slowly north and east. By the Middle Ages, parsley had been elevated from an ingredient in sauces and salads to a respected medicinal herb. Today, parsley is still used for health problems, including urinary tract infections.

In medieval Europe, parsley was an essential plant in monastery herb gardens. It was widely used for ailments associated with the liver and kidneys, including bladder infections, gout, jaundice, and **edema** (swelling). Parsley was recommended for menstrual problems and encouraging milk flow in nursing mothers. A **poultice** of crushed parsley leaves was a remedy for sprains, bruises, swellings, and insect bites. Tea made by steeping parsley seeds in hot water was given to patients suffering from indigestion, flatulence, and bloating. People freshened their breath by chewing parsley leaves, a practice that continues today in many countries.

In modern herbal medicine, parsley is recognized for its **diuretic** properties. Parsley root is suggested by herbal practitioners to help clear urinary tract disorders, such as cystitis and urethritis. Parsley is also used to treat kidney stones, ease rheumatic conditions by clearing waste products that aggravate muscle aches and stiffness, calm indigestion, and help stimulate normal menstruation. Parsley leaf preparations may calm irritated skin and eyes.

Used for centuries, all parts of parsley—leaves, roots, seeds—contain compounds for treating urinary complaints.

TIME LINE OF USAGE AND SPREAD

50-70
Greek physician Dioscorides names parsley *petros selinon*, adapted to *Petroselinum*.

CIRCA 70
Roman physician Pliny the Elder complains parsley is in every sauce and salad.

1548
Parsley is introduced into Britain.

1966
Simon and Garfunkel release now-classic album *Parsley, Sage, Rosemary, and Thyme*.

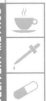

P arsley—familiar to most Americans as an often used garnish—is a biennial. It usually grows about a foot tall, though second-year seed stalks reach 2 feet or more. The leaves are divided into 3 major segments, then further divided into lobes, with sharp-toothed segments. In curly leaf parsley, the leaves are strongly crisped, giving the edges a crinkled appearance. In Italian parsley the leaves are flat. The greenish to creamy yellow, inconspicuous flowers are borne in flat-topped umbels (umbrella-like structures) with 8 to 20 rays. The seed, technically a fruit, is broadly oval.

In the **genus** there is only one other **species**, *Petroselinum segetum*, which is native to western and northern Europe but not used as an herb. The flat-leaf Italian parsley is designated *P. crispum* var. *neapolitanum*. Curly parsley is the **variety** *crispum*. A large-rooted parsley, Hamburg parsley, is var. *tuberosum*. Like Italian and curly-leaf parsleys, it is also grown for its edible and medicinal roots. Numerous cultivars of curly-leaf parsley are found in American horticulture.

Growing Habits

Parsley is another common herb, cultivated since ancient times, that has spread through cultivation and has naturalized throughout Europe. Though its exact origins are not clear, Swedish botanist Carolus Linnaeus suggested that the plant was found growing wild in Sardinia near brooks. It was found in England by 1551, and undoubtedly earlier. The leaves, roots, and seeds of parsley have all been used medicinally. The genus name *Petroselinum* is from the Greek *petros*, "rock"; *selinum* means "rock celery." Previously, parsley was classified in the same genus as celery.

Cultivation and Harvesting

Common parsley is easy to grow and is readily grown from seed, provided the gardener has one essential ingredient—patience. Parsley seed can be sown in early spring, even in the north, after the ground thaws. It is tolerant of cool temperatures. The seed, planted about ¼ inch deep, fools many gardeners into thinking that it is not viable. However, it simply takes its time to germinate, usually 4 to 6 weeks. When patience is not possible, a parsley seed's germination inhibitor can be leached out by soaking the seeds in warm water for 3 days. Parsley likes a moderately moist, but not wet, well-drained good garden loam with a slightly acidic pH.

Parsley is often grown as a fresh herb for local markets, or grown in Mexico or California for produce markets. Parsley seed is produced on a small scale in Eastern Europe.

Therapeutic Uses

+ *Kidney stones*
+ *Diuretic*
+ *Urinary tract infections*
+ *High blood pressure*

This mild-tasting herb is the plant to turn to when suffering one of the body's most excruciating conditions—the pain of kidney stones. The pain is relieved in various ways through parsley's medicinal effects. All parts of the parsley

over the (kitchen) counter MANGO PARSLEY SMOOTHIE

I n a blender, combine ½ fresh, peeled mango (or 6 or so chunks of frozen mango), ½ cup fresh, washed curly or flat Italian parsley sprigs, and 2 cups of cold water. Blend until smooth. For variety and a slightly sweeter smoothie, add half a banana along with the mango. Increase the amount of water by ½ cup or more to achieve the desired consistency.

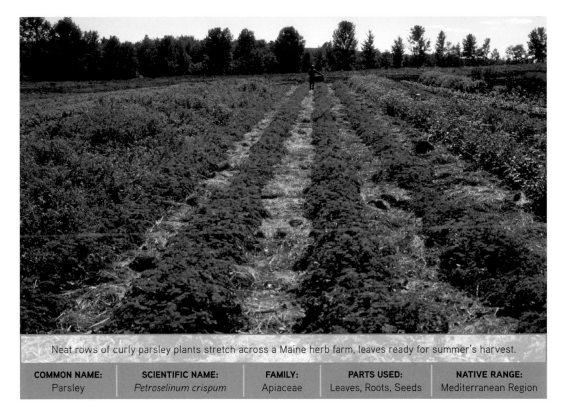

Neat rows of curly parsley plants stretch across a Maine herb farm, leaves ready for summer's harvest.

COMMON NAME:	SCIENTIFIC NAME:	FAMILY:	PARTS USED:	NATIVE RANGE:
Parsley	*Petroselinum crispum*	Apiaceae	Leaves, Roots, Seeds	Mediterranean Region

plant—leaf, root, and seeds—contain fragrant oils that have diuretic effects, may increase blood flow to the kidney, and reduce inflammation of the urinary tract. Only the root, however, has been approved for use as a diuretic by Germany's Commission E, which oversees the efficacy and effectiveness of medicinal herbs. With diuresis, and possibly through irritation of the inside of the urinary tract, the movement of kidney stones may be facilitated. Parsley's diuretic, circulatory, and **anti-inflammatory** effects also contribute to its ability to fight infections of the urinary tract, such as cystitis. In theory, parsley's diuretic properties might help in lowering blood pressure.

How to Use

FOOD: Parsley is first and foremost a food, a fresh or dried herb that is part of recipes in many cultures. It is possible that some of the medicinal effects are obtained in this way, though higher doses are usually recommended. Conditions of the urinary tract, for example, require approximately 6 g daily of parsley leaves or roots.

TINCTURE: Generally, alcohol **extracts**, or **tinctures**, of parsley are dosed at 1 to 2 ml, 3 times daily.

CAPSULES: 450 to 900 mg of parsley leaf, up to 3 times daily.

TEA: Pour 1 cup of boiling water over ¼ cup (or 2 to 3 tablespoons) fresh parsley leaves. Let stand for 5 minutes, strain, and drink, up to 3 times daily. Tea can be sweetened, if desired.

 NOTE: Different varieties of parsley have different ratios of the active compounds. The part of the plant used—leaf, root, or seed—also affects the optimal dose.

Precautions

Parsley may stimulate both menstrual flow and the uterus so it is not appropriate for pregnant women. Parsley may react with sunlight on the skin to cause a rash, particularly in lighter skinned people. The varied effects that parsley has on the kidneys warrant caution in anyone with kidney disease. Care also should be exercised if parsley is used with high-blood-pressure medications in order to prevent an unsafe drop in blood pressure.

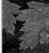

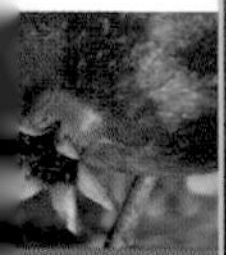

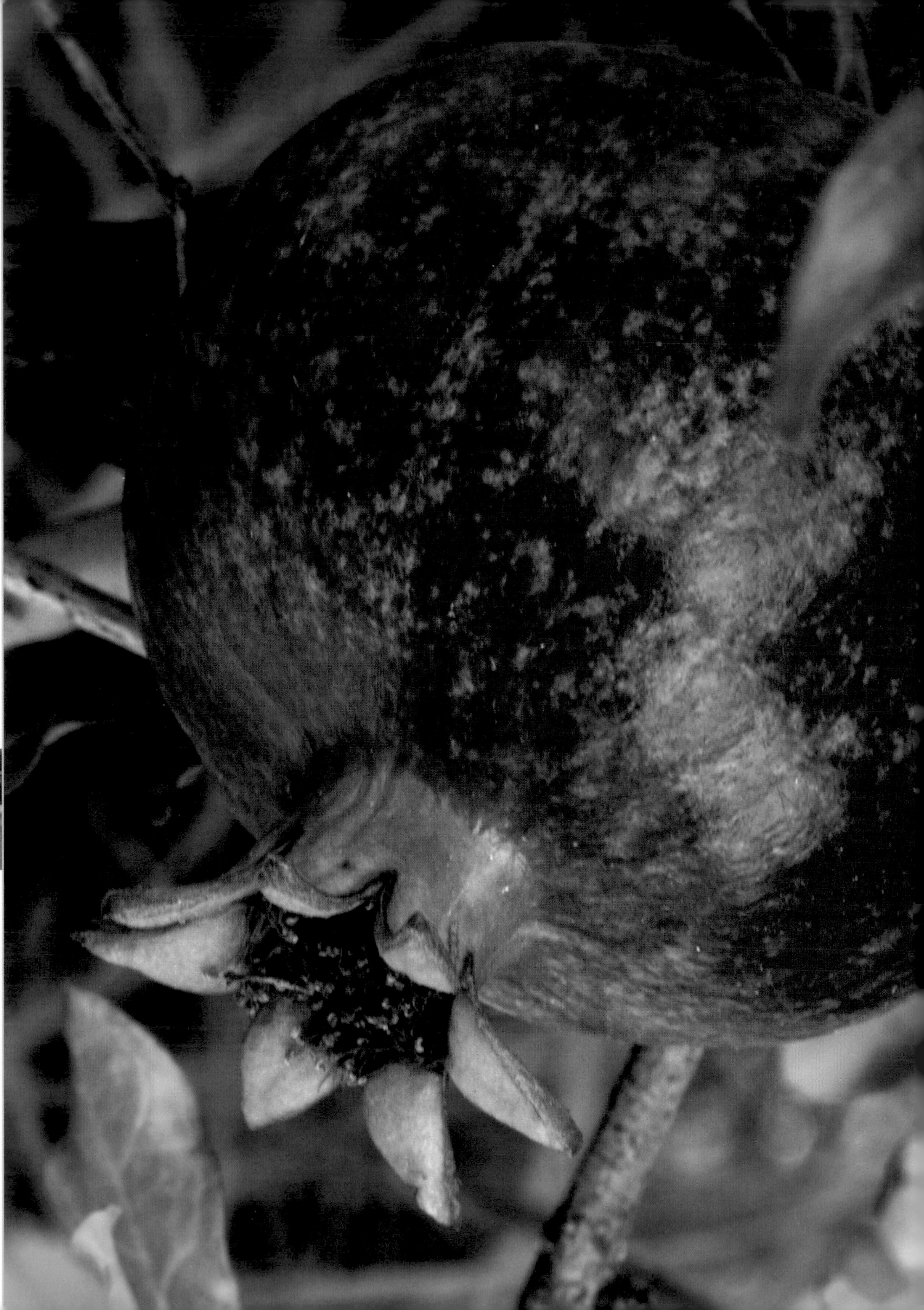

Pomegranate

❧ Punica granatum ☙

Steeped in history and romance, pomegranate is native to the mountainous Transcaucasia-Caspian Sea region, which includes northern Iraq and northwest Iran. Sumerian cuneiform records reveal that pomegranates were cultivated in the Middle East since approximately 3000 B.C. For many centuries the thick-walled fruits were carried by desert caravans as a source of nutritious, thirst-quenching juice. Pomegranate played a role in Egyptian art and mythology, symbolizing abundance and unity, as well as blood, death, and the renewal of life in early Christian, Jewish, and Islamic artistic traditions. In Greek mythology, the story is told of how Persephone, daughter of the goddess Demeter, made the mistake of eating pomegranate seeds in the underworld, and so was eternally bound to that place for part of every year. The Romans named the fruit *Punica granatum*, or "seeds from Carthage," possibly because that Phoenician city in North Africa was a source of fine pomegranates in the ancient world.

Pomegranate has enjoyed a long history of medicinal use. In addition to eating it as fruit, the Greeks and Romans used the seeds or rinds in oral contraceptives and vaginal suppositories. The medicinal use of pomegranate rind is first mentioned in the sixth-century Chinese

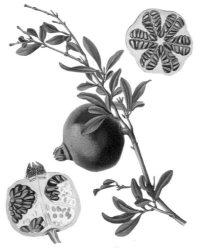

work *Ming Yi Bei Lu (Miscellaneous Records of Famous Physicians)* by Tao Hongjing. In China today, the rinds are used in preparations to relieve diarrhea and dysentery, expel intestinal worms, and stanch bleeding. Bark, fruit, root, and rind are all used medicinally in the Middle East and Asia. In the West only fruit and seed, fresh or in **extract** form, are typically used in herbal and traditional medicine.

Rich in **antioxidants**, pomegranate juice is a healthful drink, high in vitamin C, in its unsweetened form. The juice may help prevent or slow the progression of some cancers, including prostate cancer. It has been shown to lower blood pressure, improve blood flow to the heart, and inhibit plaque formation in arteries, but more research is needed.

The pomegranate's boldly beautiful crimson skin encloses delicate seeds filled with ruby-red juice.

TIME LINE OF USAGE AND SPREAD

1550 B.C.
Ebers Papyrus refers to infusion of pomegranate root to treat intestinal parasites.

A.D. 1521
Spanish missionaries plant the first pomegranate trees in the New World in Mexico.

1769
Pomegranate is introduced into California by Spanish settlers.

2002
New York Times article notes only 5 percent of Americans have tasted pomegranates.

In America the common pomegranate was a forgotten exotic tree until the last decade, when pomegranate fruit juice arrived in the produce section of every supermarket. The genus *Punica* includes only 2 species. Pomegranate is a small, thick, and bushy tree growing up to 20 feet, with many slender branches. Some twigs have sharp thorns. The opposite, narrow, lance-shaped leaves are roughly 3 inches long and half an inch wide, pointed at each end.

The beautiful vibrant orange or scarlet tubular flowers, 2 to 3 inches long, are the texture of tissue paper. Flowers are borne at the end of branches, and their base (the calyx) is thick and fleshy. Once fertilized, the flowers transform into the dark red globe-shaped fruits with the calyx at the apex. There are numerous **varieties**, primarily designated by specific fruit characteristics. Historically, the thick, leathery calyx, valued for its astringency, was dried and sold in apothecary shops.

Growing Habits

Pomegranate trees grow wild throughout much of the Mediterranean region and Middle East, making them seem like a native tree. The trees' seemingly wild nature throughout the Mediterranean region led botanists to believe it was native. In fact, it was one of the first fruit trees in prehistory to spread through cultivation. Pomegranate cultivation dates to the Bronze Age; today it is considered an ancient cultigen, or domesticated plant. Perhaps originating in the Caucasus region to Afghanistan, including modern Syria, Iraq, Iran, and northeastern Turkey, pomegranate is now grown in warm climates worldwide. It was introduced to China 1,500 years before the Christian era and known in Malaysia 2,000 years ago. Pomegranates were first grown in England in 1596. The tree was brought to California 2 centuries later.

Today, in the United States it can be found in warmer regions. It ranges from South Carolina along the Gulf Coast, through central and southern Texas, New Mexico, Arizona, and California, the largest U.S. pomegranate producer.

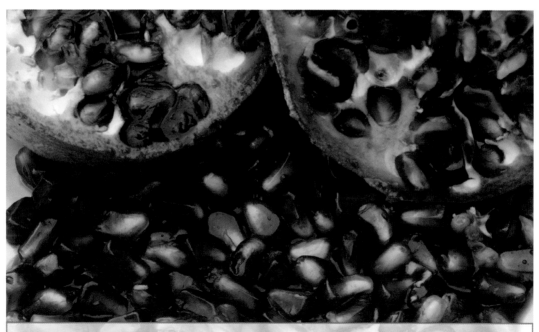

The juice of pomegranate seeds is a rich source of antioxidants that promote circulatory system health.

COMMON NAME:	SCIENTIFIC NAME:	FAMILY:	PARTS USED:	NATIVE RANGE:
Pomegranate	*Punica granatum*	Lythraceae	Fruits, Seeds	Middle East

over the (kitchen) counter POMEGRANATE PLEASURES

Heat 1 cup pomegranate juice to just under a boil. Turn off the heat. Mix in 1½ teaspoons arrowroot powder (dissolved in 2 tablespoons water to make it into a liquid). The mixture will immediately start to thicken. Add 1 to 2 tablespoons maple syrup to taste. Store in refrigerator for up to several weeks. • Add 2 tablespoons to 12 ounces sparkling water for a pomegranate spritzer. • Add 2 tablespoons to your yogurt smoothie. • Mix 2 tablespoons with ½ cup olive oil, 1 clove garlic, a dash of lemon juice, and sea salt for a yummy salad dressing.

Cultivation and Harvesting

Pomegranate grows in warmer regions; it survives light frosts of short duration but generally requires a long, hot summer for fruit ripening. Even in areas where the growing season is not long enough to produce fruit, the beauty of the flowers alone makes it worth the effort as a container plant. Pomegranate likes a well-drained, fertile loam and full sun, though it is tolerant of drought. If grown as an ornamental, pruning improves it. Large-scale production occurs in California, India, Australia, and elsewhere.

Therapeutic Uses

+ *Prostate health*
+ *Heart health*
+ *Antioxidant*

The luscious pomegranate has been cherished as food and medicine for at least 4 millennia. Compared with other common fruit juices, pomegranate is one of the richest in antioxidant activity—with roughly 3 times that of red wine and green tea! Animal studies show that pomegranate juice and pomegranate flower extract offer strong protection against the progression of **atherosclerosis**. Human studies demonstrate a modest effect on blood pressure and inflammation reduction—reasons for adding pomegranate to a heart-healthy foods list.

One of the most interesting areas of pomegranate research is prostate health. Laboratory and animal studies have shown that juice, peel, and oil all interfere with the spread of prostate cancer tumors. A 2-year human study examined the effect of 8 ounces of pomegranate juice on prostate-specific antigen (PSA) levels in 46 men who had received surgery or radiation therapy for prostate cancer. PSA is used as a marker after cancer treatment to determine if the cancer has returned. Treatments are deemed effective if they reduce PSA levels in prostate cancer patients and/or prolong the time it takes for the PSA level to double (indicating that progression of the cancer is slowing). Sixteen of 46 patients (35 percent) exhibited a decline in their PSA levels during treatment, while 4 of the 46 patients (2 percent) achieved a PSA decline of more than 50 percent. Overall, PSA doubling time was significantly delayed in a majority of the men drinking the juice. After the 2-year study, those who continued to drink pomegranate juice had lower PSA levels than those who stopped. At the conclusion of the study, the mean PSA doubling time went from 15 to 54 months, with no adverse events reported.

In men, prostate cancer is the second leading cancer-related death in the U.S. Seven government-funded studies are currently evaluating pomegranate's role in treating prostate cancer.

How to Use

JUICE: Drink 8 ounces of juice per day (the typical amount used in research studies).
CAPSULES: Generally, 2 to 3 g per day of powdered pomegranate.

Precautions

There are no known safety issues with drinking pomegranate juice or with using pomegranate juice extracts.

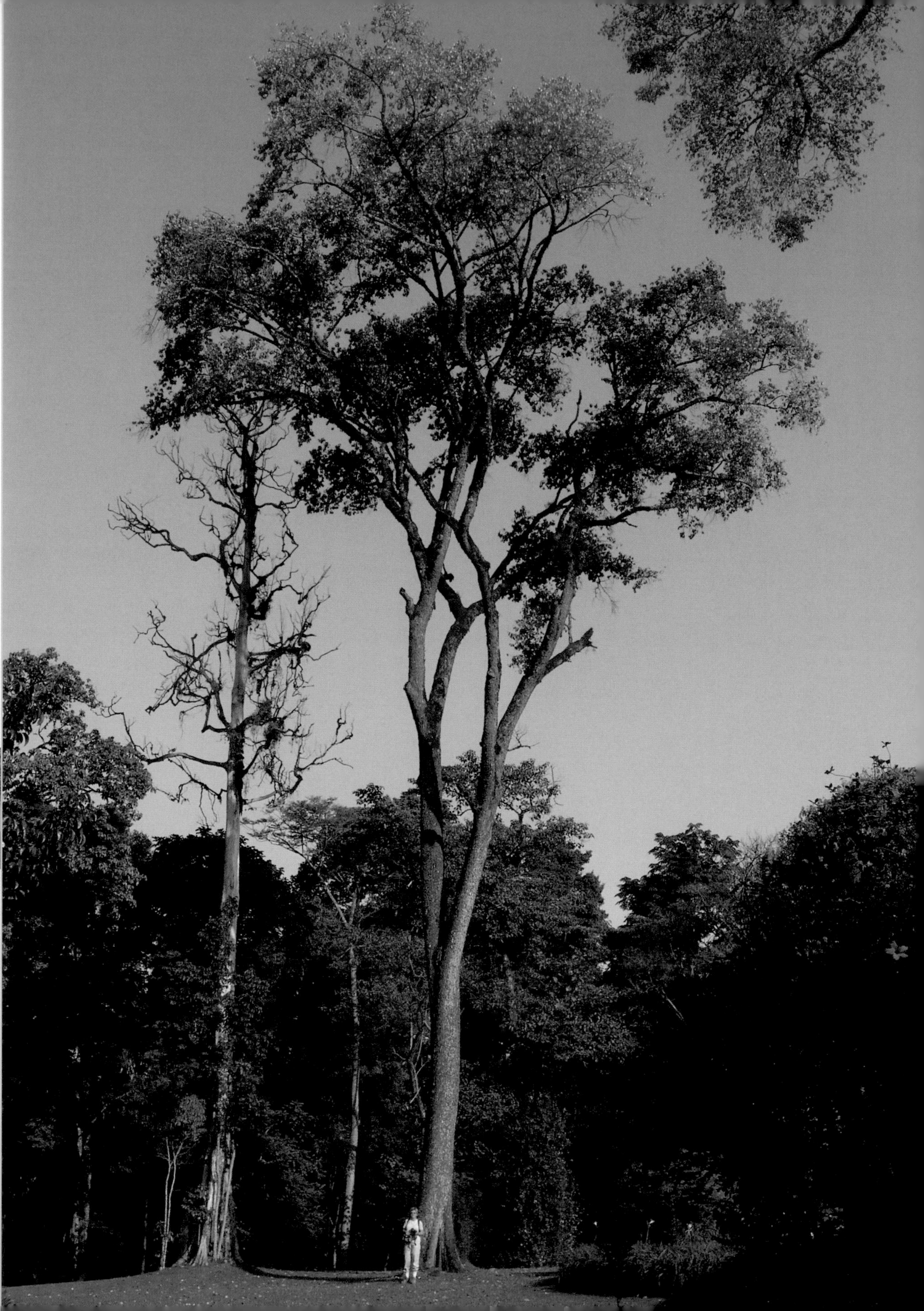

Pygeum

Prunus africana

Tall and stately, the African cherry, or pygeum, tree grows in tropical mountain forests on both eastern and western sides of the African continent, as well as on the island of Madagascar. The leaves, seeds, and fruits of pygeum are an important food source for many wild mammals and birds. People living in rural areas near forests where pygeum grows use the durable wood to make tools, carts, and household goods; they also favor it for cooking fires because it burns hot and produces little smoke. Long before the coming of Europeans to these remote forests, African tribal healers used the dark, brownish gray bark of pygeum medicinally to treat a host of ailments, including male urinary tract problems. Pygeum was introduced to Western herbal medicine in the 1960s as a treatment for enlarged prostate, the condition known as benign prostatic hyperplasia (BPH). Since that time it has become almost as popular as saw palmetto as an herbal remedy for BPH.

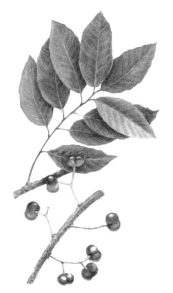

In Africa, pygeum bark has a long history in herbal medicine as a painkiller and **anti-inflammatory**. Traditionally, the bark is ground to a powder and drunk as a tea. In addition to its use as a remedy for male urinary tract problems, pygeum is routinely used to treat malaria, fever, stomach and intestinal disorders, lung ailments, kidney disease, menstrual complaints, infertility, and even mental illness. Interestingly, pygeum is also used to treat illness in animals, and is considered a singularly important plant in traditional African veterinary medicine. European interest in pygeum began in the 1700s, when explorers and settlers in both South Africa and Cameroon learned of the bark's efficacy in relieving bladder pains and other urinary tract complaints.

Some 200 years later, French physician Jacques Debat acquired the first patent on an **extract** of pygeum bark and introduced the herb to Europe. Today, in France, Germany, and Italy pygeum bark extract is widely used for relieving the symptoms of enlarged prostate. In the United States pygeum is gaining in popularity as a treatment for BPH.

International trade in pygeum bark is closely monitored, since overharvesting is threatening wild populations.

TIME LINE OF USAGE AND SPREAD

1861	1966	1994	2004
First pygeum specimens collected by Europeans in Africa's Cameroon Range.	Physician J. Debat acquires first patent on pygeum extract for treatment of BPH.	Pygeum listed in international agreement to monitor trade of species.	Pygeum bark exported from Africa to Europe estimated at 3,200 to 4,900 tons annually.

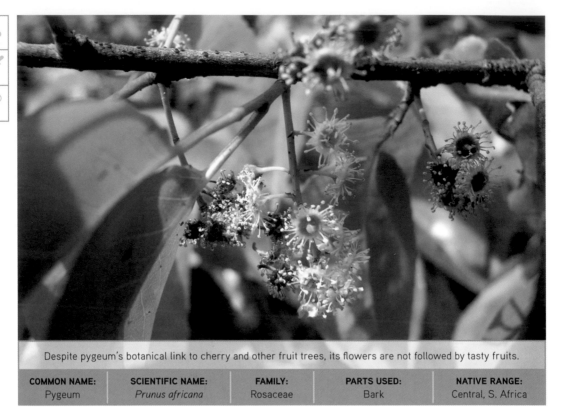

Despite pygeum's botanical link to cherry and other fruit trees, its flowers are not followed by tasty fruits.

COMMON NAME:	SCIENTIFIC NAME:	FAMILY:	PARTS USED:	NATIVE RANGE:
Pygeum	*Prunus africana*	Rosaceae	Bark	Central, S. Africa

The genus *Prunus* in the rose family is famously the source of cherries, apricots, plums, and almonds, along with species associated with herbal traditions such as wild cherry (*P. serotina*), used for wild cherry cough syrups. Of the more than 200 species of *Prunus*, most occur in the Northern Hemisphere. One species, a tall tree of African forests whose bark is known as the herbal product pygeum, is common across the southern African continent.

The small star-shaped flowers of pygeum—unlike some of its temperate climate cousins in the *Prunus* family—yield a hard, dry, unpalatable berry about ½ inch wide. The flower petals have a woolly fringe. The elliptical to ovate leaves are dark glossy green and 3 to 5 inches long, with small teeth along the margins. The reddish brown bark is the part used in herbal medicine. Like the bark, leaves, and twigs of many cherry tree relatives, those of pygeum have "cherry" or "almond" fragrances.

Growing Habits

Pygeum grows in mountain forests of central and southern Africa and islands off the African coast. It ranges from Kenya westward to Angola, south to Cape Province in South Africa.

The bark is harvested from wild populations in Kenya, Cameroon, Democratic Republic of the Congo, Uganda, Tanzania, Zaire, and Madagascar. It occurs in Tanzania, Ethiopia, Burundi, Rwanda, Malawi, and Nigeria as well. In Cameroon, it is usually found in montane forests at elevations of 3,000 to 7,000 feet. *P. africana* grows most abundantly near the upper forest and grassland boundaries in volcanic soils—primarily occurring in mountain "islands" surrounded by tropical forests. The Cameroon populations on different mountains are genetically distinct from one another. Before the bark was introduced into international trade, the tree was considered an important timber source, with a hard, beautiful cherrylike wood.

Cultivation and Harvesting

Cameroon is the largest producer of pygeum bark. Destructive harvest of the bark had raised serious conservation concerns by the late 1980s. By 1991, when more than 4,000 metric tons of the bark was processed in Cameroon alone, conservationists were alerted to a growing problem.

Most of the bark was once harvested in areas where natural habitats were protected by the cultural practices of a secret society known as the Kwifon, which had effective rules for managing sacred forests, watersheds, and plant and animal resources. Subsequently, a French company was given permits for wild harvest of the bark by the government of Cameroon. Then, to increase exports, permits were given to many commercial entities; this resulted in the breakdown of traditional conservation practices and the destruction not only of pygeum trees but also of the habitat. Concern over the trees' future led to pygeum bark being listed in CITES, the international treaty governing trade in endangered flora and fauna. The bark is allowed in commerce, but it is monitored in international trade.

Therapeutic Uses

+ *Benign prostatic hyperplasia (BPH)*

The bark of the pygeum tree is a common addition to herbal products meant to help with symptoms of benign prostatic hyperplasia. Pygeum bark has been used in France for decades, is commonly prescribed in Europe, and is now commonly sold in the U.S., often in combination with saw palmetto and stinging nettle root. Pygeum bark is most often used to help those who suffer with excessive nighttime urination, painful urination, or the sensation of a full bladder, common symptoms of BPH.

Pygeum bark is full of many **compounds** that act on the bladder and prostate, including **phytosterols** (cholesterol-like compounds found in plants) such as beta-sitosterol. These compounds may fight inflammation and decrease testosterone production, helping to shrink the prostate. Whole bark extracts have also been shown to promote bladder contraction and lower inflammation in the prostate. Moreover, pygeum does not seem to affect the **enzyme** 5-alpha-reductase, the main therapeutic mechanism in saw palmetto, another BPH remedy.

Some research on the effectiveness of whole bark extracts of pygeum shows improvements in BPH symptoms and slight shrinkage of the prostate, while other studies have shown no difference from symptoms in groups taking **placebos**. One review of 18 studies using pygeum for an average of 2 months documented a 23 percent improvement in urine flow, a 24 percent decrease in urine retained in the bladder, and 19 percent less nighttime urination—promising findings for people suffering from BPH.

How to Use

EXTRACT: Pygeum bark extracts are usually dosed at 100 mg daily, though up to 200 mg daily can be used. Extracts are often standardized to contain 14 percent sterols, including beta-sitosterol. Taking 100 mg daily in a standardized extract may have benefits for several symptoms associated with BPH.

TEA: Dried pygeum bark can be boiled for a tea, but the raw bark form hasn't been well studied.

Precautions

Adverse effects while taking pygeum are considered mild, but nausea, diarrhea, constipation, stomach upset, headache, and dizziness have been reported. Safety in pregnancy and lactation is not known.

over the (kitchen) counter COMBO COMFORT TEA

Add ½ cup dried pygeum bark (which can be bought in bulk at a health food store), ½ cup dried, stinging nettle root, and 1 cup dried, ripe saw palmetto fruit to 1 quart boiling water. Reduce heat and simmer gently for 15 to 20 minutes. Cover and steep for 1 hour. Strain and add honey to taste. Drink 2 to 4 cups of the tea daily for benign prostatic hyperplasia (BPH). Keep refrigerated.

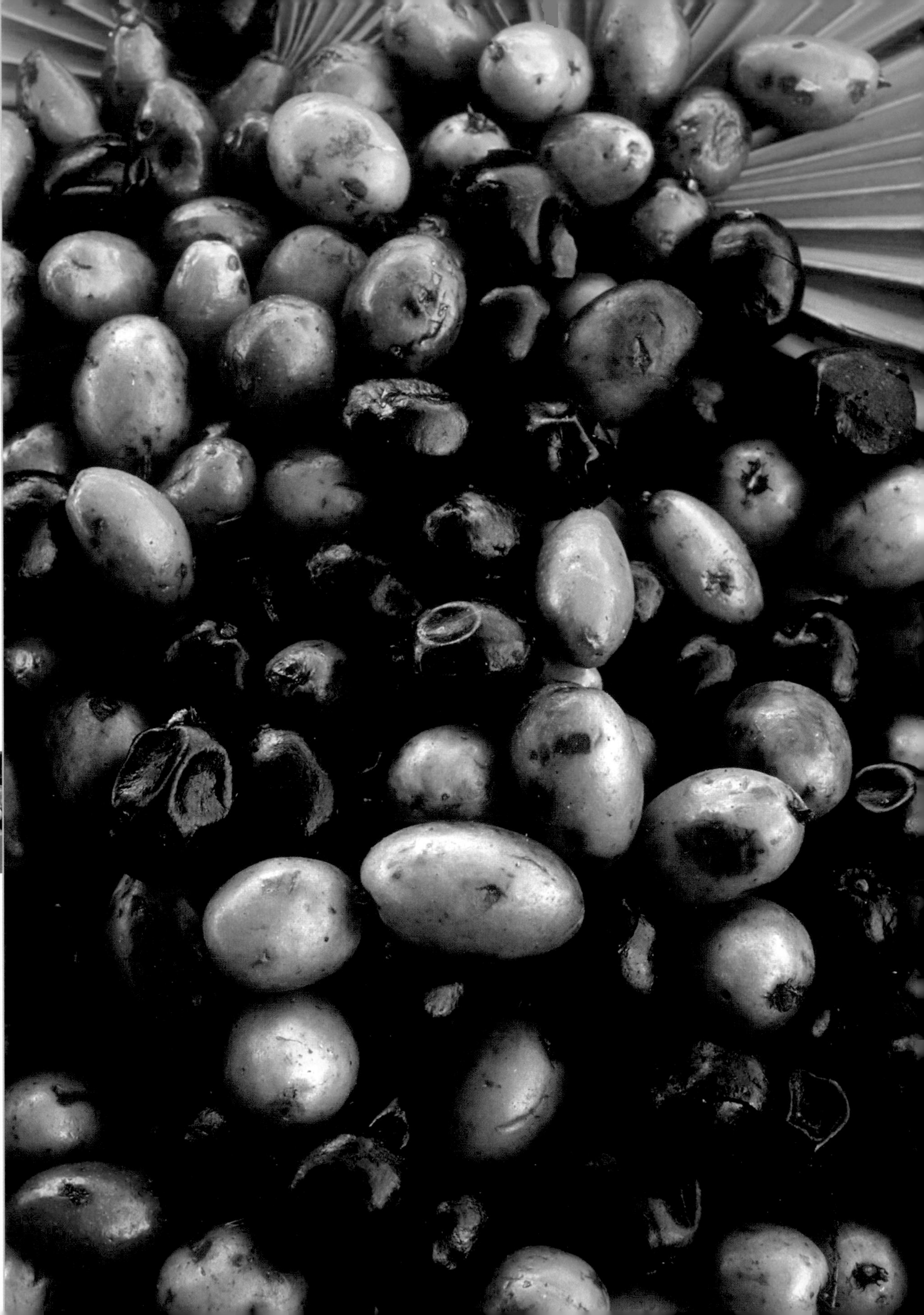

Saw Palmetto

ᏬᎦ *Serenoa repens* ᎢᏆ

Native to the southeastern United States, saw palmetto is a low-growing palm with distinctive fan-shaped leaves. Vast, unbroken tracts of saw palmetto once covered hundreds of miles of coastal land in Florida, Georgia, and other parts of this region. The density of the plants, coupled with the sawlike edges of the leaf stalks, made the tracts almost impassable. The dark purple fruits of saw palmetto—about the size and shape of olives—were an indispensable dietary staple among Native American tribes for perhaps as much as 12,000 years before Europeans set

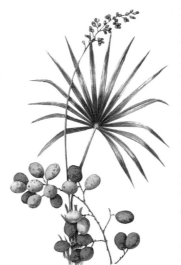

foot in this part of North America. When settlers arrived, they added saw palmetto to their diet and fed the fruits to their livestock. They also observed native tribes using saw palmetto, particularly as a remedy for urinary tract complaints. By the late 1800s, the plant had found its way into conventional medicine in the U.S. Interest in saw palmetto waned for a time, but since the 1990s it has been the herb of choice among herbal practitioners for prostate problems.

The Seminole and other tribes in the southeastern U.S. had a long tradition of using saw palmetto for urinary complaints, digestive problems, and dysentery and as an aphrodisiac, an **expectorant**, an **antiseptic**, and a tonic to improve general health. Early 20th-century conventional and American **Eclectic** physicians recommended saw

palmetto for a variety of health problems. In particular, preparations of the fruits were given to help resolve urinary tract infections and to alleviate symptoms of enlarged prostate and boost libido. While interest in herbs of all kinds had faded in the U.S. by the 1950s, saw palmetto use in Europe steadily increased. European companies were among the first to produce standardized **extracts** of saw palmetto fruit.

In modern herbal medicine, saw palmetto is primarily used to treat benign prostatic hyperplasia (BPH), an enlargement of the prostate gland. It is used by 2 million men in the United States alone. Some herbal practitioners also recommend saw palmetto for chronic pelvic pain syndrome (CPPS) in men, inflammation of the urethra, bladder disorders, and gallbladder problems.

Saw palmetto berries are the source for extracts that go into widely used herbal remedies to treat prostate problems.

TIME LINE OF USAGE AND SPREAD

1879
J. B. Read introduces saw palmetto in *American Journal of Pharmacy*.

1907
Drug firm Eli Lilly sets up saw palmetto drying facility in Vero Beach, Florida.

1926
Saw palmetto is listed in the *National Formulary* in the U.S. but dropped in 1950.

1998
Saw palmetto is relisted in the *National Formulary*.

There is only one species in the genus *Serenoa*, the saw palmetto *(S. repens)*. The primary stem is either creeping or ascending, sometimes branched at the base, growing from 3 to 9 feet in height. Leaves are about 3 feet long and broad—occurring in the familiar fan shape of the palm. Individual narrow leaflets, the length of the blade, radiate from a central base. The leaf stalks are the source of the "saw" in its name, as the edges have sharp, sawlike teeth.

The small, creamy white, fragrant flowers are crowded in large groups arising from the base of the plant. The fruits, the saw palmetto berries of commerce, are about the size of an olive, oily, green at first, changing to orange-brown, and then, if ripening on the plant, turning black.

Growing Habits

Saw palmetto is found in pine scrub, dunes, and hummocks, often in dense colonies in the southeastern United States. In Florida, palmetto-pine thickets (especially in central and southern Florida) dominate millions of acres of vegetation. Saw palmetto grows on the lower coastal plain from South Carolina to Florida, and west to southeastern Mississippi. When ripening, the fruits give off a characteristic fragrance in their habitat.

Early European travelers found them rather distasteful. An early account describes the impressions of shipwrecked Quakers on the Florida coast in 1796: "We tasted them, but not one among us could suffer them to stay in our mouths, for we could compare the taste of them to nothing else but rotten cheese steeped in tobacco juice." However, an 1898 account identifies saw palmetto as a critical food source to early inhabitants, noting that "the aborigines of the Florida peninsula depended largely upon the berries of the Saw Palmetto for food."

Cultivation and Harvesting

Given its common and abundant occurrence in Florida, saw palmetto is rarely cultivated, though wild plants are sometimes incorporated into landscape design. Millions of pounds of

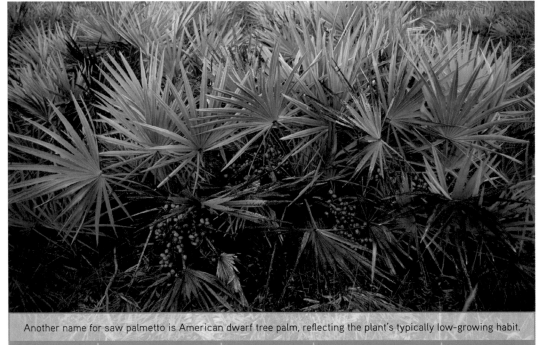

Another name for saw palmetto is American dwarf tree palm, reflecting the plant's typically low-growing habit.

COMMON NAME:	SCIENTIFIC NAME:	FAMILY:	PARTS USED:	NATIVE RANGE:
Saw Palmetto	*Serenoa repens*	Arecaceae	Fruits (berries)	Southeastern U.S.

In a saucepan, mix 2 tablespoons dried saw palmetto berries and 2 cups water. Cover, boil, and turn off heat. Let stand 1 hour, then strain. Stir in 1 tablespoon honey and ¼ teaspoon vanilla extract. Fill a microwavable teacup with the mixture and microwave for about 1 minute, or until hot. Enjoy!

saw palmetto berries are harvested each year mostly in Florida, but also in southern Georgia and adjacent Alabama. Palmetto thickets are nearly impenetrable because of the sharp, saw-toothed leaf stem margins that easily rip clothing. Eastern diamondback rattlesnakes rest in the shade of saw palmetto and wasps build large nests in the center of the shrub, making berry harvest a daunting task in the heat and humidity of late summer. The harvest season lasts from late July to mid-September.

Migrant farmworkers from Latin America and the Caribbean harvest the berries. A team of 3 pickers can gather a half ton of berries in a morning. They are transported to a central buying facility, where they are cleaned and dried. In recent years, extract operations have been set up in Florida. Container loads, each holding about 20,000 pounds of dried berries, are shipped to Europe for extraction, then back to the U.S. as finished extracts or packaged products.

Therapeutic Uses

+ *Benign prostatic hyperplasia (BPH)*

Saw palmetto's blue-black, single-seeded berries are used to make the premier herbal medicine for treating prostate problems. Extracts of the berries act to inhibit an **enzyme**, 5-alpha-reductase, that stops the formation of a potent, prostate growth-enhancing form of testosterone. Saw palmetto also may have effects on **estrogen, progesterone**, and testosterone and their receptors in the body, other mechanisms for slowing the growth of the prostate. All of these effects translate into easing the symptoms of BPH by enhancing urinary flow rates, reducing pain with urination, and decreasing nighttime urination. In most clinical studies,

saw palmetto, used as a standardized extract of 320 mg daily, relieves BPH symptoms as effectively as the pharmaceutical finasteride; however, finasteride more effectively decreases the size of the prostate. Whereas finasteride decreases testosterone levels in the blood, saw palmetto does not seem to affect blood test results for testosterone, other sex hormones, or PSA (prostate specific antigen, a marker for prostate cancer and BPH).

Much research has been done on saw palmetto, and the research has undergone rigorous analysis in which researchers compiled results from many studies. The results have been mixed, probably due to flaws in research models, a range in the type of extracts used, and the length of time supplements were taken.

How to Use

EXTRACT: Studies have used a specific extract, standardized at 80 to 90 percent fatty acids and sterols—the **compounds** most effective for BPH symptoms—and dosed at 160 mg, twice daily.

TINCTURE: 1 to 2 ml, 3 times a day.

CAPSULE: Follow manufacturer's guidelines.

NOTE: It may take 1 to 2 months of using saw palmetto to begin to experience the full benefits of the herb.

Precautions

Saw palmetto can cause mild stomach upset, constipation, diarrhea, headache, high blood pressure, and itching. Rarely, saw palmetto can cause impotence or decreased sex drive. Due to its possible hormonal effects, saw palmetto is not recommended for those on hormone therapy, nor during pregnancy. However, women are not likely to take this herb.

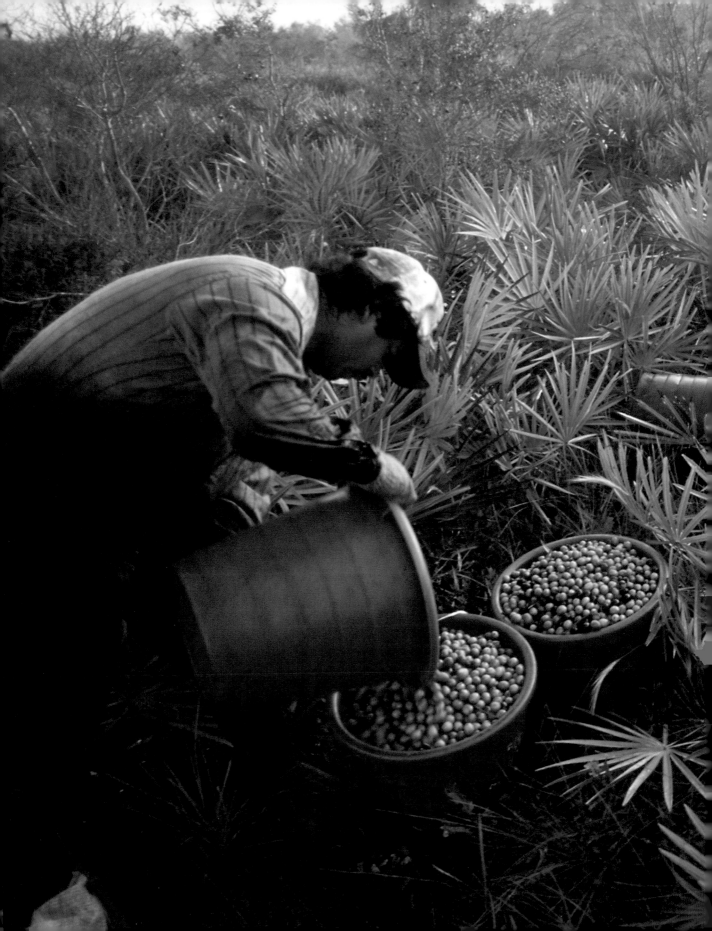

Saw Palmetto Harvest

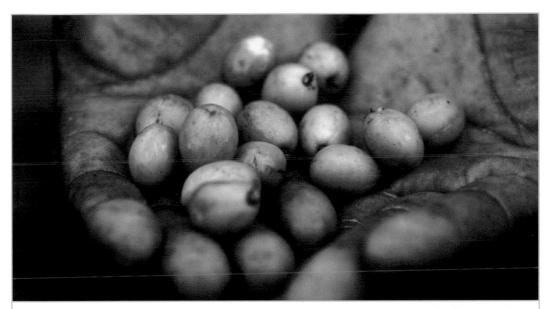

A picker (opposite) consolidates a morning's efforts of gathering saw palmetto berries from wild plants in southern Florida. Saw palmetto thickets, source of the majority of berries harvested for commercial trade, cover millions of Florida acres. Despite high heat and humidity, pickers wear long sleeves and leather gloves for protection against the razor-sharp spines edging the plants' leaf stalks. Ripe berries (above), rich in extractable compounds, range from yellow-green to dark blue-black. Freshly picked berries (below) await drying at a Florida facility. Dried berries are shipped to extractors, mostly in Europe; extracts return to the U.S. for incorporation into products.

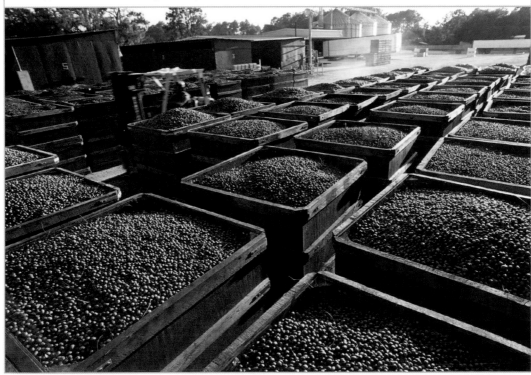

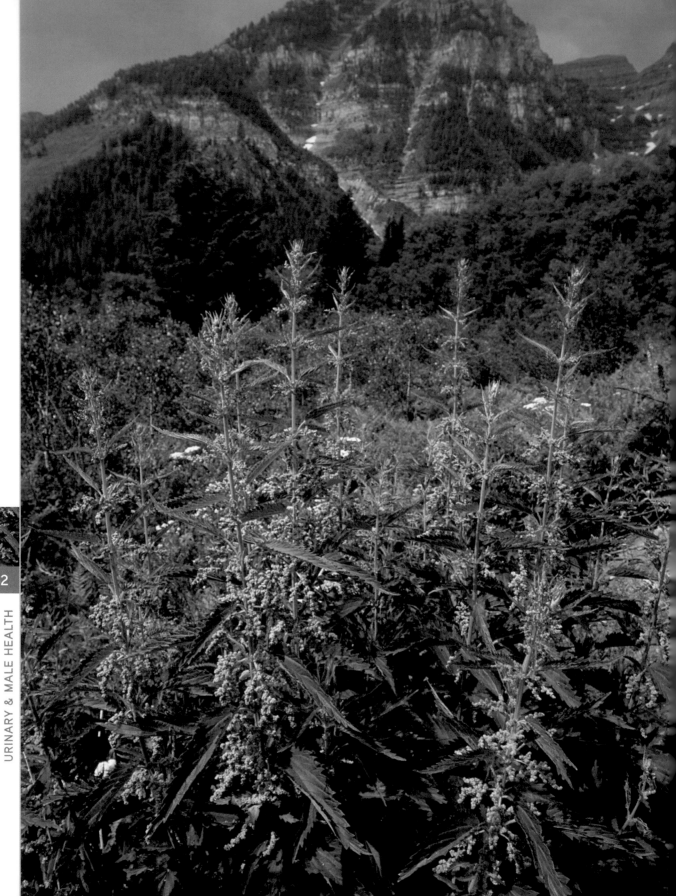

Stinging Nettle

✿ *Urtica dioica* ✿

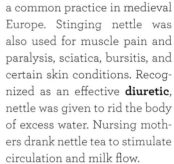

An encounter with stinging nettle is not soon forgotten. Except for the roots, the entire plant bristles with nearly invisible, needle-sharp hairs that penetrate skin at the slightest touch. The pain is both instantaneous and persistent. Its source is a chemical cocktail released from the hairs that causes an intense burning sensation and swelling of the skin. The result is a rash similar to poison ivy, only much more painful. Someone lost in antiquity discovered something quite remarkable about stinging nettle. Apply it to a body part that's already in pain, and the original pain will dissipate. Scientists believe nettle does this by lowering levels of certain inflammatory chemicals in the body, and possibly by interfering with the way pain signals are transmitted. Stinging nettle's unique ability to fight pain with pain has made it a valuable addition to herbal medicine in treating arthritis, rheumatism, and several other painful conditions.

The ancient Romans were well aware of stinging nettle's properties. Its **genus** name, *Urtica*, comes from the Latin *urere*, meaning "to burn." Roman troops fighting in Europe and England lashed themselves with stinging nettle brought from Italy to feel warmer during northern winters. Lightly flogging the skin over arthritic joints with bundles of freshly cut nettles—or urtication, as it came to be called—was a common practice in medieval Europe. Stinging nettle was also used for muscle pain and paralysis, sciatica, bursitis, and certain skin conditions. Recognized as an effective **diuretic**, nettle was given to rid the body of excess water. Nursing mothers drank nettle tea to stimulate circulation and milk flow.

Modern herbal practitioners recommend nettle preparations—some taken internally, others externally—to treat rheumatism, joint pain from osteoarthritis, strains and sprains, tendonitis, and more. Nettle is an aid to reduce sneezing and itching in people with hay fever. Stinging nettle is widely used in Europe to treat symptoms of early stage enlarged prostate, or benign prostatic hyperplasia (BPH). It is also given for urinary tract infections and chronic skin problems, including eczema and psoriasis.

A clump of wild stinging nettle flourishes in Utah's Wasatch Mountains; both leaves and roots are used medicinally.

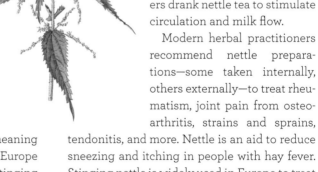

TIME LINE OF USAGE AND SPREAD

3000–2000 B.C.
Burial shrouds dating to the Bronze Age are found to be made of nettle fibers.

4TH CENTURY B.C.
Hippocrates and other healers of his day describe 61 remedies using nettle.

1914–1918
Germany uses nettle as a substitute for cotton in German army uniforms.

1939–1940
British government requests 100 tons of nettles for camouflage uniforms in WWII.

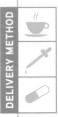
Anyone who goes out gathering any of the various species of stinging nettle knows to go well armed: long sleeves, long pants, sturdy shoes, socks, and gloves. There are about 40 species of stinging nettle, occurring nearly worldwide. Four species are found in North America. There are 3 subspecies of *Urtica dioica*, the species used in herbal medicine. Subspecies *dioica* has male and female flowers on separate plants, with rough, hairy stems, and leaves with stinging hairs above and below. In **subpecies** *gracilis,* male and female flowers are usually on the same plant, stems are mostly smooth, and there are relatively few stinging hairs. Another subspecies, *holosericea,* which occurs only west of the Continental Divide, has softly hairy stems, but the stinging hairs are still there. Stinging nettle is an **herbaceous** perennial, growing from 2 to 6 feet tall and spreading by a creeping **rhizome**, often creating relatively large patches.

Growing Habits

Typical *Urtica dioica* (subspecies *dioica*) is native to Eurasia and widespread around the world, where it has spread as a weed. Flowering spring to fall, it is found at the edges of fields, along fencerows, and at the edge of **deciduous** woods. It grows in the eastern U.S., is generally absent from the interior of the continent, and occurs in West Coast states.

It was long believed that all North American stinging nettle was a Eurasian weed, but genetic evidence shows that subspecies *gracilis* is a North American native, occurring in habitats similar to those of its European cousin. It is native to Canada, the eastern U.S., and the mountains of the Carolinas and eastern Tennessee. It is also occurs in the West.

Cultivation and Harvesting

Cultivate stinging nettle? Why not? Not only does it have valuable herbal properties, but the young shoots as they emerge in the spring are an excellent vegetable. Nettles can be grown from seed, cuttings, or root divisions. Divisions are best made in autumn, after the leaves have died back. It does best in a damp, rich soil under full sun. The herb can be cut back three or four times a year to encourage new growth.

Historically, the leaves of stinging nettle were the plant part most used in herbal medicine. Today, however, the roots are widely used as well. When nettle leaves are harvested, the herb is cut and dried before flowering. The root is harvested in autumn, after vegetative growth has died back. Most commercial production of stinging nettle takes place in Eastern Europe. But there are limited commercial plantings in western Europe and the United States. China has recently emerged as a supplier.

Therapeutic Uses

+ *Benign prostatic hyperplasia (BPH)*
+ *Allergies*
+ *Arthritis*

Extracts of the root of stinging nettle have been shown to be useful for symptoms associated with prostate enlargement, such as

over the (kitchen) counter STINGING NETTLE PESTO

Wearing leather gloves, gather enough tender nettle leaves to make 6 cups. Blanch leaves in boiling water for 1 minute to deactivate the "sting." Drain, pat dry, and roughly chop the blanched leaves. Combine the nettle leaves, 1/3 cup olive oil, 1/2 cup grated Parmesan cheese, 1/3 cup pine nuts or walnuts, 3 cloves minced garlic, 1/2 teaspoon salt, and 1/8 teaspoon pepper in a food processor and blend until smooth. Use with pasta, meat, fish, or good homemade bread.

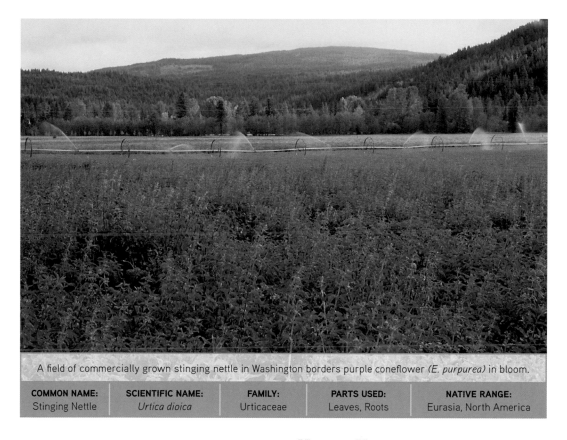

A field of commercially grown stinging nettle in Washington borders purple coneflower *(E. purpurea)* in bloom.

COMMON NAME:	SCIENTIFIC NAME:	FAMILY:	PARTS USED:	NATIVE RANGE:
Stinging Nettle	*Urtica dioica*	Urticaceae	Leaves, Roots	Eurasia, North America

decreased urinary flow, nighttime urination, and retained urine. It is possible that **compounds** in stinging nettle interfere with the conversion of testosterone through an **enzyme** called aromatase; other compounds in stinging nettle also are **anti-inflammatory**, inhibit cell growth, and block the enzyme ATPase—all contributing to how stinging nettle may stop the growth of the prostate. The compounds in nettle root most likely responsible for these effects are the **lignans**, **polysaccharides**, and **lectins**. In one trial, men taking 600 mg of a stinging nettle root extract daily had increased urinary flow after 6 weeks.

Therapeutic use of the leaves of stinging nettle—rather than the root—results in different effects, possibly providing relief from allergies and from arthritis. Extracts of stinging nettle leaf have been studied in osteoarthritis patients. Findings seem to indicate that herbal treatments using stinging nettle leaves both decrease pain and increase quality of life. Stinging nettle leaves and seeds are also used as a diuretic.

How to Use

TEA: Steep 1 teaspoon dried nettle leaves in 1 cup boiling water for 2 to 5 minutes. Strain.

DECOCTION: Boil 5 g of chopped, dried root in 2 cups water for 10 minutes. Strain, cool, and consume throughout the day.

CAPSULE: Dried, powdered root extracts in capsule form can be taken in doses of 300 to 800 mg daily, depending on the formulation. Freeze-dried nettle leaf capsules are also available for management of hay fever.

TINCTURE: Use 1 to 3 teaspoons daily of an alcohol-based liquid extract of the root.

EXTRACT: Standardized extracts are available. Some combine stinging nettle root and saw palmetto berries; others contain pumpkin seed oil. Follow manufacturer's dosage guidelines.

Precautions

Side effects include upset stomach, rash, and impotence. Those taking medicines for diabetes, high blood pressure, anxiety, or insomnia should exercise caution with stinging nettle preparations because interactions are possible.

Tomato

Lycopersicon esculentum

They are one of the world's most popular fresh vegetables—although botanically, tomatoes are fruits. Today they come in more than a thousand different varieties, ranging in color from brown, green, and purple to yellow, orange, and, of course, brilliant red. Native to western South America, tomatoes were first domesticated in Mexico and later cultivated by the Aztec. These ancient plants produced small, cherry-size fruits—not the large, meaty beefsteaks so common at farmers markets and in grocery produce aisles. Spanish conquistadores carried

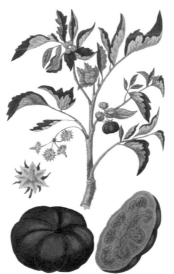

tomato seeds from Mexico back to Spain in the 1500s, and so introduced the tomato to Europe. They also introduced the plant to the Philippines, and tomato cultivation soon spread throughout Asia. In Europe, tomatoes were initially viewed with suspicion, as they were known to belong to the nightshade **family**, which includes a number of poisonous plants. Tomato's **genus** name, *Lycopersicon*, means "wolf peach" in Latin and reflects the early belief that like a wolf, they were dangerous. Gradually, though, tomatoes moved from ornamental plantings to kitchen gardens, becoming an essential ingredient in many European cuisines.

The tomato found its way into North America in the early 1700s. As in Europe, Americans were initially slow to accept the idea of eating tomatoes. By the late 1820s, cookbooks included a few recipes with tomatoes as an ingredient. Around this time, a number of American physicians began espousing the virtues of tomato for treating diarrhea, indigestion, and liver complaints. Within a decade, tomato pills appeared on the scene and were promoted as a tonic, a gentle laxative, and general cure-all. Over time, tomatoes became a popular food in the U.S. Yet their medicinal value was hotly debated up to the early 1900s.

Modern research reveals that tomatoes are indeed a healthful food, rich in vitamins and other nutrients. They also contain lycopene, a plant pigment with **antioxidant** and cancer-preventing properties. Recently, tomato consumption has been shown to be associated with a lower risk of prostate cancer.

Ripe tomatoes are bold, beautiful, and packed with lycopene, a plant pigment that may lower risk of prostate cancer.

TIME LINE OF USAGE AND SPREAD

1544
Botanist Pietro Mattioli pens the first botanical description of tomato.

1692
The first cookbook to mention tomatoes is published in Italy.

1784
D. Landreth Seed Company is one of the first in America to sell tomato seeds.

1876
Heinz ketchup makes its official debut in America.

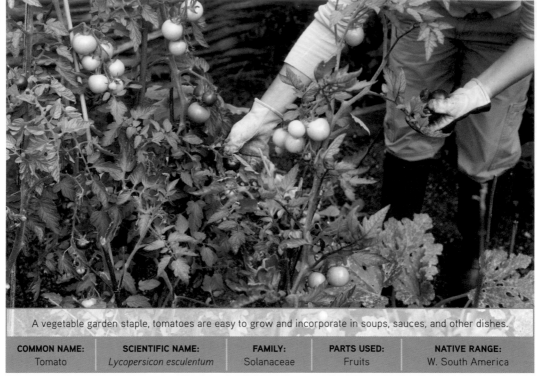

A vegetable garden staple, tomatoes are easy to grow and incorporate in soups, sauces, and other dishes.

COMMON NAME:	SCIENTIFIC NAME:	FAMILY:	PARTS USED:	NATIVE RANGE:
Tomato	*Lycopersicon esculentum*	Solanaceae	Fruits	W. South America

In the never-ending shift of scientific names by botanists, tomato is either placed in the small genus *Lycopersicon*, which includes only 7 species, or among the 120 species of the genus *Solanum*. This genus also includes eggplants and potatoes, among food plants, along with a number of potentially toxic plant species. The tomato, as it is known to most, is a cultigen that has evolved in cultivation over the past 500 years. It is a tender perennial, but grown as an annual, with erect or sprawling stems reaching to 10 feet. The leaves, up to 18 inches long, are divided into 5 to 9 coarsely toothed leaflets, with margins often curled or crisped. The flower clusters have up to 20 lobed yellow flowers an inch in diameter and length. The fruit is the familiar red, rarely yellow or orange, tomato that comes in a variety of sizes, shapes, and colors.

Growing Habits

The wild relatives of tomato occur in a narrow area of western South America including Ecuador, Peru, Bolivia, and Chile, with one **endemic species** from the Galápagos Islands. But are these wild relatives the actual genetic source of the plant we have come to know as tomato?

Plant geographers have advanced 2 basic theories. One theory is that the tomato that we know today originated in Peru, and another is that the tomato originated elsewhere in the Americas, particularly Mexico. It is thought that cultivated tomatoes spread from the vicinity of Veracruz and Puebla in Mexico. There is no evidence for pre-Columbian cultivation of tomatoes in South America.

The name "tomato" itself is derived from an Aztec Nahuatl word, *tomatl*, first recorded in a 1572 work. In the mid-16th century, tomato was a curious botanical specimen grown by herbalists in Europe, who were anxious to receive new plants from exotic lands. Given its resemblance to extremely poisonous nightshade family members, the tomato was not regarded as a potential medicinal plant, and the possibility of eating the fruit was far from herbalists' minds. Although grown in the gardens of Thomas

Jefferson and George Washington, it is fairly unlikely that tomatoes adorned their salads. The tomato was mostly a curiosity for the collector. By the mid-19th century, a Dr. Hand of Maryland introduced a tomato breed called Trophy, for many decades a standard **variety** that became the parent of our modern tomatoes.

While some may argue over whether a tomato is a fruit or a vegetable, given recent scientific studies and findings on its potential health benefits, that argument is easily resolved in favor of simply calling a tomato an herb.

Cultivation and Harvesting

Tomato culture is too well known to every gardener to describe cultivation in detail. Suffice it to say that it is an annual, easily grown from seed. It is not frost tolerant and enjoys warm temperatures and brilliant sunshine in a rich, well-drained garden soil.

Therapeutic Uses

+ *Prostate cancer prevention*

The red color of tomatoes probably comes from a **compound** called lycopene, also found in watermelons, red peppers, and red grapefruit—and now known to be important for prostate health. Lycopene is one of the family of **carotenoids**, powerhouse antioxidants found in fruits and vegetables. In addition to its antioxidant properties, lycopene may act in several different ways to inhibit the growth of cancer cells and affect inflammation or immune system function. Tomatoes also contain vitamin C and other carotenoids that make it a healthful food beneficial for many medical conditions.

Research suggests that consuming tomatoes and tomato products—and hence lycopene—lowers risk for developing prostate cancer. One estimate is that lycopene may lower prostate cancer risk by 25 to 30 percent. Lycopene has been used to treat prostate cancer, in some cases helping to lower prostate specific antigen (PSA) levels; in other cases, it showed no benefit. The medicinal use of lycopene is still being debated and defined. The varied effects of lycopene are also of interest to researchers for the treatment or prevention of liver, breast, pancreatic, lung, and gastric cancers.

How to Use

Tomatoes, and in particular cooked tomato products—tomato sauce, tomato juice, tomatoes baked, stir-fried, or boiled—provide lycopene and other nutrients relevant to prostate cancer prevention. One estimate is that 10 servings per week of cooked tomatoes provides the best benefit for prostate cancer prevention. In addition, capsules containing 5 to 15 mg of lycopene can be taken once a day.

Precautions

Some antioxidants are of concern for people undergoing chemotherapy or radiation therapy. It is unclear whether lycopene or tomatoes fall into this category. Some basic research indicates that lycopene may be of benefit during chemotherapy or radiation therapy. Check with a health care provider before adding lycopene to any cancer treatment protocol.

over the (kitchen) counter QUICK 'N EASY TOMATO SAUCE

In a heavy saucepan, combine 1 tablespoon olive oil, ½ cup finely chopped onion, ¼ teaspoon freshly ground black pepper, and 3 cloves garlic, minced. Cook over medium heat, stirring frequently, for about 5 minutes. Mix in a 28-ounce can crushed tomatoes. Simmer 10 minutes. Add ¼ cup chopped fresh basil and 2 tablespoons chopped fresh oregano. Simmer 5 minutes more. Salt to taste. Serve over cooked pasta or meat loaf or chicken breasts for a healthful, maybe even cancer-preventing, meal.

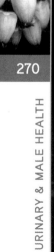

Uva Ursi

Arctostaphylos uva-ursi

Found as far north as the Arctic Circle, uva ursi—also known as bearberry—is a slow-growing, prostrate evergreen shrub that flourishes in alpine forests in the Northern Hemisphere. The tongue-twisting genus name, *Arctostaphylos*, is derived from the Greek words *arctos staphyle*, meaning "bear's grapes." The species name, *uva-ursi*, is the Latin equivalent of the same phrase. Both the scientific name and the common name bearberry are a reference to the herb's shiny red or pink berries, which bears apparently love despite their mouth-puckering sour taste. In North

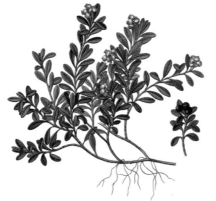

America, Native Americans were the first to use uva ursi as a healing herb. They also smoked a mixture of bearberry leaf and tobacco, and sometimes other herbs, during religious ceremonies. Across the Atlantic, uva ursi was little used until its medicinal merits as a remedy for kidney and bladder problems were noted in a Welsh herbal from the 1200s. By the 1700s, uva ursi had become one of the best available natural remedies for urinary tract infections. Sulfa drugs and antibiotics largely replaced it in conventional medicine in the past century. Yet uva ursi remains a respected herb for treating urinary tract infections.

Native Americans used uva ursi leaves and stems to treat inflammations of the bladder and other parts of the urinary tract, as well as kidney aliments, and as a tonic to maintain both kidney and bladder health. Externally, salves of the herb were rubbed on sores, rashes, boils, and burns. In Europe, the leaves were used medicinally—brewed into a tea taken for urinary tract inflammation and kidney ailments.

Today, uva ursi has known **astringent** and antibacterial properties, making it effective in reducing inflammation and fighting infection. In modern herbal medicine, uva ursi leaf is primarily used to treat inflammations of the urinary tract, including chronic cases that have become resistant to conventional antibiotics. Herbal practitioners sometimes recommend uva ursi leaf for vaginitis and chronic diarrhea. In Germany, the leaf is available as a standardized medicinal tea. Externally, preparations of uva ursi are used to bathe cuts and scrapes, to treat cold sores, and to ease back pain.

Uva ursi's pale pink flowers draw the eye, but it is the herb's leaves that herbalists prize for urinary tract remedies.

TIME LINE OF USAGE AND SPREAD

1200s	1601	1788	1791
Bearberry is first documented as a medicinal herb by Welsh physicians.	Bearberry is mentioned as medicinal herb by C. Clusius, pioneering Flemish doctor.	Bearberry makes its first appearance in the *London Pharmacopoeia*.	Physician W. Lewis mentions uva ursi in *An Experimental History of the Materia Medica*.

The modern reach of the genus *Arctostaphylos* includes 66 species of diverse shrubs or trees primarily native to the Northern Hemisphere, including North America, Central America, Europe, and Asia. The vast majority of *Arctostaphylos* species occur in western North America. Uva ursi is the most widespread species, and the only one that occurs outside of North America. Though often associated with European herbal traditions, uva ursi, along with all of its cousins, is predominantly found in North America.

Uva ursi is a prostrate, mostly evergreen woody perennial. In the wild it often forms mats, which typically cover large areas. The leaves are oblong and somewhat spatula shaped, or they may also be elliptical. They are a dark shiny green and an inch or so in length. The drooping, urnike flowers are whitish, pink, or with reddish streaks. The dry, inedible fruit is globe shaped, looking somewhat like a large pea, except for its beautiful, clear red hue. Within uva ursi's tough, leathery skin lie 5 stone-hard seeds.

There is considerable variation among the diverse **species** in this widespread plant. This is not surprising, given that it grows in such distinctly different habitats.

Growing Habits

Uva ursi is found growing among coastal dunes and on inhospitable mountaintops at elevations of more than 7,000 feet. In some areas, uva ursi sprawls entirely in the open, while in other regions it is a plant of boreal, or northern, forests. It thrives in acidic, sandy, or rocky soils. Primarily associated with cooler climates, uva ursi occurs from east to west in the northern reaches of the United States and on southward to Virginia. It also flourishes throughout the mountainous areas of the West in warmer regions, and it ranges even as far south as the mountains of Guatemala in Central America. Its range also includes not only the northern reaches of Europe and Asia but also the peaks and cool mountain habitats that stretch across the southern part of Europe.

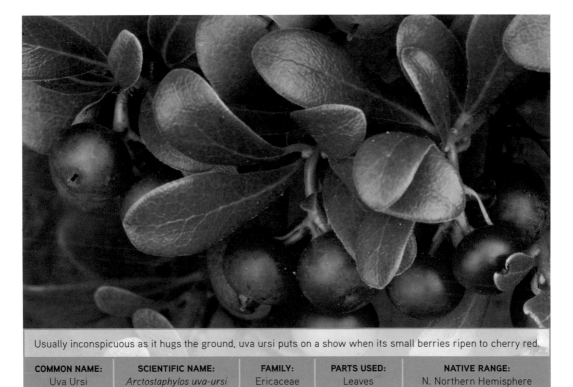

Usually inconspicuous as it hugs the ground, uva ursi puts on a show when its small berries ripen to cherry red.

COMMON NAME:	SCIENTIFIC NAME:	FAMILY:	PARTS USED:	NATIVE RANGE:
Uva Ursi	*Arctostaphylos uva-ursi*	Ericaceae	Leaves	N. Northern Hemisphere

An infusion of uva ursi can be made using hot or cold water. Steep 1 teaspoon of dried uva ursi leaf in 1 cup water. Let stand for approximately 10 minutes and then strain. Drink up to 4 times daily for a urinary tract infection. Herbalists recommend a cold-water infusion for those prone to stomach problems because the tannin compounds, at times irritating to the stomach, have a less harsh effect in cold water.

Cultivation and Harvesting

Uva ursi is propagated from cuttings or layering (where stems touch the ground and form roots) in the early spring, summer, or fall. Cuttings of this slow-growing plant take about twice as long to root as most woody-stemmed herbs. The best growing parts to use for cuttings are the side branches from the middle area of the plant. Two- to 6-inch-long cuttings can be placed in sand, with a bottom-layer heat of 72°F. Cuttings should be misted and dipped in an appropriate rooting hormone to stimulate root growth.

Uva ursi can also be grown from seed, but the seeds have impermeable seed coats and dormant embryos. To make germination most likely, it is best to leave the process in the hands of the specialist.

Uva ursi is happy in a poor, gravelly, acidic soil, with a pH of 5 or less, and generally grows in full sun. Thriving on cool, rocky slopes, the plant likes coastal breezes as well as cold mountain habitats and is hardy to -50°F. It is grown extensively as a ground cover particularly in the Pacific Coast states.

Herbalists in its North American range harvest uva ursi on a small scale. Some commercial harvesting occurs in Canada. But the vast majority of the world's supply of uva ursi comes from the wild-harvesting that takes place in the mountains and valleys of Eastern Europe.

Therapeutic Uses

+ *Urinary tract infections*

Despite the fact that bearberry is another common name for uva ursi, it is not the plant's berries but its leaves that are important in herbal medicine. An effective antibacterial for the kidneys and urinary system, uva ursi leaves contain arbutin and related **compounds**, **glycosides** that have been shown to inhibit many different types of bacteria. Arbutin exerts its urinary antibacterial effect only after undergoing changes in the liver and then traveling through the kidneys. There is substantial debate as to whether taking small amounts of sodium bicarbonate daily or making dietary changes in order to make the urine more alkaline and arbutin more effective in fighting the infection—are a necessary complement to uva ursi treatment.

Despite the long-standing traditional use of uva ursi for urinary tract infections—and convincing data for how this works—there is a lack of human clinical research to back it up. A product using dandelion in combination with uva ursi has been found to be of some benefit in preventing urinary tract infections.

How to Use

TEA: Generally, a common dose of uva ursi dried leaf is 1 teaspoon dried herb steeped in 1 cup boiling water. The tea can be taken 3 to 4 times per day.

CAPSULE: Standardized **extracts** of 700 to 1,000 mg, taken 3 times daily.

TINCTURE: Generally, 5 ml (1 teaspoon), taken 3 times a day.

Precautions

Herbalists recommend taking uva ursi for no longer than 2 weeks at a time. Uva ursi is not recommended for children, pregnant women, lactating mothers, or those with renal failure. The **tannins** in uva ursi can cause stomach upset, nausea, vomiting, and constipation.

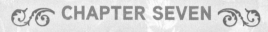

CHAPTER SEVEN

Female Health

Plants *and* Women's Health

❧◦❧

Anyone browsing various histories of medicine might easily conclude that all the great Greek, Roman, Indian, and Chinese healers of antiquity, along with the herbalists of the Middle Ages, were men. Yet there is little doubt that throughout history, many women were also skilled in the healing arts, whether as herbalists, midwives, or physicians. Yet startlingly few of these women have secured a place in history, and only a handful of names have come down through the ages. Merit Ptah, believed to be the first female doctor mentioned by name, was a "chief physician" who practiced in Egypt almost 5,000 years ago. During China's Song dynasty (960-1279), the title of An Guo Lady (the Lady Who Brought Relief to the Nation) was conferred on a female physician after she cured the empress dowager of a serious illness. In England and Europe during the Middle Ages, the chief medical activities of most women revolved around midwifery. But in certain Christian religious orders, women treated

all manner of sickness and disease. In fact, medieval monasteries and convents were often the only places where the sick and afflicted could find medical care. The German abbess Hildegard von Bingen (1098-1179), a remarkably talented and unconventional woman who founded two Benedictine convents, was renowned for her healing work and her original theories of medicine. In her encyclopedic book *Physica*—also known as *Liber Simplicis Medicinae (The Book of Simple Medicine)*—Hildegard described more than 200 plants used to treat a wide range of health complaints that commonly grew in the woods and fields around her convents or were cultivated in their gardens. It isn't difficult to imagine that women, in particular, may have sought Hildegard's medical advice, or the skills of her nuns.

Women and men share many body systems, and therefore many similar health problems. But women also have their own health issues, which deserve special consideration. Most of these involve the female reproductive system. Its major organs consist of the ovaries, which

produce egg cells and various hormones; the uterus, a muscular-walled structure characterized by an extensive blood vessel system; and the oviducts, or fallopian tubes, which essentially connect the ovaries to the uterus and provide a passageway down which eggs can move. Women's lives are also governed, and their health often affected, by a number of physiological conditions and events. These include the hormonally controlled menstrual cycle, pregnancy, and menopause.

Historically, life was often difficult for women. Aside from the risks posed by disease, women typically became wives and mothers just as they were emerging from their own childhoods. Multiple pregnancies in quick succession often led to serious health problems, and complications of childbirth were frequently fatal. For thousands of years, herbal medicines were the only remedies available for treating problems associated with pregnancy and childbirth and other complaints, such as menstrual cramps, breast pain, problems nursing or lack of breast milk, symptoms of menopause, and infertility.

Many women today still turn to herbal medicine to help alleviate some of these problems, along with other women's health issues. Herbal remedies for the irritability, nervousness, cramps, bloating, and headaches that accompany premenstrual syndrome (PMS), for example, have become increasingly popular. So have herbal alternatives to hormone replacement therapy (HRT) as a way to alleviate hot flashes, insomnia, mood swings, and other symptoms associated with menopause. This chapter highlights 8 herbs in the modern herbal pharmacopeia used primarily to treat women's health-related issues. Most have a long history of traditional use. Several have been, and continue to be, the subject of laboratory tests and clinical research trials; results of a few of these investigations support some of the actions claimed to be associated with use of these herbs.

The first herb in this chapter, black cohosh *(Actaea racemosa)*, has become remarkably popular in the United States in recent years as an herbal remedy for both menstrual and menopausal complaints; it is often recommended by herbalists as an alternative to HRT. Black haw *(Viburnum prunifolium)*, like black cohosh a native North American herb, is also commonly recommended for alleviating menopausal symptoms as well as calming uterine spasms that may lead to miscarriage. Chaste tree *(Vitex agnus-castus)* may be far less familiar to the average American woman than either black cohosh or black haw. Thought in ancient times to dull sexual desire, chaste tree is used in modern herbal medicine primarily to help correct menstrual disorders and ease symptoms of PMS.

Urinary tract infections are a common problem for some women, and downing a glass of cranberry juice to help keep them at bay is a practice that dates to at least the last century. Research on cranberry *(Vaccinium macrocarpon)* has documented that the fruits of this herb contain substances that interfere with the ability of bacteria to cling to the lining of the urinary tract, thus preventing infection. Dong quai *(Angelica sinensis)* is an ancient herb used in traditional Chinese medicine to treat a variety of women's health problems. Herbalists in the West recommend it for a wide variety of menstrual conditions. They recommend raspberry leaf *(Rubus idaeus)* as a pregnancy herb, to relax uterine muscles prior to and during labor. Shatavari *(Asparagus racemosus)* has its origins in Ayurvedic medicine, where it has been used for centuries as an herb with rejuvenating properties, one that can help women cope with stress, stimulate the body's defenses, and strengthen the organs and activities of the female reproductive system. Western herbalists often suggest shatavari to strengthen the uterine wall, bring relief from PMS, and improve chances of conception. The last herb presented in Chapter 7, soy *(Glycine max)*, may be more familiar to many as a food. Because soy is a source of isoflavones—plant "estrogens" that are chemically similar to the female hormone estrogen—some women use soy to help relieve the more troublesome symptoms of menopause. However, many medical professionals caution that soy should be used with care by women who have a history of breast cancer or are at high risk for the disease, as isoflavones may stimulate the estrogen receptors of breast cancer cells, causing them to grow.

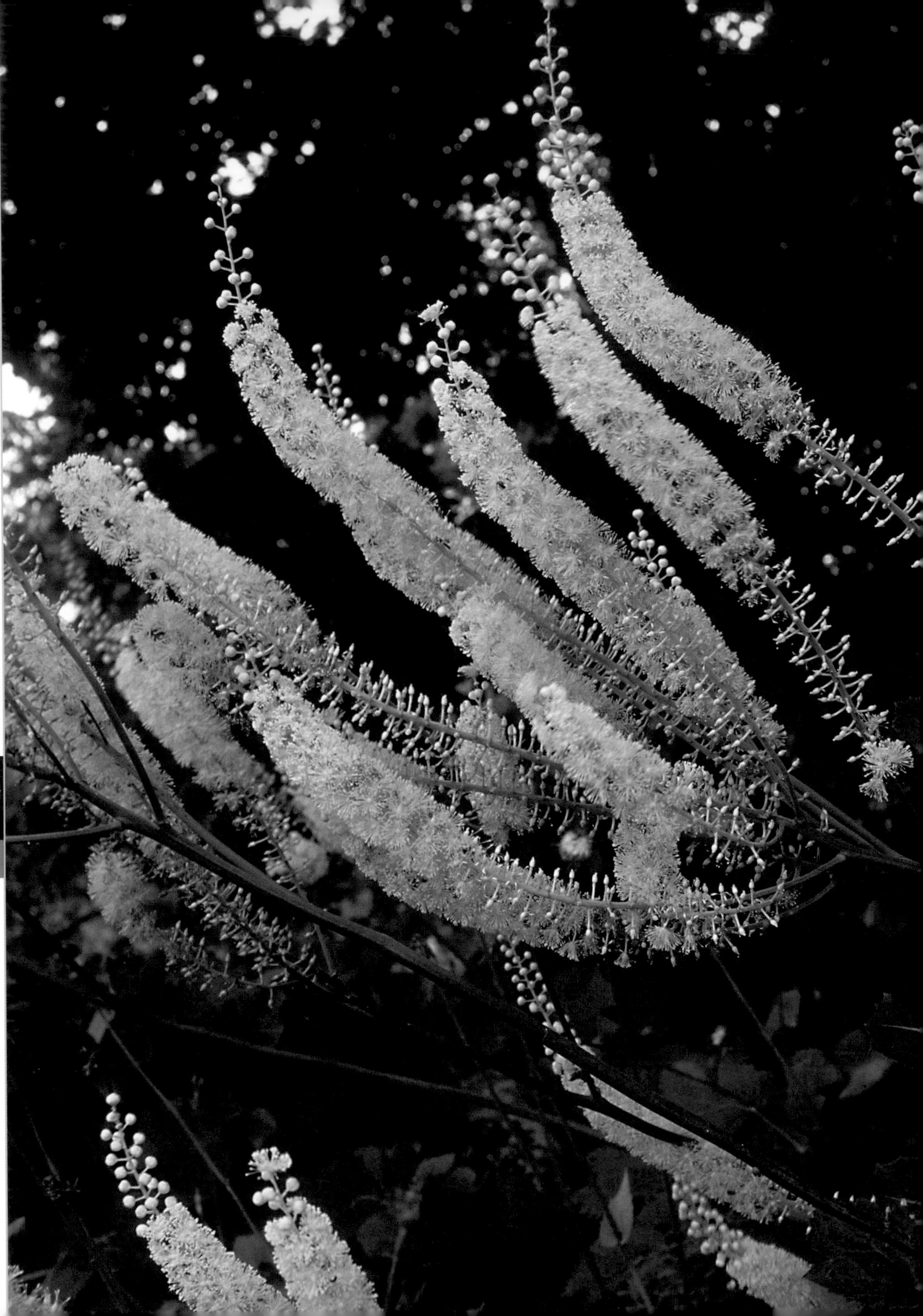

Black Cohosh

Actaea racemosa

Native to eastern North America, black cohosh thrives in moist, shaded woodlands. Over time, it has also become a popular garden perennial, where it rarely goes unnoticed. Shortly after midsummer, black cohosh begins sending up tall flower stalks covered with tiny, pearl-shaped buds. As the buds open, the stalks take on the look of soft, white bottle brushes towering above the dark green foliage. The fact that honeybees scorn the flowers, but flies and beetles love them, may be the source of at least 2 of black cohosh's other common names, bugbane and

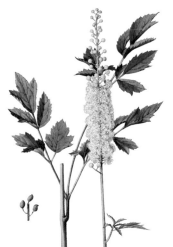

bugwort, respectively. Another is black snakeroot. To understand its source, dig around the base of the plant and expose its twisted **rhizomes**, like dark little snakes.

For many centuries, Native Americans throughout the eastern U.S. prized these sinuous roots. The Delaware, for example, used the roots in herbal mixtures drunk as women's tonics. The Iroquois applied it externally to ease the pain of aching joints; the Algonquin took it internally for kidney problems. The Cherokee used black cohosh as a **diuretic** and to treat fatigue and tuberculosis. European settlers to the eastern United States observed how native tribes used black cohosh and incorporated the plant into their own herbal medicine chest. Preparations of the roots were a cure for fevers, sore throat, malaria, and general malaise, but they were most widely used to treat rheumatism, menstrual irregularities, and pain following childbirth. Nineteenth-century doctors recommended black cohosh for arthritis pain relief and nervous tension; it was also incorporated into a variety of patent medicines and pills promoted for "women's complaints." Yet by the 20th century black cohosh was all but forgotten in the U.S., but not in Europe.

For at least 40 years, black cohosh has been widely prescribed in Europe for menstrual cramps, premenstrual discomfort, and menopausal symptoms. In the U.S., it has recently experienced a comeback. Herbal practitioners recommend it for hot flashes, night sweats, and vaginal dryness, as well as irritability, mood swings, and anxiety. It may be an effective alternative for women who cannot or will not take hormone replacement therapy.

Feathery plumes sway above black cohosh's dark foliage; its roots are used to allay troubling menopausal symptoms.

TIME LINE OF USAGE AND SPREAD

1705
Black cohosh is first described by botanists.

1820
Black cohosh is listed in the *Pharmacopeia of the United States* as "black snakeroot."

1876
Lydia Pinkham sells black cohosh patent remedy for menstrual complaints.

1955
Black cohosh is marketed in Germany under the trade name Remifemin.

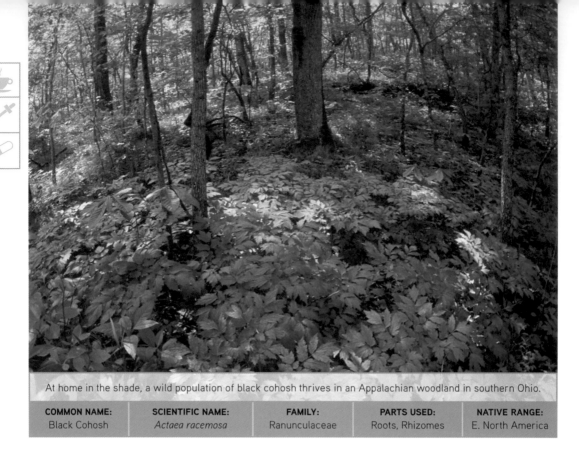

At home in the shade, a wild population of black cohosh thrives in an Appalachian woodland in southern Ohio.

COMMON NAME:	SCIENTIFIC NAME:	FAMILY:	PARTS USED:	NATIVE RANGE:
Black Cohosh	*Actaea racemosa*	Ranunculaceae	Roots, Rhizomes	E. North America

Black cohosh is a bold, beautiful woodland wildflower, long placed in the genus *Cimicifuga* but now included among the 12 species of *Actaea*. This native North American perennial grows from about 1½ feet before blooming to a graceful 7 feet in flower. The leaves are divided in 3 parts. The terminal leaflet on each leaf group is tri-lobed, with the middle lobe the largest. The leaf base is more or less heart shaped or triangular, and the margins on the upper half of the leaflets have sharply serrated teeth. The delicate flowers are without petals but have showy displays of numerous white stamens. The flowers are borne on long, slender wands easily spotted from a distance. Populations of dozens of individual plants may include only a few blooming plants. In the southern part of its range, black cohosh begins flowering in late May; blooming continues in the north into early September.

Growing Habits

Black cohosh, like goldenseal and American ginseng, is a plant of rich habitats in the eastern **deciduous** forest. Generally found on slopes and at the edge of bottomland forest, black cohosh ranges from southern Ontario south to the Appalachians in northern Georgia, west to Arkansas, north to Wisconsin. Though usually found in the deep shade of forests, in woods that have been clear-cut, black cohosh will continue to grow for several years, sometimes even in full sun.

The **genus** name *Actaea* comes from *aktara*, a classical name referring to elms. The reference is to the superficial resemblance of the leaflets to elm leaves.

Cultivation and Harvesting

Black cohosh is relatively easy to grow, given a moderately rich, somewhat moist, shady situation. Propagation is achieved by sowing seeds in a well-prepared seedbed as soon as they are ripe in autumn, for germination in spring, or by dividing roots in early spring, or autumn. Plants should be given a spacing of 2 feet. The plant thrives under cultivation and is adaptable to relatively poor, acidic, rocky woodland soils despite its preference for moist woodland soil. It makes a good back border for a lightly shaded area in an herb garden.

In the late 1990s concern arose over large-scale harvest of wild black cohosh in Appalachia. However, at about the same time, the primary manufacturer of black cohosh **extracts** in Europe developed efficient propagation methods for large-scale plantings and started growing it as a field crop in northern Europe without shade. Today the root is supplied from Europe and China and wild-harvested in the Appalachians and Ozarks.

Therapeutic Uses

+ *Menopause*
+ *Premenstrual syndrome*
+ *Menstrual cramps*
+ *Arthritis*
+ *Mild depression (melancholy)*

The primary use for black cohosh is to treat menopause-related symptoms. Germany's health authorities recognize its use for menopausal symptoms (hot flashes, night sweats, sleep disturbances), as well as for premenstrual syndrome and menstrual cramping. Early studies suggested that black cohosh acted like a natural **estrogen,** or **phytoestrogen**, gently reducing hot flashes and vaginal dryness. But newer research has found no hormonal effects of black cohosh in menopausal women.

More than 20 published clinical trials have evaluated the effectiveness of black cohosh for menopausal hot flashes. While some studies show a modest reduction in symptoms, not all clinical trials have been positive. There may be added benefit when black cohosh is combined with St. John's wort. One clinical trial of 301 women reported a 50 percent reduction in symptoms with the combination compared with 19 percent reduction in the **placebo** group. At this time, it is impossible to determine the effectiveness of black cohosh for hot flashes.

Scientists at the University of Illinois at Chicago have demonstrated that **compounds** in black cohosh act as antidepressants and reduce pain sensitivity, lending support to the traditional use of black cohosh as a treatment for melancholy, or depressed mood, as well as its widespread use as a remedy for arthritis and menstrual pain. No clinical trials have evaluated its effectiveness for these conditions.

How to Use

TEA: Simmer 2 teaspoons of chopped root and rhizome in 2 cups water for 10 minutes. Strain. Drink ¼ cup, 2 to 3 times per day.
CAPSULES: 40 to 200 mg of dried rhizome taken daily, in divided doses.
TINCTURE: Generally, 1 to 2 ml, 3 times per day.
STANDARDIZED EXTRACT: 20 to 40 mg black cohosh extract twice daily. Products are often standardized to provide 1 to 2 mg of 27-deoxyactein.

Precautions

Except for minor gastrointestinal upset, clinical trials have shown black cohosh to be free of side effects. A few reports have suggested black cohosh may, in rare cases, cause damage to the liver, prompting European, Australian, Canadian, and British health authorities to require product labels suggesting conferral with a health care provider by anyone with any type liver disease. Safety during pregnancy and breast-feeding is not known.

---

over the (kitchen) counter MENOPAUSE TINCTURE

Mix ½ ounce black cohosh rhizome, ½ ounce shatavari, and ½ ounce chaste tree fruit in a coffee grinder. Grind herbs and place in a quart jar. Pour 6 ounces vodka or brandy over herbs and stir well. Close lid tightly and shake gently. Let sit for 14 days and then strain liquid through cheesecloth or a piece of muslin. Put strained liquid in a dark glass jar. This tincture can be used during the menopausal transition. Take 5 ml (1 teaspoon) morning and night.

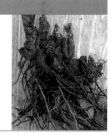

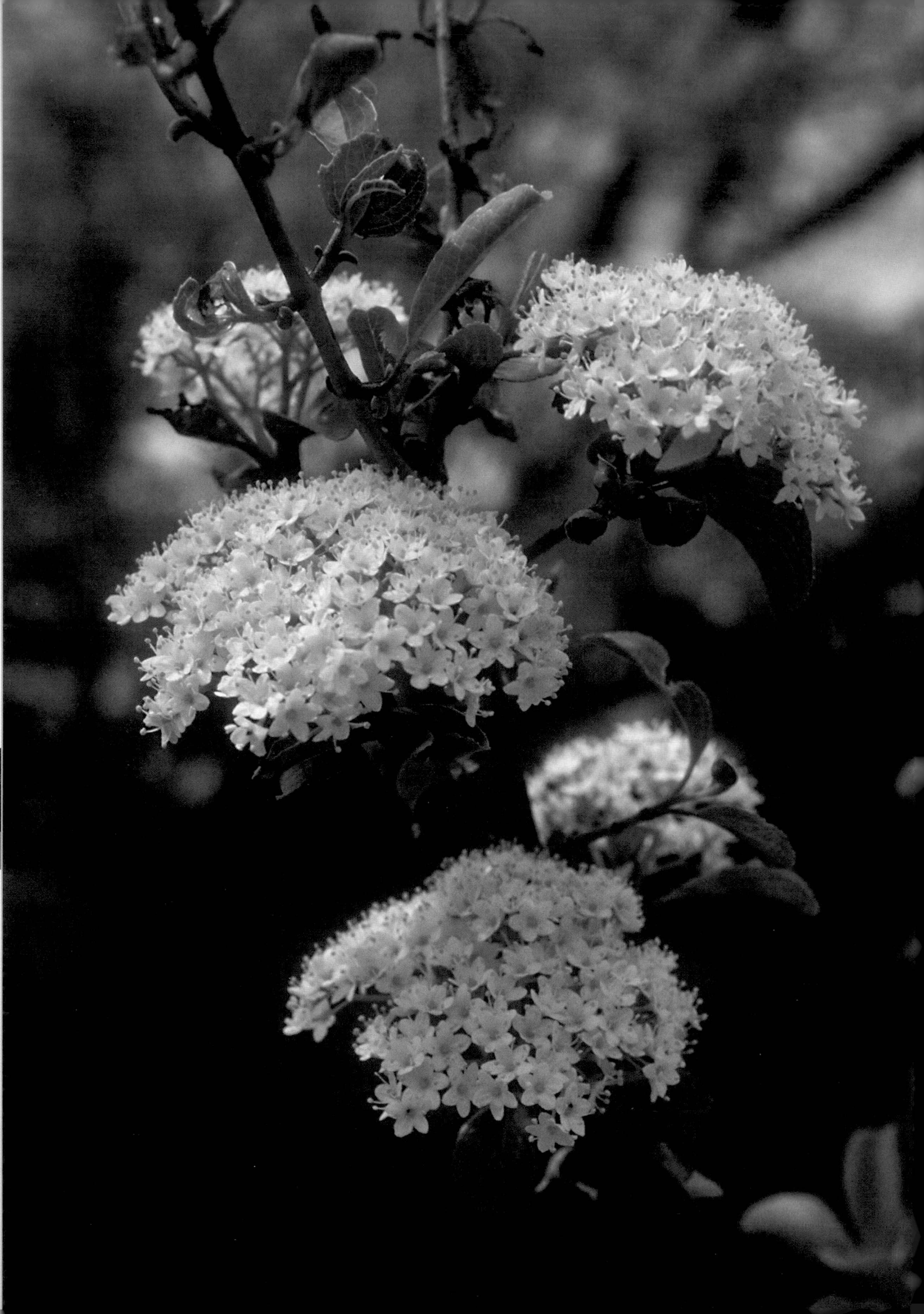

Black Haw

❦ Viburnum prunifolium ❦

The glossy green leaves of black haw turn to a brilliant reddish-purple in autumn, a transformation that turns these large, woody shrubs into beacons of color in moist woods and thickets of eastern and central North America. The "haw" in black haw refers to the sweet, olive-size, blue-black fruits that hang in pendulous clusters and persist well into winter. Where black haw grows abundantly, the fruits are eaten fresh and made into jams and jellies, sauces, and drinks. Centuries ago, Native Americans valued these forest fruits that were available for such an

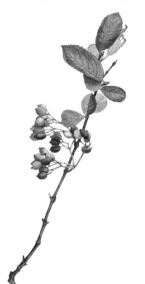

extended season. They also used the fawn-colored bark of black haw roots, stems, and branches medicinally. The Cherokee and other tribes brewed a tea from black haw bark that women drank to ease menstrual cramps, prevent miscarriage, and calm uterine spasms after childbirth. Black haw preparations were also remedies for muscle spasms, fever, and smallpox.

Black haw was quickly adopted as a medicinal by European settlers, primarily as a remedy for menstrual complaints. It was frequently called crampbark, because it successfully relaxed muscle cramps—especially muscles of the uterus. Not until the middle of the 1800s, however, did black haw catch the serious attention of the American medical community. In the 1860s, physician D. L. Pares began promoting black haw as a tonic for toning muscles of the uterus and to prevent miscarriage and abortion. It was also given to regulate irregular menstruation and alleviate pelvic discomfort. Although not all physicians believed in black haw's medicinal value, it was added to the *United States Pharmacopeia* in 1882, where it remained until 1926.

Herbal practitioners and **naturopathic** doctors still recommend black haw, primarily to ease menstrual pain and cramping. They also suggest it to treat menopausal symptoms and calm uterine muscles, particularly in cases where muscle spasms might lead to miscarriage. Black haw preparations are also taken to treat uterine prolapse, morning sickness, and heavy menstruation. Black haw's antispasmodic properties are helpful in treating asthma, lowering blood pressure, and alleviating cramping pains in the digestive and urinary tracts.

Used for centuries in folk medicine, black haw bark contains compounds that relax muscles in the uterine wall.

TIME LINE OF USAGE AND SPREAD

1597
Herbalist J. Gerard suggests black haw-related species for swelling and inflammation.

1866
Black haw is introduced into U.S. medicine by E. W. Jenks of Detroit, Michigan.

1878
American Eclectic physician J. King notes black haw's use in preventing miscarriages.

1883
Physicians question black haw's medicinal value in the *U.S. Pharmacopeia.*

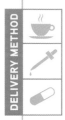
Viburnums are small trees and shrubs represented by many horticultural selections grown for their impressive displays of white flowers, attractive fruits, and bold fall leaf colors. Of the 210 species of *Viburnum*, 3 are found in Europe, with the greatest genetic diversity split between South America and eastern Asia. China has some 70 *Viburnum* species. In eastern North America more than a dozen species are common.

Black haw is a **deciduous** shrub or small tree, from 6 to 30 feet tall. The opposite, elliptical, or oval dull green (not glossy) leaves are finely toothed, papery, and mostly smooth (without hairs). The white flowers, in showy flat clusters, bloom March to May. The small fruits are bluish black when ripe. European *V. opulus* var. *opulus,* or crampbark, used like black haw, is a shrub that grows to 12 feet with maplelike leaves and bright red berries.

Growing Habits

Black haw is widespread in the eastern United States, growing in pastures and forest bottomlands, dry upland forest bluffs, and along riverbanks and brooks, roadsides, and fencerows. It occurs from Connecticut south to Georgia, west to Texas, north to Wisconsin. The European *V. opulus* var. *opulus* is found throughout much of Europe and North Africa. Much cultivated as an ornamental shrub, it has become naturalized but is infrequent in disturbed areas and thickets near urban areas in North America.

Cultivation and Harvesting

Viburnums are among the most widely planted shrubs, valued for their showy flowers, and in some **species** highly ornamental fruits. Black haw was adopted in European horticulture nearly 300 years ago, favored as a deciduous hedge as well as a small tree that can be pruned to form an excellent screen. Its edible blue-black fruits are both beautiful and sweet,

FEMALE HEALTH

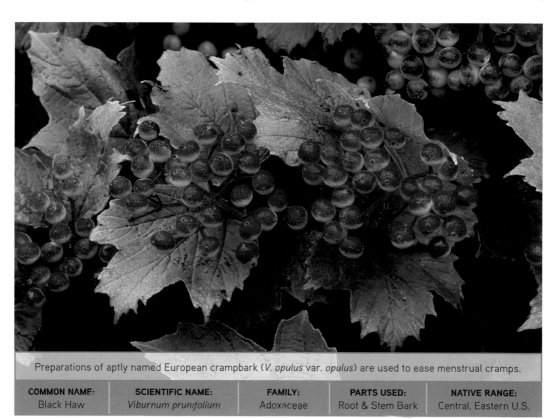

Preparations of aptly named European crampbark (*V. opulus* var. *opulus*) are used to ease menstrual cramps.

COMMON NAME:	SCIENTIFIC NAME:	FAMILY:	PARTS USED:	NATIVE RANGE:
Black Haw	*Viburnum prunifolium*	Adoxaceae	Root & Stem Bark	Central, Eastern U.S.

Combine ½ ounce black haw root bark with ¼ ounce ginger root. Grind the herbs in a coffee grinder and place in a 1-quart jar. Add 4 ounces vodka or brandy. Stir well. Close tightly and shake gently. Let sit for 14 days and then strain the liquid through cheesecloth or a piece of muslin. Put liquid in a dark glass jar. This tincture can be used to ease menstrual cramping. Take 5 ml (1 teaspoon) every 4 to 6 hours as needed.

sometimes used to make jams and jellies. Propagation is by softwood cuttings in early summer. Most species of *Viburnum* prefer a relatively rich, moist soil, but the adaptable black haw is tolerant of dry soils.

The branch and trunk bark of black haw is the part used in herbal medicine, sourced from wild trees in the eastern and central U.S. It is likely, however, that other *Viburnum* species enter the commercial supply of wild-harvested material, given their occurrence in similar habitats. Traditionally, the bark of crampbark is used like black haw, but crampbark is considered an adulterant to commercial supplies of black haw.

Therapeutic Uses

+ *Menstrual cramps*
+ *Intestinal cramps*
+ *Muscle cramps*

Black haw was widely used in folk medicine to ease muscle cramping, menstrual cramping, and intestinal cramping; to prevent miscarriage; to relieve pain after childbirth; and to treat asthma. In the mid-19th century, American **Eclectic** physicians regarded black haw as a valuable uterine tonic. Midwives and early physicians recommended to women prone to miscarriage that they drink black haw tea daily to quiet what was known as an irritable womb. It was used to ease menstrual cramping, especially when the cramping was accompanied by heavy bleeding. American Indian women also used it to ease the heavy bleeding that sometimes accompanied menopause.

Black haw is still widely used by many midwives in the traditional ways—to relieve pain

following a birth and, to a lesser extent, to prevent miscarriage. Many herbal products in the modern marketplace designed to ease menstrual cramping contain black haw or its close relative crampbark *(Viburnum opulus)*. Animal studies have confirmed that **compounds** in the bark of the root and stems relax the uterus, trachea, and small intestine by interacting with beta-adrenergic receptors in the smooth muscles—the same mechanism that many prescription drugs work to relax these tissues. Yet, despite the praise of practitioners, both past and present, and the animal data, there are no human studies evaluating the antispasmodic effects of black haw.

How to Use

TEA: Simmer 2 teaspoons dried root or stem bark in 1 cup water for 5 to 7 minutes. Strain. Drink ¼ cup every 2 to 3 hours, to 2 cups daily.
CAPSULES: Typically, 1,000 mg is taken 3 times per day.
TINCTURE: Take 5 to 10 ml of the **tincture** 3 times per day.

Precautions

No adverse effects from the use of black haw are reported in medical literature. Black haw appears to be safe for short-term relief of menstrual or intestinal cramping. Black haw may contain small amounts of **salicin**, a compound related to aspirin. Those allergic to aspirin could theoretically be allergic to black haw, though this has not been reported. Black haw should not be used during pregnancy except under the direction of a health care professional.

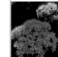

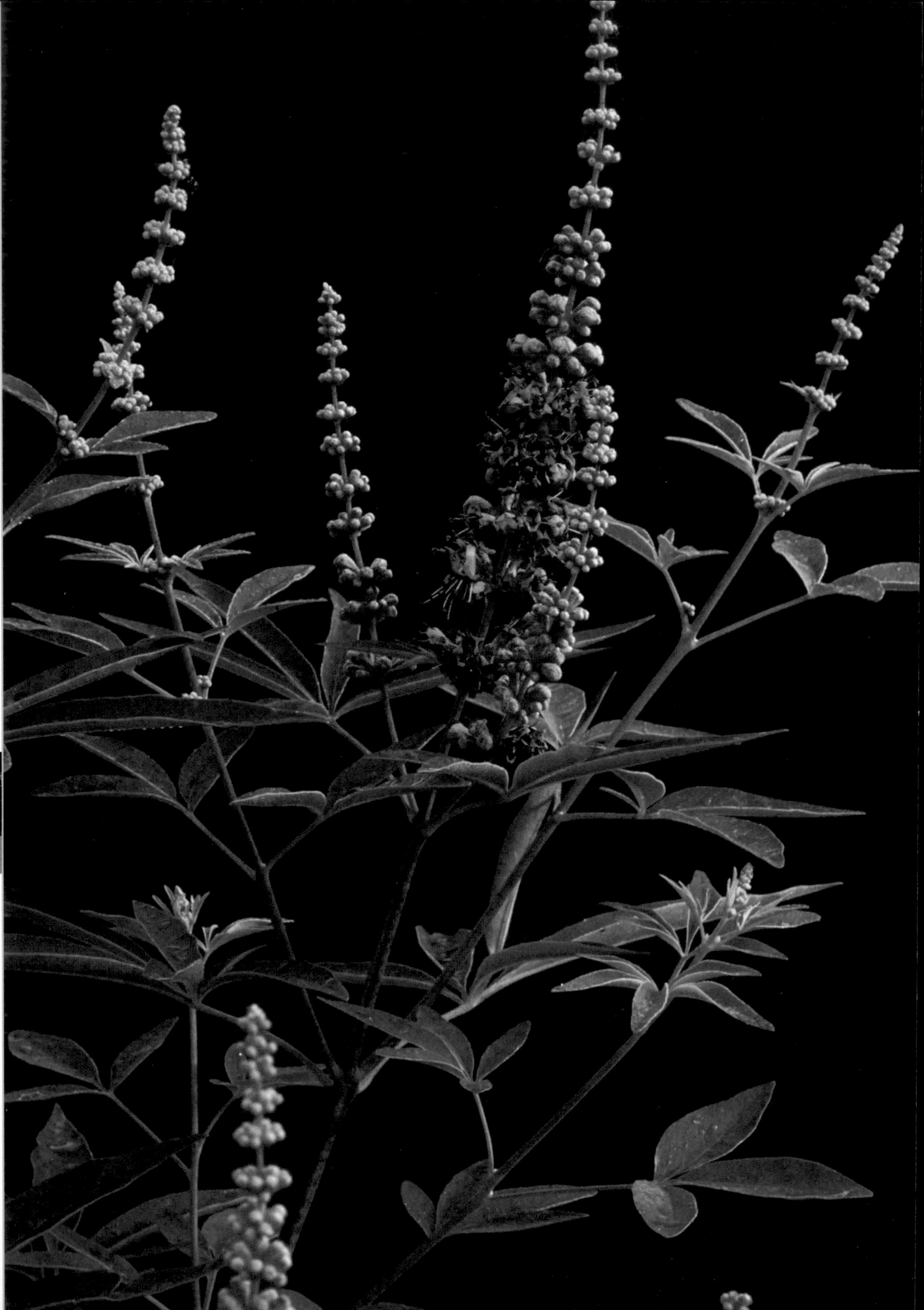

Chaste Tree

❧ *Vitex agnus-castus* ☙

Chaste tree often suffers from mistaken identity. People may do a double take when they first glimpse the leaves of this small tree, as their resemblance to the leaves of marijuana *(Cannabis sativa)* is striking. A blooming chaste tree is also frequently thought to be butterfly bush *(Buddleia)*, because both plants produce long clusters of violet flowers beloved by bees, butterflies, and hummingbirds. The flowers are followed by small, fleshy fruits that contain dark brown seeds easily mistaken for peppercorns, both in appearance and taste. These seeds are

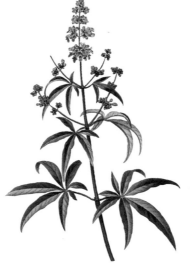

chaste tree's link to chastity, forged more than 2,500 years ago. In ancient Greece, chaste tree was thought to calm sexual passion. It was an important component of festivals held to honor Demeter, the goddess of agriculture, fertility, and marriage. Women who remained chaste during the festival adorned themselves with the tree's fragrant blossoms. The vestal virgins of ancient Rome carried twigs of chaste tree. As a symbol of purity, chaste tree was later adopted by the Catholic Church in medieval Europe. Novitiates entering a monastery followed a path strewn with chaste tree blossoms. Chaste tree seeds, believed to suppress sexual desire, were ground and served in monastery dining halls to encourage celibacy—thus the common name, monk's pepper.

Chastity and celibacy aside, chaste tree has been used for several thousand years to treat gynecological problems. Ancient physicians, including Pliny the Elder, Dioscorides, and Theophrastus, wrote of chaste tree's value for easing menstrual difficulties and for stimulating production of breast milk. In the Middle Ages, women took chaste tree for menstrual problems. In the mid-1900s, German researchers demonstrated how the herb helps balance hormones associated with gynecological health.

Today, European gynecologists and Western herbal practitioners recommend chaste tree preparations to manage menstrual disorders, including premenstrual syndrome (PMS). Women also take the herb to relieve some of the symptoms of menopause, such as hot flashes.

Since medieval times, herbalists have used chaste tree fruits to ease menstrual and menopausal problems.

TIME LINE OF USAGE AND SPREAD

4TH CENTURY B.C.
Greek physician Hippocrates notes chaste tree's use for menstrual conditions.

A.D. 1570
Chaste tree is introduced to English gardens.

1633
Herbalist J. Gerard suggests chaste tree and pennyroyal to stimulate menstruation.

1950s
German researcher develops a patent medicine containing chaste tree extract.

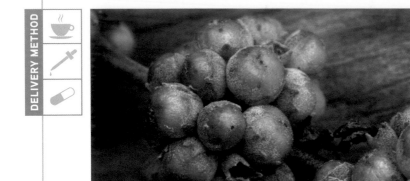

Borne in compact clusters, chaste tree fruits turn dark when ripe and are easily mistaken for peppercorns.

COMMON NAME:	SCIENTIFIC NAME:	FAMILY:	PARTS USED:	NATIVE RANGE:
Chaste Tree	*Vitex agnus-castus*	Verbenaceae	Fruits	SW Asia, S. Europe

FEMALE HEALTH

There are more than 250 tropical species in the genus *Vitex*, but only 1 species, *Vitex agnus-castus,* is found in Europe. Chaste tree is a highly aromatic shrub or small tree ranging from 3 to 18 feet in height. The fruit-bearing twigs are densely covered with short, resinous hairs, sticky to the touch. The leaves are palmate (leaflets radiating from a central point), with usually 5 to 9 nearly lance-shaped to elliptical leaflets, pointed at both ends, up to 6 inches long, and less than an inch wide. The leaf margin is without teeth or has wavy edges. The leaves are grayish green and mostly smooth above; beneath, the leaves are lighter in color, with dense hairs. The small tubular, lavender to lilac, 5-lobed flowers are crowded into triangular groupings up to a foot in length. The flowers, blooming from May through October, are about ¼ inch long. The seeds (fruits) are light brown when ripe and smaller than a peppercorn. They closely hug the stem in whorled clusters.

Growing Habits

Native to southwestern Asia and southern Europe, chaste tree has been grown since ancient times and has spread throughout Europe, cultivated in England as early as 1570. Introduced to American horticulture in the early 19th century, it is today naturalized in much of the South, west to Texas, north to Arkansas and southeastern Oklahoma.

Vitex derives from an ancient designation, *vei,* meaning to "wind," "bend," or "twine," referring to the use of the tough, flexible branches in constructing woven wattle fences. The **species** name *agnus-castus* derives from a historical misinterpretation of the original Greek name, *ágnos,* first applied by Roman physician Dioscorides and translated as "holy," "pure," or "chaste." *Castus* derives from the Latin *castitas,* meaning "chastity. "

Cultivation and Harvesting

Chaste tree is one of the few species in the **genus** that grows in warm, temperate climates. It will survive freezing temperatures to –20°F. It does well if placed in a warm area, against a stone wall or foundation, as far north as southern Missouri or Maryland. Chaste tree prefers full sun and likes a moderately fertile, well-drained, light soil.

The fruits are the part used. Commercial production occurs on specialized farms in Italy, and chaste tree is now also commercially grown in China. The leaves are **deciduous**, and the small fruits cling to the branch once the leaves drop. The seeds are easily stripped from the stem by hand, or a modified combine can be run through a plantation where plants are coppiced, or cut back, from 3 to 6 feet in height to facilitate mechanical harvest.

Therapeutic Uses

+ *Premenstrual syndrome (PMS)*
+ *Breast tenderness (mastalgia)*

Premenstrual syndrome (PMS) involves a number of physical, psychological, and emotional symptoms occurring 5 to 10 days before a woman's menstrual period. It is estimated that up to 90 percent of women experience occasional PMS. The dried fruits of chaste tree have repeatedly been shown to dramatically improve the symptoms of PMS. Germany's health authorities recommend the herb for the treatment of PMS, menstrual irregularity, and mastalgia, or breast tenderness.

A three-month study published in the *British Medical Journal* evaluated the effectiveness of chaste tree in 178 women with PMS. Chaste tree users showed a significant improvement in PMS symptoms such as irritability, moodiness, anger, headache, and breast fullness. Overall, the reduction in PMS symptoms was 52 percent for women taking chaste tree versus 24 percent for those taking **placebo**.

Another randomized placebo-controlled study of chaste tree was conducted in Beijing, China, involving 208 women with PMS. Women taking a 40-mg chaste tree **extract** had a significant reduction in PMS symptoms compared with those taking placebo.

When the psychological symptoms of PMS are more severe (premenstrual dysphoric disorder), the condition is typically treated with antidepressant medication. A randomized controlled trial found that chaste tree was roughly equivalent to fluoxetine (Prozac) for improving psychological and physical symptoms.

Chaste tree is sometimes recommended for women having difficulty conceiving. Chaste tree extracts, used daily for at least 3 months, have been shown to restore **progesterone** levels, which may improve female fertility. However, more investigation needs to be done before recommendations can be made.

How to Use

TEA: Steep ½ teaspoon of the dried chaste tree fruit in 1 cup of hot water for 5 to 7 minutes. Strain. Drink 1 cup each morning. Note: The tea is somewhat spicy and acrid in taste.

CAPSULES: 250 to 500 mg of dried chaste tree fruit taken once per day.

TINCTURE: 2 to 3 ml of **tincture** taken daily each morning.

STANDARDIZED EXTRACT: 20 to 40 mg of chaste tree extract taken once per day.

Precautions

Chaste tree appears to be extremely well tolerated in clinical trials. While no adverse effects have been reported in pregnancy, women should consult a health care provider before using chaste tree for infertility.

over the (kitchen) counter CHASTE TREE FRUIT TEA

Combine ½ cup dried chaste tree fruits and 1 cup dried motherwort (*Leonurus cardiaca*). Add to 2 to 3 cups boiling water. Reduce heat and simmer gently for 10 minutes. Cover and steep for about 15 minutes. Strain. Add honey. Drink 2 to 4 cups daily for menstrual irregularities or for premenstrual syndrome (PMS).

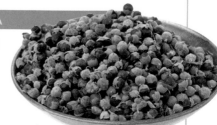

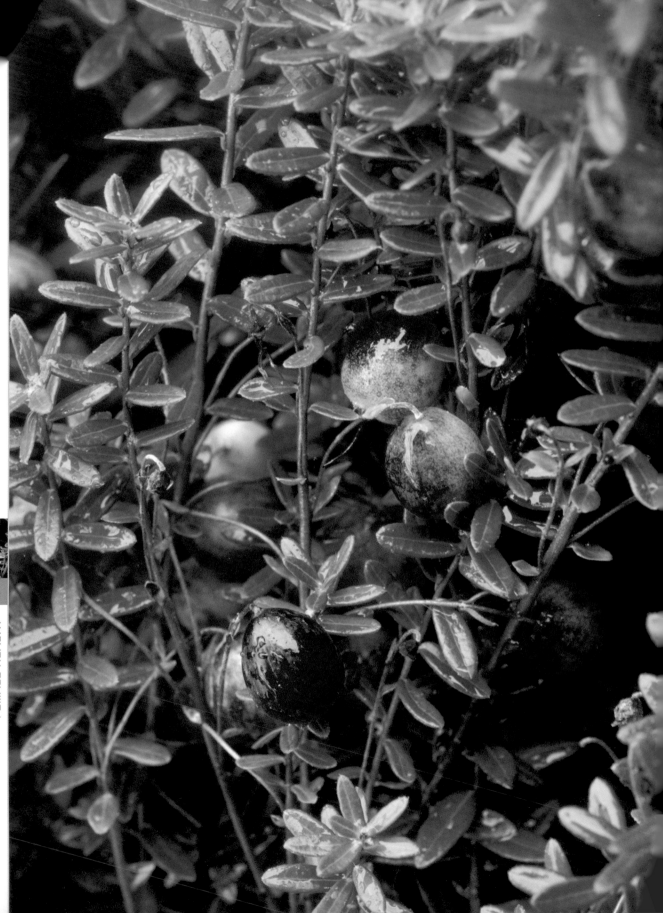

Cranberry

Vaccinium macrocarpon

Ruby red and exceedingly tart, the American cranberry is native to the swamps and bogs of northeastern North America. It can still be found growing wild in parts of its native range, which extends from eastern Canada south to the mountains of Georgia and west as far as Minnesota. Most of the cranberries that now find their way into foods and drinks—and grace millions of Thanksgiving tables—are cultivated on large commercial farms. Cranberry shares the genus *Vaccinium* with a number of other popular berries, including blueberry, huckleberry, and bilberry.

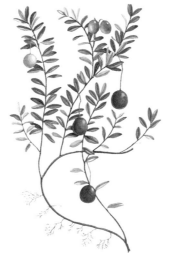

The word "cranberry" is probably derived from "crane berry," a term coined by Dutch and German colonists either because the flowers looked to them like the head and neck of a crane or because cranes flocked to cranberry bogs when fruits were ripe.

Cranberries were an important food for Native Americans. They ate the berries cooked and sweetened with maple syrup or honey and as an ingredient in pemmican, a nutritious, high-calorie mixture of dried venison, fat, and dried fruit that was an essential winter staple. The Indians also employed cranberry medicinally; it was applied as a **poultice** for cuts and abrasions and arrow wounds, and as a cure for indigestion, kidney diseases, and lung ailments. Native Americans introduced the cranberry to European colonists, who quickly adopted it as both food and medicine. It became a remedy for digestive problems, gallbladder attacks, blood disorders, and kidney stones. In the same way that British sailors used limes, New England sailors and whalers ate cranberries while at sea to prevent scurvy.

In the late 1800s, cranberry gained popularity to treat urinary tract complaints. Research revealed that the herb keeps bacteria from adhering to the lining of the bladder and urethra. In herbal and conventional medicine today, cranberry is widely used to prevent—not treat—urinary tract infections. Herbal practitioners also recommend it for kidney and bladder stones, incontinence, and prostate problems. It also may help prevent bacteria-induced stomach ulcers, lower **LDL** ("bad") **cholesterol** in the blood, and, in the lab, inhibit growth of some types of cancer cells.

Tasty but tart, cranberries have bacteria-fighting substances with proven power to prevent urinary tract infections.

TIME LINE OF USAGE AND SPREAD

1647
The word "cranberry" first appears in a letter written by missionary John Eliot.

1816
Cranberries are first cultivated in the U.S. by Henry Hall on Cape Cod.

1860s
Cranberry production skyrockets because of demand during the Civil War.

1930
Ocean Spray Cranberries is formed as a grower-owned marketing cooperative.

Cranberry, an edible fruit and the stuff of jelly and juice, is also a medicinal herb. The genus *Vaccinium* encompasses about 140 species, including other familiar fruits such as blueberries. Much like *Aloe vera*, cranberry juice is a quintessential American folk remedy and, in the popular mind, a sure cure for urinary infections. That folk belief prompted scientists to begin to investigate cranberry's medicinal potential nearly a hundred years ago.

Cranberries do not grow on trees. In fact, the largest feature of the small shrub is the fruit itself. A mostly evergreen shrub, cranberry grows to scarcely 6 to 8 inches tall. The small elliptical, leathery leaves are about a half inch long. The white to pink, urnlike flowers hang like tiny bells. The bright familiar fruits are the cranberries of commerce.

Growing Habits

Cranberry grows in wet, acidic habitats, notably sphagnum moss bogs, as well as in swamps, heathlands, and wet freshwater shores in much of the Northeast and upper Midwest. It ranges from Newfoundland to Manitoba, through New England south to Virginia, westward to Ohio, northern Illinois, Wisconsin, and Minnesota. It is also found in the mountains of North Carolina and Tennessee. It is naturalized in the West, in Washington, Oregon, and British Columbia in Canada, following introduction for commercial cultivation.

The designation "large-fruited" cranberry distinguishes our supermarket cranberry from the small cranberry *V. oxycoccos*, a diminutive plant that occurs throughout the northerly regions of the Northern Hemisphere, notably the north of Europe but also North America in bogs south to New Jersey, Pennsylvania, and Minnesota. It has considerably smaller fruits, which turn brownish red and are not as visually appealing as the common cranberry; it is mostly available in Europe.

The **genus** name *Vaccinium* comes from an ancient Greek word derived from prehistoric Mediterranean languages, referring to berry-producing shrubs. The **species** name, *macrocarpon*, is a reference to its large fruits.

Cultivation and Harvesting

Cranberry is a specialty crop grown in bog habitats in the United States as a highly specialized farming enterprise. The primary cranberry fruit production states are Wisconsin, Massachusetts, Oregon, New Jersey, and Washington. As a fresh produce specialty fruit, once harvested it is measured in barrels rather than tonnage. On average, 6 to 7 million barrels of fresh cranberries are harvested in the main cranberry production states. Since it is such a small plant, and each plant produces only a few fruits, cranberries are grown in wet soils that can be flooded with a few inches of water at harvest time. The berries, which are still attached to the plant, float on the water's surface, where they can be harvested by hand with specialized rakes or harvested with machinery specifically designed for the task.

over the (kitchen) counter CRANBERRY TEA

In a large pot, combine 12 cups water and a 12-ounce package of cranberries and bring to a boil. Reduce heat and simmer, covered, for 30 minutes. Add 1½ cups sugar, the juice of 2 oranges and 2 lemons, 10 cloves, and 3 cinnamon sticks. Turn off heat and steep, covered, for 1 hour. The tea (or juice, if you prefer) can be consumed hot or cold. It is not as sweet as many juices, is less expensive, and is a great source of vitamin C. This cranberry drink will keep in the refrigerator for 7 days.

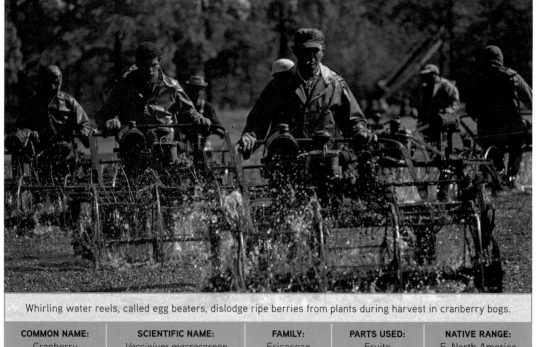

Whirling water reels, called egg beaters, dislodge ripe berries from plants during harvest in cranberry bogs.

COMMON NAME:	SCIENTIFIC NAME:	FAMILY:	PARTS USED:	NATIVE RANGE:
Cranberry	*Vaccinium macrocarpon*	Ericaceae	Fruits	E. North America

Therapeutic Uses

+ *Bladder infections (prevention)*

The herbal remedy most associated with maintaining a healthy urinary tract is the delicious, native North American cranberry. Originally it was thought that cranberry prevented urinary tract infections by acidifying the urine; however, scientists have shown that **compounds** known as **proanthocyanidins** prevent harmful bacteria such as *Escherichia coli* from adhering to the cells that line the bladder and urethra. This is good news given that *E. coli* is responsible for 90 percent of all urinary tract infections.

In 2008, researchers reviewed 7 studies of cranberry juice along with four studies of cranberry **extract** tablets. They concluded that both modes of delivery reduced the risk of a urinary tract infection developing by 35 percent in people who had a history of frequent infections compared with control groups. This research is significant, especially given the statistic that roughly 25 percent of all women will have a recurrent urinary tract infection in their lifetimes.

While the evidence is very strong for the use of cranberry to prevent urinary tract infections, there is, on the other hand, very little evidence that it is an effective treatment once a urinary tract infection is contracted. The best treatment for an acute bladder infection is antibiotics.

Cranberry juice or tablets can also be a very effective urinary deodorant for those who are incontinent.

How to Use

JUICE: Cranberry juice is an easy and tasty way to prevent urinary tract infections. One well-designed study used 10 ounces per day of Ocean Spray cranberry juice.

EXTRACT: Cranberry extract in tablet form has been shown to be as effective, better tolerated, less expensive, and lower in calories when compared with the juice. The dose of concentrated juice extract is 300 to 500 mg, taken twice a day.

 NOTE: Don't like cranberries? Try adding blueberries or blueberry juice to your diet! Blueberry (*Vaccinium angustifolium*) contains similar active ingredients.

Precautions

Given the widespread use of cranberry by the general public, it is safe to say that there are virtually no adverse effects associated with its use. Cranberry is safe during pregnancy and lactation and for children. Although several case reports have indicated a concern for a potential interaction between cranberry juice and warfarin, used to prevent blood clots, human studies have documented no adverse interactions.

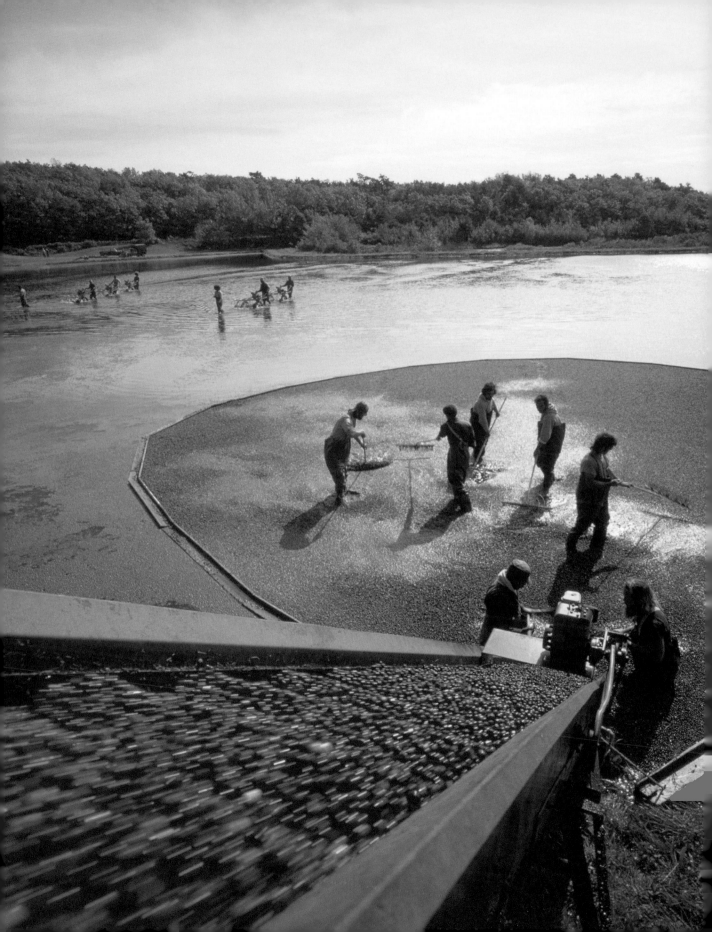

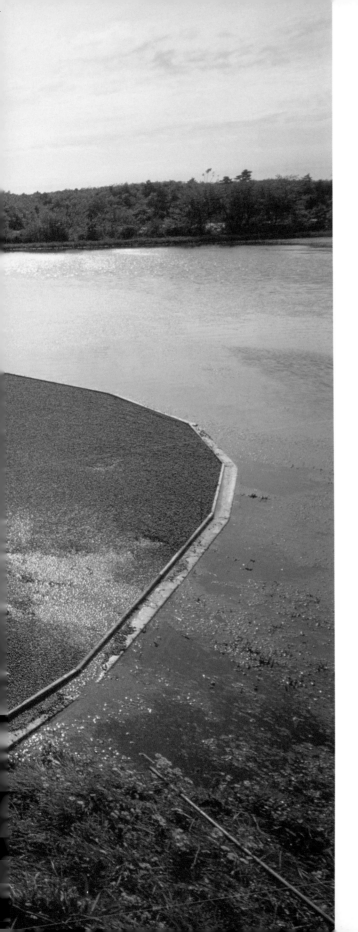

Cranberry Harvest

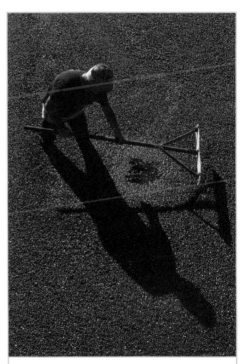

In cranberry-raising regions of the U.S. and Canada, ground-hugging cranberry plants grow in sandy fields called bogs. Because cranberry fruits contain pockets of air, they float in water. As a result, "wet harvesting" is the most common way to gather ripe cranberries. In late autumn, the bogs are flooded with water, typically to a depth of 6 to 8 inches above the tops of the plants. Harvesters move through the bogs driving water reels, machines that agitate the water to help remove the berries from the plants (see p. 293). As berries float to the surface, harvesters such as this cranberry farmer in Oregon (above) use rake-like "brooms" to corral the berries in a corner of the bog (left). Cranberries ride a conveyor belt out of an Oregon cranberry bog as workers keep them consolidated inside the corral. Trucks will carry the berries to cleaning facilities. Wet-harvested cranberries go into making juice and sauce and ingredients in other foods. A small percentage of cranberries are dry-harvested with machines that comb the berries off the plants; these are sold as fresh produce.

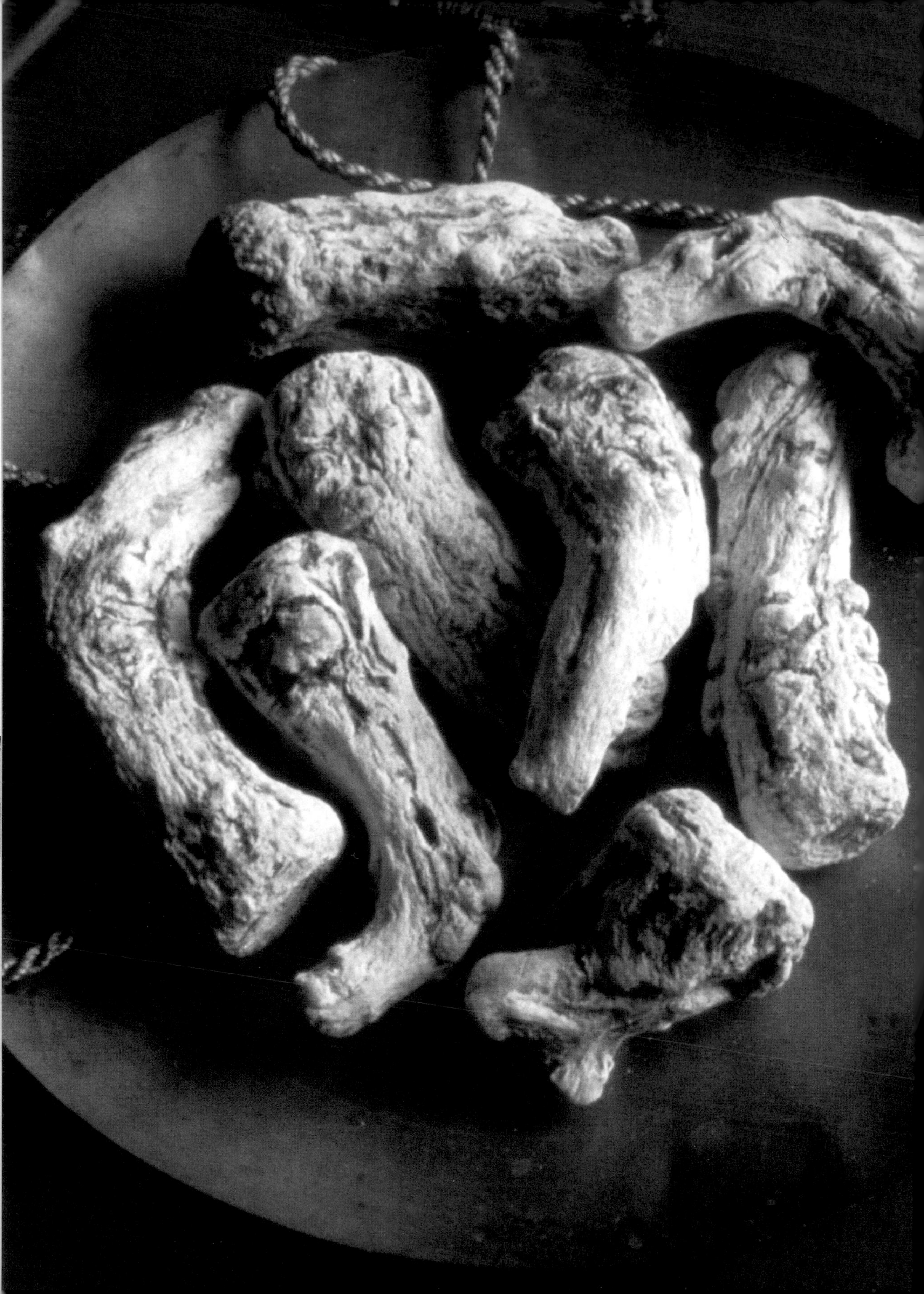

Dong Quai

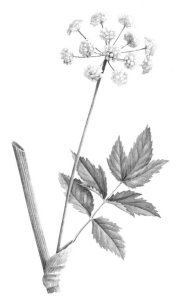 *Angelica sinensis*

Dong quai, also called Chinese angelica, is a member of the celery family native to cold, mountainous regions of central China. It has been used in Chinese, Korean, and Japanese traditional medicine for millennia. According to legend, dong quai made its medicinal debut as a result of a man's desire to prove himself. He set out for the mountains, where he hoped his ability to survive in the wild would attest to his strength and resourcefulness. Before he left, the man told his devoted wife that if he had not returned after 3 years, she should consider him dead and take another husband. Of course, that is precisely what happened. And shortly after the wife had remarried, the man returned. Heartbroken, she fell deathly ill. During his mountain pilgrimage, the man had collected the root from a plant he'd never seen before. He prepared it as a medicine, gave it to his wife, and she was fully restored to health. The name dong quai is often translated as "return to order," because the herb is thought to help restore normal, healthy function to various body systems, and the body as a whole. Dong quai is one of the most widely prescribed herbs in Chinese medicine and is used—typically in combination with other herbs—primarily to treat health problems in women. For this reason, it is sometimes referred to as female ginseng.

In Chinese traditional medicine, different parts of the dong quai root are used. The uppermost part is thought to have anticoagulant properties, the main part tonic actions, and the root tip the ability to prevent blood stagnation. For centuries, Chinese herbalists have used mixtures containing dong quai to treat circulatory, respiratory, and reproductive conditions. Herbal preparations are also taken for strengthening *xue*, "the blood"; relieving headache, infection, and inflammation; improving circulation; and lowering blood pressure.

In the West, herbal practitioners recommend dong quai for women's reproductive problems, including premenstrual syndrome (PMS). Some women also take dong quai to relieve hot flashes and other symptoms of menopause.

Widely used in Asia, dong quai is now popular in Western herbal medicine for treating women's health complaints.

TIME LINE OF USAGE AND SPREAD

CA 1ST CENTURY
First record of use in China in *Divine Farmer's Classic of the Materia Medica.*

1061
Botanical description of dong quai is recorded in *Illustrated Classic of the Materia Medica.*

1596
Ben Cao Gang Mu (Herbalist's Manual) records 27 remedies containing dong quai.

1899
Drug firm Merck introduces dong quai as a "female tonic" called Eumenol.

One of the most famous and most widely used of all Chinese medicinal plants, dong quai is a member of the genus *Angelica*, which includes 110 Northern Hemisphere species, about half of which are from China. Dong quai is a perennial, growing up to 39 inches in height. The ribbed stem is green or purplish. Leaf stems on lower leaves have oval paper sheaths encasing the stem. The much divided leaves, up to about a foot long and 10 inches broad, have numerous divided ovate, lance-shaped leaflets. The leaflets are lobed, with irregularly sharp-toothed margins. The tiny white (rarely purple) flowers are borne on a crowded umbel (umbrella-like) rounded flower-head, with 10 to 30 rays radiating from a central axis. The fruits (seeds) have lateral wings broader than the main part of the fruit. Flowering is from June to July; fruiting, in August and September. All parts of the plant are aromatic.

Growing Habits

Dong quai grows at forest edges and in shrubby thickets, mostly in higher mountain habitats at elevations of 6,000 to 10,000 feet, in central and southern China in Gansu, Hubei, Shaanxi, Sichuan, and Yunnan provinces. It is also cultivated within its natural range. Dong quai is found wild in deep, ancient forests in Gansu, the province best known for dong quai production.

The Chinese name *dang-gui* essentially translates to "proper order" in reference to the herb's health benefits. The English name dong quai is a phonetic spelling of the Chinese name. *Angelica* is the classical name for the plant group, held in high esteem for medicine, flavoring, and fragrance.

Cultivation and Harvesting

Dong quai, which grows at elevations well over a mile high in its native habitat, is a plant with growing conditions that the home gardener in the West would find exceedingly difficult to duplicate. It is not surprising that dong quai is very rare in Western horticulture, and North American-grown plants identified as dong quai

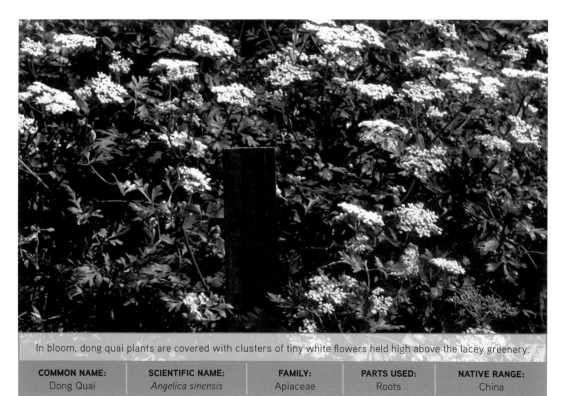

In bloom, dong quai plants are covered with clusters of tiny white flowers held high above the lacey greenery.

COMMON NAME:	SCIENTIFIC NAME:	FAMILY:	PARTS USED:	NATIVE RANGE:
Dong Quai	*Angelica sinensis*	Apiaceae	Roots	China

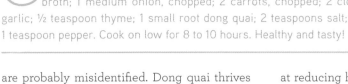
Combine in a Crock-Pot the following: 1 pound skinless, boneless chicken breasts (hormone free); 8 cups water or organic chicken broth; 1 medium onion, chopped; 2 carrots, chopped; 2 cloves garlic; ½ teaspoon thyme; 1 small root dong quai; 2 teaspoons salt; and 1 teaspoon pepper. Cook on low for 8 to 10 hours. Healthy and tasty!

are probably misidentified. Dong quai thrives in a rich, moist, sandy loam. Propagation is by seeds, which must be fresh.

Large-scale cultivation was first described in A.D. 650. The roots are harvested in the second or third autumn of growth. The roots are carefully dug by hand. Subject to bruising, they are delicately rinsed and handled as if they were as fragile as eggs. If the roots become too wet in cleaning, they will turn black on the outside and may be subject to rotting. Dong quai is not dried in the sun in central China, as sunlight causes the roots to harden. In some regions, where roots were once partially dried in the shade, they are tied in small bundles and dried under smoke over a fire. Specialized handling practices have evolved over many centuries.

Therapeutic Uses

+ *Women's tonic*
+ *Premenstrual syndrome (PMS)*
+ *Menstrual cramps*
+ *Kidney tonic*

Dong quai root has been used for millennia as a spice and medicine in China, Korea, and Japan. It is still one of the most popular herbs used in traditional Chinese medicine. Dong quai is well known for treating women's health problems, such as painful menstruation, as well as relieving fatigue and strengthening mothers after childbirth. It gained popularity in the West in the late 1800s when Merck introduced Eumenol, an **extract** of dong quai, to Europe to treat gynecological complaints.

Studies suggest that dong quai may have weak **estrogenic** activity, and it is often recommended for symptom relief in menopause. In a randomized, **double-blind**, **placebo**-controlled clinical trial of 71 postmenopausal women, however, dong quai was no better than placebo

at reducing hot flashes. This study was widely criticized for using dong quai by itself instead of in combination with other herbs, which is how it is used in traditional Chinese medicine. When an herbal mixture containing *Angelica sinensis* root, *Paeonia lactiflora* root, *Ligusticum* **rhizome**, *Atractylodes* rhizome, *Alisma orientalis* rhizome, and *Wolfiporia cocos* was studied in menopausal women, it reportedly reduced hot flashes by 70 percent. Herbal combinations are the rule rather than the exception in many traditional systems of medicine, and clinical trials using just 1 herb may erroneously lead us to judge an herb as ineffective.

Dong quai has been used in combination with astragalus (*A. membranaceus*) to tone and strengthen the kidneys, as well as to enhance the immune system. One study found that this combination significantly reduced the deterioration of renal function and damage in animals with chronic kidney damage.

Dong quai and other *Angelica* **species** are known to contain psoralen, which is sometimes used in combination with ultraviolet therapy as a treatment for psoriasis. Studies have shown that this approach improves psoriasis in 40 to 66 percent of patients.

How to Use

TEA: Simmer 1 to 2 teaspoons root in 1 cup water for 5 to 7 minutes. Strain. Drink 1 cup, 2 to 3 times per day.
CAPSULES: 1 g, taken 2 to 3 times per day.
TINCTURE: 3 to 5 ml, taken 2 to 3 times per day.

Precautions

Those with bleeding disorders or taking anticoagulants should not use dong quai, as it may increase risk of bleeding. Use should be avoided during pregnancy. The psoralen in dong quai could, in theory, cause photosensitivity.

Raspberry Leaf

❦ *Rubus idaeus* ❦

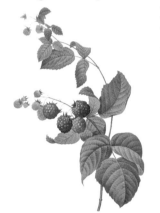

Biting into a plump, perfectly ripe red raspberry is a sensory experience. The initial explosion of fragrant sweetness is underscored by a subtle, pleasant tartness. A raspberry is actually an aggregation of very tiny fruits—the "bumps" on the berry—neatly arranged around a hollow, central cavity. *Rubus idaeus* is native to Asia Minor. Botanical lore suggests that the ancient Greeks discovered the plant in the first century B.C., when they encountered raspberries growing on the slopes of Mount Ida in Phrygia (now Turkey). This legend may be the basis of raspberry's species name, *idaeus*. Alternatively, Ida, a nymph from Greek mythology, may have been the source. According to the myth, raspberries were white until Ida pricked her finger while picking raspberries for the infant Zeus. From that point on, the fruits were tinged red with her blood. By the fourth century A.D., the Romans were cultivating raspberry plants. As they conquered various parts of Europe and England, they brought raspberries with them. Archaeologists have unearthed raspberry seeds at excavated Roman forts in Britain. In the Middle Ages, raspberry plants were cultivated in Europe and England. By the late 1700s, cultivars of *Rubus idaeus* were being exported to the colonies in North America.

It is likely that the Greeks and Romans grew raspberry as much for medicinal purposes as for food. All parts of the plant were used to treat various ailments. The fruits, eaten in large quantities, acted as a laxative, helped increase sweating, and eased both rheumatism and indigestion. In the 1597 edition of his *General Historie of Plantes*, English herbalist John Gerard recommended boiling the leaves of raspberry (he called it raspis) with honey, alum, and white wine to make a "most excellent lotion or washing water," and said the same **decoction** "fastneth the teeth." Raspberry leaf tea made an effective gargle for sore mouths and throats; applied to the skin it cleansed wounds and skin ulcers; and it was given during pregnancy.

Raspberry leaf remains a pregnancy herb in modern herbal medicine. Herbalists recommend raspberry leaf preparations to strengthen, tone, and relax smooth muscles of the uterus and pelvis; shorten labor; and ease delivery. Raspberry tea may also help regulate menstrual cycles and decrease heavy menstrual flow.

Everybody loves the berries, but it is raspberry leaves that are prized in herbal medicine as a pregnancy aid.

TIME LINE OF USAGE AND SPREAD

1ST CENTURY B.C.	1548	1771	1941
Greeks discover wild raspberries in foothills of Caucasus Mountains.	A description of raspberry cultivation appears in an English herbal.	British begin exporting raspberry plants to the American colonies.	British journal *Lancet* reports raspberry leaves contain a uterine relaxant.

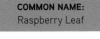

FEMALE HEALTH

Not only the succulent berries but also the raspberry plant's leaves are hand-picked from wild plants.

COMMON NAME:	SCIENTIFIC NAME:	FAMILY:	PARTS USED:	NATIVE RANGE:
Raspberry Leaf	*Rubus idaeus*	Rosaceae	Leaves	Eurasia

There are few among us who are not familiar with the delectable flavor of raspberry fruits; the use of raspberry leaf, however, is limited to the herbal realm. There are more than 250 species in the genus *Rubus*, the source of thorny shrubs such as raspberry and blackberry and their numerous cultivated varieties. Primarily found in the Northern Hemisphere, brambles such as raspberry are widespread in cultivation. A deciduous shrub, the raspberry has an erect, round stem from 3 to 6 feet tall, which produces numerous suckers. The stems are covered with many sharp prickles. The leaves usually have 5 to 7 lobes. The coarse, sharp-toothed leaves have short stalks and are mostly smooth above, with white, hoary-soft hairs beneath. The drooping, white, 5-petaled flowers have short petals. The red or amber drupe is the familiar raspberry of commerce. It flowers from June to August.

Growing Habits

Typical raspberry is found in fields and along fencerows and woodland edges throughout Europe. In China, where it is also widespread, raspberry is found in forests, thickets, river valleys, and forest margins, mostly in northeastern China and adjacent Russia, as well as Japan. In North America, raspberry is absent from the southeastern tier of states and from Texas, Kentucky, and Kansas; otherwise, it is found throughout North America and Canada. In the Northern Hemisphere, raspberry is nearly as widespread as human settlement.

Cultivation and Harvesting

Raspberry is a plant that does best in a moderately rich, somewhat moist soil. It is easy to grow and can be propagated by replanting the suckering shoots around the perimeter of the plant. It must be given a situation where it can spread, although careful training in rows or along a fence will help keep it under control.

Raspberry is occasionally planted for leaf production, but usually in small plantings in North America or western Europe for specialized markets to supply small quantities of certified organic leaf. Most of the leaf material in international commerce is wild-collected in central and Eastern Europe, including Bulgaria, Macedonia, and Romania. Relatively low in moisture content, the leaves are easily dried in the shade, then rubbed and sifted to remove stem material or prickles.

Therapeutic Uses

+ *Women's tonic*
+ *Pregnancy tea*
+ *Diarrhea*

Raspberry has long been referred to as a woman's herb. The leaf was often taken as tea by young women to regulate menstrual cycles and ease menstrual cramping and has a long tradition of use during pregnancy. Raspberry leaf has been used as nourishment during pregnancy and preparation for labor since ancient times, most likely back to the sixth century. It was said to tonify, or strengthen, the uterus.

Today, it is found in many popular pregnancy teas; surveys indicate 15 to 25 percent of women in the U.S., Canada, and Australia have taken raspberry during pregnancy. A survey of 172 certified nurse-midwives found 63 percent using herbal preparations recommended red raspberry leaf.

There is scant modern evidence available to determine what benefit, if any, raspberry offers during pregnancy. A small group of midwives in Australia reviewed medical charts of women taking raspberry leaf during pregnancy and failed to find negative outcomes for mother or infant compared with pregnant women who had not taken raspberry. This was then followed by **double-blind,** **placebo**-controlled clinical trials of 192 women, identified as having low-risk pregnancies, in Sydney, Australia. They were given either 1,200-mg raspberry leaf capsules twice daily or a placebo, from 32 weeks' pregnancy until labor. The study found no difference between the 2 groups in length of pregnancy or adverse effects on the baby. Women taking the raspberry leaf had a slightly shorter second stage of labor (when the cervix is fully dilated until the birth of the baby), and a lower rate of forceps delivery than those in the placebo group. The study suggested raspberry leaf is unlikely to prevent premature labor, as is sometimes claimed in the lay literature.

Raspberry leaf contains **tannins**, which act as a mild **astringent** and can help ease diarrhea. This might also explain its traditional use as a remedy for sore throat and tonsillitis.

How to Use

TEA: Steep 1 to 2 teaspoons dried raspberry leaves in 1 cup water for 5 minutes. Strain. Add honey and/or lemon as desired. Drink 1 cup 2 to 3 times per day. To **extract** the tannins to ease sore throat or diarrhea, the tea must be steeped for a longer period, 15 to 30 minutes. Generally, the dose is ⅓ cup taken 3 to 4 times per day as needed.

CAPSULES: 500 to 600 mg dried raspberry leaf, 2 to 4 times daily.

TINCTURE: 5 ml taken 2 times per day, or follow manufacturer's directions.

Precautions

Raspberry leaf appears to be quite safe, and no significant adverse effects were noted in the clinical studies published in the medical literature. However, women should always check with a health care practitioner before using herbal remedies during pregnancy.

---

over the (kitchen) counter RASPBERRY BLISS TEA

Pour 4 cups boiling water over 6 teaspoons dried raspberry leaves and 2 teaspoons dried spearmint leaves. Steep for 5 to 7 minutes. Strain. Add ½ cup fruit juice—apple, grape, or raspberry. The tea will keep in the refrigerator for 3 to 4 days.

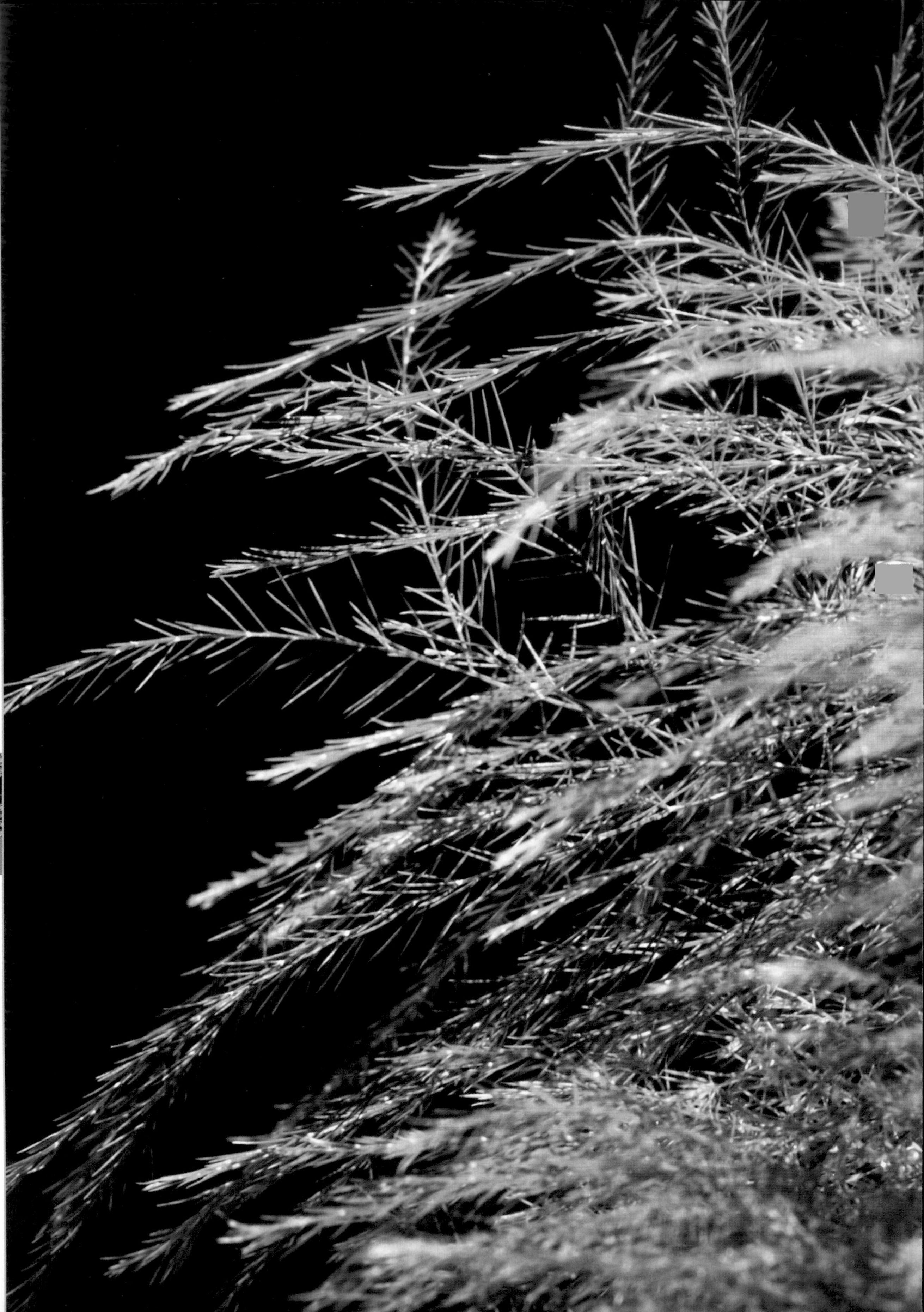

Shatavari

Shatavari is a branching, climbing perennial with tiny spines that lurk beneath feathery foliage. It grows wild throughout tropical and subtropical parts of India and in the Himalaya at lower elevations. Shatavari shares a genus with *Asparagus officinalis*, whose fleshy green spears are prized as a vegetable. Parts of shatavari are also edible. Its tender young shoots are eaten cooked or made into preserves. The fleshy, whitish brown, tuberous roots—actually highly divided rhizomes that may grow to 3 feet or more in length—have a slightly sweet flavor and are

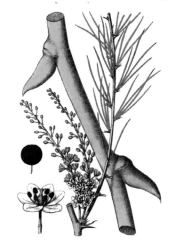

also eaten as a vegetable. Shatavari's profusion of roots are reflected in its name; "shatavari" comes from Sanskrit, meaning "plant of a hundred roots." The dried and processed roots of shatavari have been used in traditional Indian **Ayurvedic medicine** for many centuries, primarily for rejuvenating female reproductive organs and treating conditions relating to women's health and fertility.

Shatavari is arguably the most important herb in Ayurvedic medicine for women, a sort of female counterpart to ashwagandha *(Withania somnifera),* which is used, among other things, to enhance sexual potency in men. Traditionally, Ayurvedic practitioners have valued shatavari as a nourishing, soothing, and cooling herb that can help in treating conditions in which the body and mind are depleted or out of balance. Shatavari has been prescribed for women complaining of infertility, loss of libido, threatened miscarriage, and menopausal symptoms and for the stimulation of breast milk production. The herb has a long history of use as a rejuvenating tonic with **adaptogenic** properties for improving health, vitality, and well-being.

Today, shatavari has become popular in Western herbal medicine as an herb that may raise fertility levels and increase conception in women as well as strengthen reproductive tissues in both men and women. Shatavari has been shown to relax muscles in the uterine wall, and it may provide relief from symptoms of premenstrual syndrome (PMS) and menopause. The herb is also used to soothe indigestion and is still used to promote breast milk production.

Shatavari's filamentous foliage is striking, but it's the roots of this tropical plant that are used medicinally.

TIME LINE OF USAGE AND SPREAD

2000 B.C.	**A.D. 1960s**	**1993**	**2001**
Shatavari used medicinally at least 4,000 years ago.	Studies explore shatavari's role as a milk promoter in animals.	Research shows shatavari increases white blood cell activity to fight infection.	Wild shatavari stocks are considered vulnerable in India due to overharvesting.

When one mentions asparagus, visions of buttery spears, nestled beside steamy baked salmon may come to mind. These are the spring stalks of the European *Asparagus officinalis*. Shatavari (*A. racemosus*) is *not* that asparagus, but rather a quite different-looking plant used in herbal medicine. In fact, despite *A. officinalis,* most of the 120 members of the genus *Asparagus* are somewhat woody plants with thorny stems, like *A. racemosus.*

Shatavari is a woody, much branched perennial climbing to more than 20 feet in height, and usually clambering over other vegetation. The branches have distinct striated ridges. One feature of most *Asparagus* **species** is that they lack leaves in the traditional sense; rather, their stems are chlorophyll-producing parts, and the small, leaflike structures extending from the stems are actually modified stem structures called cladodes (one of which is a cladophyll). In shatavari, these structures are in groups of 3 to 6, linear and flat with a distinct midrib. The stems have straight or backward-curved spines, nearly an inch long on the main stem; on lateral stems the spines are shorter, up to ⅜ inch long. The small, mostly white flowers occur in crowded groups. In bloom, they become conspicuous, sweetly fragrant white masses, imparting their heady scent some distance. The plant has red berrylike fruits.

Growing Habits

Shatavari is widespread in broad-leaved forests, appearing along streams or in mountain valleys at elevations up to 6,000 feet. *A. racemosus* is found in southern Tibet, Nepal, Bhutan, Myanmar, Pakistan, India, Africa, Madagascar, and Australia. It requires a warm climate. In many areas where it is native or naturalized it is a common plant of thickets. It is available in both American and European horticulture, primarily as a collector's specimen plant.

The perennial tubers, the part used in herbal medicine, grow in bunches; they are 6 to 8 inches long and about ½ inch in diameter. They are covered with a thin, light brown skin removed before use, almost like a potato peel.

Cultivation and Harvesting

In various parts of India, the root is wild-collected for use, or it may be grown as an ornamental around homes for the sprays of fragrant flowers. Sometimes commercially cultivated for medicinal use, it is propagated from side roots at the base of the plant. To give the plants a nutrition boost before planting, the roots are dipped in cow dung slurry and planted about a day later. The saplings are then planted in beds.

Indian agronomists have recommended spraying the herbicide 2,4-D on the crop plant to thwart development of lateral leaflike cladodes so that the roots will grow larger—not exactly the vision conjured by a back-to-nature organic herb.

Therapeutic Uses

+ *Tonic*
+ *Premenstrual syndrome (PMS)*
+ *Menstrual cramps*
+ *Breast milk production*
+ *Menopause*
+ *Indigestion*
+ *Stomach ulcer (preventive)*

Ayurvedic practitioners commonly recommend shatavari to maintain the function of the female reproductive organs. The plant is said to enhance fertility and is often used to normalize

over the (kitchen) counter SHATAVARI KALPA STIR

Combine 1 ounce shatavari root with 2 tablespoons ghee (clarified butter) in a skillet on low to medium heat and roast until root turns light brown. Add 2 tablespoons sugar and ¼ teaspoon cardamom and stir until well mixed. Take one teaspoonful per day during menstruation, menopause, or after childbirth as a rejuvenating tonic.

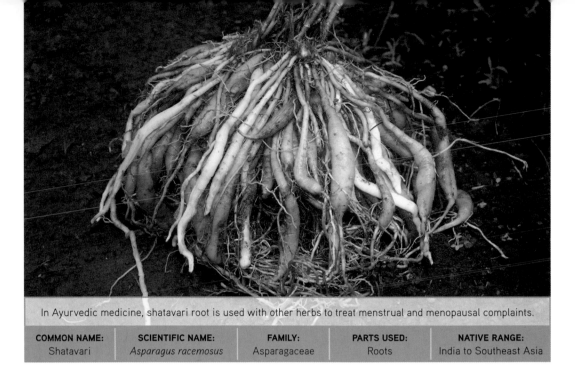

In Ayurvedic medicine, shatavari root is used with other herbs to treat menstrual and menopausal complaints.

COMMON NAME:	SCIENTIFIC NAME:	FAMILY:	PARTS USED:	NATIVE RANGE:
Shatavari	*Asparagus racemosus*	Asparagaceae	Roots	India to Southeast Asia

irregular menstrual cycles, especially when they are caused by stress or illness. One open study found that a formulation containing shatavari eased menstrual cramps, regulated uterine bleeding, and improved symptoms of premenstrual syndrome (PMS) in a small group of women. At this time, the mechanism(s) of action is not clearly understood.

Women often use shatavari kalpa (see opposite page), a combination of shatavari and cardamom, after childbirth to regain strength and promote production of breast milk. A small number of animal and human studies suggest that shatavari in combination with other herbs enhances the production of breast milk, but one randomized controlled study of the single herb in women with poor milk production failed to find any benefit.

Shatavari, often in combination with other herbs, is popular for relieving menopausal symptoms such as hot flashes, night sweats, and vaginal dryness. This beneficial effect is thought to result from the **estrogen**-like **compounds** present in the herb's root. Despite its widespread use in Ayurveda and the public demand for more natural approaches to alleviating menopause-related symptoms, there have been no published clinical trials to determine the effectiveness of shatavari during menopause.

There are, however, a handful of studies confirming the protective effect of shatavari on the gastrointestinal tract. Animal studies show that shatavari is as effective as ranitidine (Zantac), a commonly used ulcer medication, in protecting against ulcer formation, possibly by reducing the production and release of hydrochloric acid in the stomach. A study with human volunteers found that shatavari increases contractions of the stomach and small intestine, thus helping to hasten the passage and digestion of food. Shatavari was shown to be equivalent in effectiveness to metoclopramide, a prescription medication that is used as a treatment after meals for sluggish digestive function that is also accompanied by nausea, heartburn, and indigestion.

How to Use

TEA: Simmer 1 teaspoon dried root in 1 cup water for 15 minutes. Strain. Drink 1 to 2 cups per day.

CAPSULES: Generally, 500 mg, 1 to 2 times daily.

TINCTURE: Take according to manufacturer's recommendations.

Precautions

Shatavari appears safe and generally well tolerated if used appropriately. However, shatavari is not recommended for use during pregnancy.

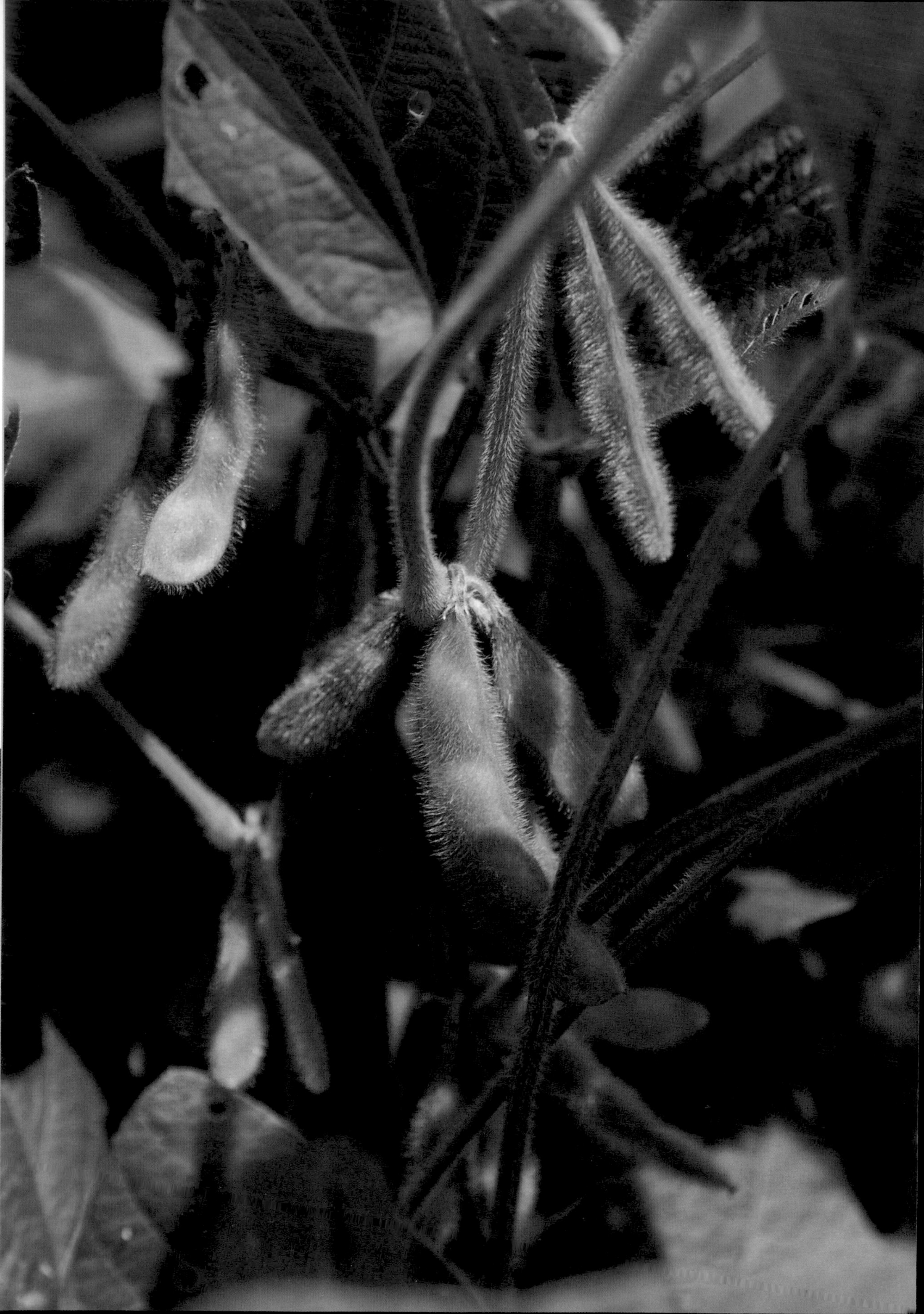

Soy

❧ *Glycine max* ❧

Miso, soy sauce, tempeh, tofu—these and other foods derived from soybeans have been a cornerstone of Asian cuisine and nutrition for centuries. Native to central and eastern Asia, wild soybeans are thought to have been domesticated around the 11th century B.C. in northern China. By the first century A.D., soybeans were being cultivated throughout China, as well as in Korea, Japan, northern India, Nepal, and many countries in Southeast Asia. European traders and visitors to China and Japan in the 1500s encountered many foods and sauces made

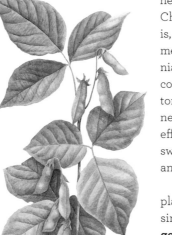

from soybeans and brought the news back to the West. Yet soybeans weren't planted in Europe until the 1730s. Even then, they were grown in greenhouses and botanic gardens for display and study. Several decades later, soybeans reached North America. They gradually gained acceptance as a forage crop for livestock, and as a legume that improved agricultural soils. Not until World War II, however, were soybeans widely grown in the U.S. as a substitute for other protein-rich foods and as a source of edible oil. Since then, soybeans and soybean oil have become standard ingredients in many foods, and traditional Asian soy dishes are commonplace almost everywhere.

In the West, soy is often thought of strictly as a food. Yet soy has a long history as a medicinal herb in the East and as an ingredient in many healing preparations in ancient Chinese texts. Soy was, and still is, used in traditional Chinese medicine to treat fever, insomnia, headaches, anxiety, and lung conditions. It is considered a tonic for the heart, liver, and kidneys. Soy sprouts have a laxative effect and are eaten to reduce swelling, ease painful urination, and promote sweating.

Soy is rich in **phytoestrogens**, plant **compounds** chemically similar to the hormone **estrogen.** Hence, herbalists suggest soy **extracts** to help relieve menopausal symptoms, including hot flashes and night sweats. However, because soy may increase risk of breast cancer in some women, use of extracts for menopausal symptoms remains controversial. Soy lecithin, a fatty substance extracted from soybeans, may help lower cholesterol levels in blood.

Packaged inside fuzzy green pods, the seeds of soy—soybeans—are a source of food products and extracts.

TIME LINE OF USAGE AND SPREAD

712
Earliest Japanese reference to soybeans noted in *Kojiki* (*Records of Ancient Matters*).

1665
Friar Domingo Navarrete describes tofu as common inexpensive food in China.

1739
Soybean seeds from missionaries in China planted in Jardin des Plantes, Paris.

1765
The first soybeans are planted in the United States.

Soy is a member of the pea family, an annual growing up to 6 feet (though usually much shorter). Its 3 oval leaflets have a prominent midrib and are on short stalks. The terminal leaflet usually has the longest stalk and is slightly larger than the other leaflets. Depending on the cultivated variety, leaflets are from 2 to 5 inches long. Flowers are rather small, pealike, and inconspicuous, whitish to mauve in clusters in leaf axils. The fruit, when ripe, is a brown, hair-covered pod, about the size and shape of a pea pod, containing the familiar soybeans of commerce. The seeds (soybeans) range from white to black depending upon the **variety**. Unripe soybean pods are known as edamame in Japanese cuisine. Soy (*Glycine max*) is considered a cultigen, having evolved in cultivation from its parent, wild Asian soy, sometimes botanically deemed *Glycine soja*. Wild soy differs from cultivated soy in being a twining annual vine with slender stems. Like soy, it is covered with brownish hairs.

Growing Habits

Soy is primarily an agricultural crop grown on a large scale in the United States, and now naturalized in most states east of the Mississippi, except for New England. Its wild relative is commonly found in lowland thickets throughout Japan, Korea, eastern Siberia, Taiwan, and much of eastern China. Soy has been cultivated in China for at least a thousand years.

Cultivation and Harvesting

Soybeans may be grown on a small scale in the vegetable garden, but the plant is absent from most gardening books. The space it takes to grow a few soybeans in the home garden is hardly worth the effort when soybeans and soy-based products are so widely available and relatively inexpensive wherever food products are sold. The most widely grown legume in the world and an important source of protein, soybeans thrive in fertile, well-drained soil and grow in full sun. The seeds are planted as soon as danger of frost has passed in spring.

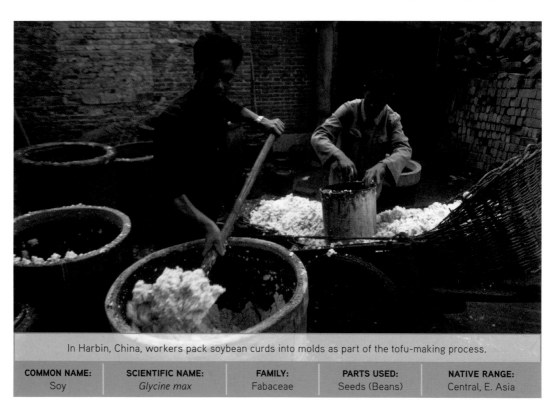

In Harbin, China, workers pack soybean curds into molds as part of the tofu-making process.

COMMON NAME:	SCIENTIFIC NAME:	FAMILY:	PARTS USED:	NATIVE RANGE:
Soy	*Glycine max*	Fabaceae	Seeds (Beans)	Central, E. Asia

Combine 6 ounces soy milk, a dash of vanilla, ½ cup strawberries or blueberries, ½ banana. Add ½ cup ice cubes. Mix ingredients in blender for 10 to 15 seconds. Serve immediately. Yum!

The United States is a major producer of soybeans. In 2008 about 3 billion bushels of soybeans were produced on an estimated 75 million acres of farmland. Some 40 percent of the United States soybean crop is exported; China, the European Union, Mexico, Japan, and Taiwan are the largest recipients of the American export crop. Among the top producing states are Iowa, Illinois, Minnesota, Indiana, and Nebraska. Soy production represents a $27 billion crop in the U.S. alone, more than 5 times the value of the highest estimates of the combined retail value of all herb products sold in all U.S. market segments.

Therapeutic Uses

+ *Protein source*
+ *Heart health*

Soy is widely consumed in the Asian diet. Soybean contains a full complement of essential **amino acids**, making it a complete protein. Thus, it is a very useful part of any vegetarian or vegan diet. Of any plant, soy contains the highest concentration of **isoflavones**, a class of phytoestrogen compounds that are structurally similar to estrogen. Large epidemiologic studies in Asian countries have shown that lifelong traditional consumption of soy may offer some protection against menopausal symptoms, breast cancer, and osteoporosis.

Studies in non-Asian populations have yielded conflicting results. There have been scores of studies on soy for health, and more than 2 dozen on soy for hot flashes, some showing an effect and others not, making it difficult to arrive at any definitive conclusion. When looking at the totality of the evidence, most reviewers have concluded that the data are just too contradictory to come to any conclusion regarding the effectiveness of soy, or isoflavones, for relieving hot flashes, preventing bone loss, or protecting the heart.

In 2006, an American Heart Association review concluded that there is little evidence to support the use of soy to relieve hot flashes or protect against cancer; however, the authors noted that "soy products such as tofu, soy butter, soy nuts, or some soy burgers should be beneficial to cardiovascular and overall health because of their high content of polyunsaturated fats, fiber, vitamins, and minerals and low content of saturated fat. Using these and other soy foods to replace foods high in animal protein, which contains saturated fat and cholesterol, may confer benefits to cardiovascular health."

One area of concern with soy is its safety in women with breast cancer, as it contains compounds that can mimic estrogen. Some human studies showing positive effects of soy indicate that early consumption of soy might be important for protection against breast cancer later in life. Less is known about soy consumption in women at high risk or those who currently have breast cancer. Some studies indicate that it may prevent recurrence, while others suggest that it might increase risk or reduce the effectiveness of tamoxifen, used in treatment. Many oncologists recommend that women limit soy to 1 to 2 servings per day or limit intake to the amounts consumed in the Asian diet, which provides 50 to 90 mg of soy isoflavones per day.

How to Use

Soy foods should be part of a wholesome diet. Avoid processed soy "junk" food and focus on edamame, soy nuts, miso, and tempeh.

EXTRACTS: 50 to 90 mg per day soy isoflavones.

Precautions

Soy is healthful when consumed as part of a varied, wholesome diet and is an excellent source of protein. Until more is known, breast cancer survivors should not combine soy extracts with tamoxifen (or should avoid therapeutic doses) because of possible plant-drug interactions.

Glycine max

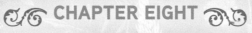

CHAPTER EIGHT

Wellness *and* Perception

Plants *and* Wellness

❦

One of the great heroes of Chinese culture, the legendary—and divine—Shen Nong, is said to have lived around 3000 B.C. One translation of his name, the Divine Farmer, refers to his role in teaching the Chinese people how to use plants and cultivate food. According to the legend, Shen Nong personally sampled hundreds, if not thousands, of different plants in order to determine which were good to eat or had medicinal properties, and which were poisonous and should be avoided. Some versions of the tale relate that Shen Nong had a transparent belly, so he could witness firsthand the effects on his internal organs of whatever he consumed! Sometime around the first century A.D., an unknown Chinese scholar penned the *Shen Nong Ben Cao Jing (The Divine Farmer's Materia Medica)*, a manuscript attributed to Shen Nong that describes 365 Chinese medicines, of which 252 are derived from plants. The *Shen Nong Ben Cao Jing*, considered to be the earliest complete Chinese pharmacopoeia,

contains the first written account of Asian ginseng *(Panax ginseng)*. It states that ginseng is used for "repairing the five viscera, quieting the spirit, curbing the emotion, stopping agitation, removing noxious influence, brightening the eyes, enlightening the mind, and increasing wisdom." Continued use of ginseng, the text states, leads to "longevity with light weight."

A sound, healthy body. A calm spirit. A mind enlightened, focused, and at ease. These are key elements of what we, in the West, call "wellness." Of course, wellness can mean different things to different people. But most would probably agree that wellness is much more than simply the absence of disease. In the 1950s, Halbert L. Dunn, a biostatistician and one of the first people to use the term, defined wellness as an integrated way of living that focuses on maximizing one's potential. Wellness involves balancing the physical, intellectual, emotional, social, occupational, spiritual, and environmental aspects of life, and emphasizes the state of a person's interconnected being and ongoing development. Optimal wellness makes it

possible to achieve goals and find meaning and purpose in life while overcoming whatever hardships life brings our way. For most people, wellness also involves proactively making choices toward a healthier lifestyle.

In traditional Chinese and Indian Ayurvedic medicine, a number of herbs stand out as being particularly in tune with the concept of wellness. For thousands of years, practitioners of these healing traditions have treated patients with such herbs, not necessarily to cure a particular complaint, but to strengthen the body's ability to correct problems and heal itself. These herbs, often referred to as *rasayanas*, qi tonics, or rejuvenating herbs because of their restorative powers, were believed to normalize body systems and functions and foster healing of the body as a whole. Several were particularly prized for their ability to enhance mental function and perception as well.

These herbs continue to play an integral role in Ayurvedic and traditional Chinese medicine. A number have also found a respected place in Western herbal medicine, where

314

WELLNESS & PERCEPTION

rather than being called tonics or rejuvenative herbs, they are typically called adaptogens. The Soviet scientist Nikolai Lazarev coined the term "adaptogen" in 1947 to describe herbs that increase the body's resistance to stress resulting from trauma, anxiety, and fatigue. Many modern herbalists might extend the list of stressors to include infection, heat or cold, exertion, sleep deprivation, overwork, strained personal relationships, pivotal life events, psychological duress, and exposure to toxic substances or radiation. In short, adaptogens are thought to help the body "adapt" to the many, often negative, influences it encounters every day, and to restore balance in all of its systems.

This chapter highlights 8 herbs believed to promote wellness and improve perception. Among them are several of the most well known adaptogens in ancient, and modern, herbal medicine. Scientific investigations have yet to confirm, beyond all doubt, many of their purported effects. But the fact remains that many of these herbs have been employed medicinally for several millennia and their popularity has not faded in that time.

Ashwagandha *(Withania somnifera)*, native to India, has been widely used in Ayurvedic medicine for several thousand years. It is considered by many herbal practitioners a first-rate stress-relieving adaptogenic herb with gentle sedative properties. Recent research reveals that it may also be useful in treating various forms of dementia. Historically, bacopa *(Bacopa monnieri)* also has its roots deep in Ayurvedic healing and is now recommended by Western herbalists as an anxiety-relieving herb that may also improve cognitive functions, including memory and attention span.

Ginseng, both Asian *(Panax ginseng)* and American *(Panax quinquefolius)*, has played such a pivotal role in traditional Chinese medicine throughout the centuries that it has often been called the king of herbs. Thought to help restore all the body's systems—and to have anti-cancer properties—ginseng is also prized in modern Western herbal medicine for improving mental clarity.

Both goji *(Lycium barbarum and Lycium chinense)* and gotu kola *(Centella asiatica)* are mild adaptogens in Chinese and Indian traditional medicine, respectively. Both are relatively new to Western herbal medicine, and somewhat controversial, as extravagant claims made about their healing properties remain unsubstantiated. Research is under way, however, to shed light on their therapeutic value.

Rhodiola *(Rhodiola rosea)* is also relatively new to American herbal medicine, but it is widely use in China, Russia, and Scandinavia to combat fatigue and enhance both physical and mental performance. Practitioners of traditional Chinese medicine were the first to use schisandra *(Schisandra chinensis)*, an adaptogen that has since been incorporated into Russian conventional medicine and is now used in Western herbal medicine as a stamina-promoting stress reliever with numerous applications.

Finally, this chapter ends with stevia *(Stevia rebaudiana)*, which is not an adaptogen but a sweet-tasting herb native to South America that has been developed as a sugar substitute. Proper nutrition, regular exercise, and a life of balance and moderation are fundamental to wellness, and for those who need to reduce their intake of sugar, stevia may represent an aid to reaching their healthy goals.

Ashwagandha

Withania somnifera

A small, woody shrub and member of the nightshade family, ashwagandha is native to the drier regions of India, North Africa, and the Middle East. In Sanskrit, the name ashwagandha means "the smell of a horse," which may refer to the pungent odor of the plant's fresh roots. Alternatively, it may imply that the roots can impart a horse's strength and vigor. Ashwagandha has played a central role in traditional medicine in India for more than 4,000 years. Practitioners of Ayurvedic, Unani, and Siddha healing have traditionally prescribed ashwagandha

as a strengthening tonic to speed healing during and after an illness. The herb is sometimes called Indian ginseng, because like ginseng *(Panax ginseng)* used in traditional Chinese medicine, ashwagandha is an **adaptogen** that boosts the immune system and helps the body adapt to stress. Unlike ginseng, which has pronounced stimulating effects, ashwagandha has calming properties. Its sedative effect is reflected in the Latin **species** name, *somnifera*, which means "to induce sleep."

Ashwagandha is one of the most commonly used herbs in Indian traditional medicine. Practitioners often combine it with other herbs, because it is believed to work synergistically to produce effects not possible with a single herb. For centuries, people have taken ashwagandha as a sedative to calm nervous tension and combat insomnia, as a **diuretic**

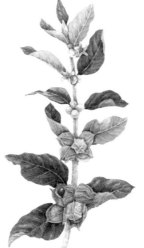

and **anti-inflammatory**, and as a restorative for increasing energy, strength, and longevity. It is a common home remedy throughout India as a geriatric tonic. Preparations of the roots and fruits are given for dementia as well. Ashwagandha is used to treat respiratory conditions, tumors, and high blood pressure, and has long been considered an aphrodisiac.

Modern herbalists use **extracts** of ashwagandha to combat stress and boost the immune system. Preparations may be as effective as some prescription medications in relieving anxiety, insomnia, even depression. With its proven anti-inflammatory properties, it is an ingredient in many pain relief formulations, particularly for arthritis and rheumatism pain, and may protect against cartilage damage associated with osteoarthritis. It is also taken for cognitive disorders and Parkinson's disease.

Western herbalists recommend root extracts of ashwagandha, an Indian medicinal herb, for relief from stress.

TIME LINE OF USAGE AND SPREAD

2000 B.C.
Ashwagandha is being used medicinally in India.

CA 327 B.C.
Alexander the Great drinks wine made with ashwagandha as a tonic.

A.D. 2002
Law prohibits labeling *W. somnifera* or any non-*Panax* herb as "ginseng."

2006
Japanese researchers show ashwagandha extracts curb growth of cancer cells.

Usually associated with Ayurvedic traditions of India, the genus *Witha-nia* includes about 20 species native to the Old World. One rare species from the south Atlantic island of St. Helena, believed extinct since 1875, was rediscovered in 1998. Ashwagandha is a perennial shrub growing up to 3 feet tall. The entire plant is covered with silver-gray, felted hairs, though in some variations the plant is nearly without hairs. The opposite leaves are broadly oval, and about 2 to 6 inches long, The small yellow-green, star-shaped flowers are up to a half inch wide and long. The bright red, globular berry is enclosed within the remnants of the papery calyx. There is considerable variation between wild plants and cultivated plants, including differences in the flowers, mature fruits and seeds, and size of the roots. The stout, fleshy root is the part used in herbal medicine.

Growing Habits

Ashwagandha is not limited to India but occurs throughout drier regions of the Mediterranean, from the Canary Islands to southern Europe and North Africa, southward on the African continent and throughout the Middle East to India, where it has been used for centuries. In China it is found mainly in Gansu province.

Cultivation and Harvesting

Commercial cultivation began in the late 19th century. In India, where most of the world's supply originates, commercial cultivation occurs on soils unsuitable for other crops. In much of its natural range, the plant also grows in inhospitable conditions where other plants do not thrive. It is not fertilized in commercial production, as this encourages leafy growth and thwarts development of the root. The plant does not require irrigation and does best if the soil is dry but well drained.

The roots are harvested after the first year of growth. The entire plant is uprooted and the tops are cut off. Before drying, the roots are cut into smaller pieces. Ashwagandha is easily grown from seed. For the home garden, ashwagandha makes an interesting specimen plant.

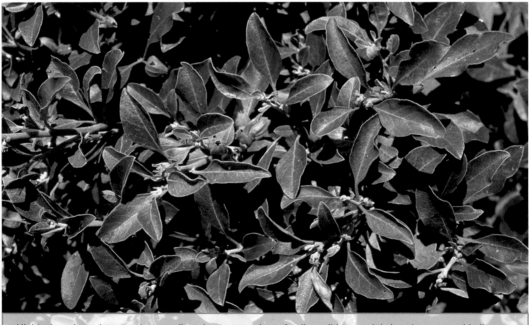

Highly drought resistant, ashwagandha tolerates a variety of soil conditions and thrives in warm, arid climates.

COMMON NAME:	SCIENTIFIC NAME:	FAMILY:	PARTS USED:	NATIVE RANGE:
Ashwagandha	*Withania somnifera*	Solanaceae	Roots	Egypt to Pakistan

Simmer 1 to 2 teaspoons powdered ashwagandha in 2 cups milk over low heat for 15 minutes. Add 1 tablespoon raw sugar and ⅛ teaspoon cardamom and stir until well mixed. Turn off heat. Drink a cup once or twice a day for a pick-me-up.

Therapeutic Uses

+ *Rejuvenating tonic*
+ *Anti-inflammatory*
+ *Antianxiety*

An herb used for so many conditions—from increasing vitality to treating fatigue, anxiety, and skin conditions—invites skepticism. But modern science has confirmed that specific **compounds** in the ashwagandha root exhibit **antioxidant**, anti-inflammatory, immune system modulating, neuroprotective, and anti-stress activity. In the West, however, there has been scant research on adaptogens such as ashwagandha, in part because there is no equivalent to an "adaptogen" in Western medicine and no rigorous research model to test the theory.

Ashwagandha is almost always used in combination with other herbs in **Ayurvedic** medicine, and most research has been conducted on traditional formulations. Ashwagandha was historically used to treat arthritis and has been shown to exhibit antiarthritic properties. A randomized controlled study of 90 patients with osteoarthritis of the knee found an **extract** containing ashwagandha, boswellia, ginger, and turmeric superior to **placebo** for relieving pain and improving function in the patients. This same combination was also shown to reduce joint swelling in patients with rheumatoid arthritis.

Modern research has found that the plant, rich in iron, may help treat anemia. In one randomized study, 58 children were given 2 g per day of ashwagandha or a placebo for 60 days. The children receiving ashwagandha had significant increases in **hemoglobin** and **serum albumin** and no adverse effects. A similar trial was conducted in 101 adults given 3 g daily of ashwagandha or placebo for 12 months. Those taking the herb had an increase in hemoglobin and red blood cell counts and reported improved libido and sexual performance. Though difficult to interpret, these studies suggest that ashwagandha may well be a useful tonic for those with anemia.

Interest in the use of ashwagandha in the area of cancer treatment is burgeoning. Early research suggests it might increase the effectiveness of radiation therapy and chemotherapy, while reducing side effects. Animal studies suggest that ashwagandha can slow tumor growth and prolong survival. A study in mice found it prevents immune-suppressing effects of the chemotherapy drug paclitaxel. More research is needed to determine if these results can be replicated in human clinical trials.

How to Use

TEA: Simmer 1 teaspoon of powdered root in 1 cup water for 10 minutes. Strain. Drink ⅓ cup 3 times per day.

CAPSULE: 1 to 6 g per day of the dried root, taken in 2 to 3 divided doses.

EXTRACT: Standardized extracts containing 2.5 percent anolides, taken at doses of 500 mg 2 to 3 times daily.

TINCTURES: 2 to 4 ml, taken 3 times daily.

Precautions:

Ashwagandha is safe and generally well tolerated, though it can cause sedation, nausea, and diarrhea. Some evidence suggests it may stimulate thyroid hormonal activity, so it should be used cautiously by those taking thyroid medication. Ashwagandha should not be used during pregnancy, as it can stimulate the uterus. Do not use with sedating medications, because of potential interactions.

Withania somnifera

319

ASHWAGANDHA

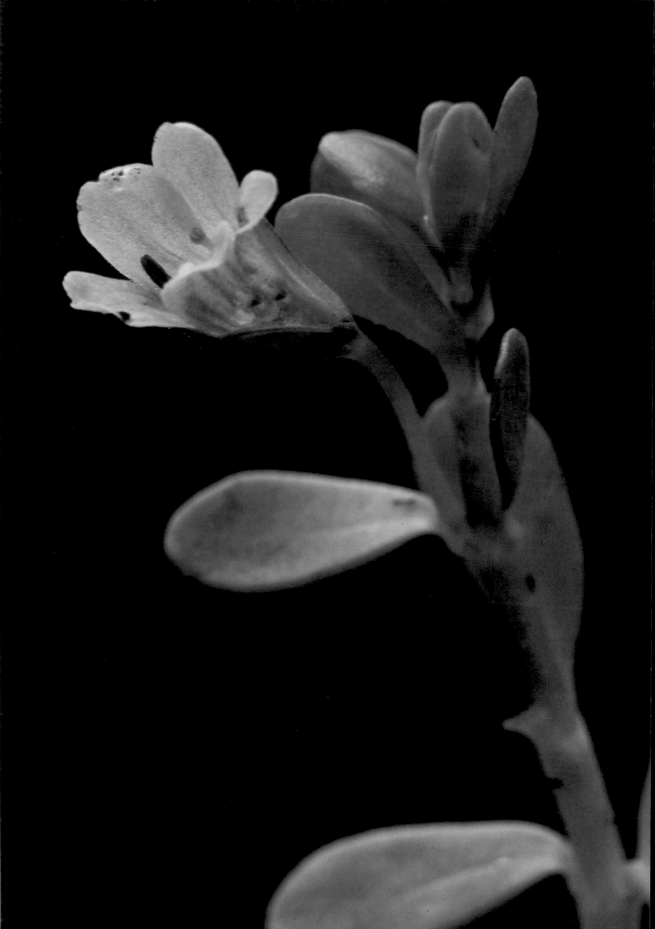

Bacopa

Bacopa monnieri

Bacopa is a marsh lover. This perennial creeping herb with small succulent leaves and delicate mauve flowers thrives in wetlands and along muddy shores in India and many parts of Asia. Crushed bacopa leaves have a distinctive, lemony scent. In English, the plant is also known as coastal water hyssop, but in Hindi it's often called *brahmi*. This unassuming herb has been used in Indian Ayurvedic medicine for at least 3,000 years to treat a number of conditions, but notably to improve memory and cognitive ability. Two ancient Vedic texts, the *Caraka Samhita*

and the *Sushruta Samhita*, document bacopa's use for enhancing comprehension, learning, and memory. In accordance with tradition, newborn infants in India are ceremonially anointed with bacopa to open the gateway of intelligence. Bacopa teas and syrups are also routinely given to Indian children to enhance their intellectual prowess.

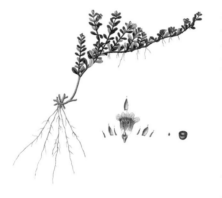

Historically, **Ayurvedic** practitioners have used bacopa to improve a patient's memory and mental abilities, as a nerve tonic to ease anxiety, as a treatment for asthma, and as an aid to healthy heart and lung function. The herb is also considered a blood purifier and a remedy for diarrhea, bronchitis, and fevers. Juice from the leaves can be applied to inflamed joints to relieve pain. Over the past few decades, bacopa has captured the interest of herbal practitioners in the West—and medical researchers in many countries. Studies have shown that bacopa appears to help people process visual information quickly, learn faster, and consolidate new material into memory more effectively. It may improve memory and learning by relieving anxiety, as well as by enhancing nerve impulse transmission, which in turn improves cognitive functions.

In modern Western herbal medicine, bacopa is used to relieve tension and prevent stress. It may help people focus, lengthen attention span, increase concentration, and improve memory and other cognitive functions. Herbal practitioners also recommend the herb for promoting emotional well-being, physical endurance, and a healthy immune system. Bacopa may also aid cognitive ability in the elderly.

Dainty bacopa's leaves, stems, and flowers are a source of memory-boosting extracts that may also reduce anxiety.

TIME LINE OF USAGE AND SPREAD

6TH CENTURY B.C.
Texts note use of bacopa to boost mental function and treat mental disease.

A.D. 1960s
Indian researchers are the first to isolate some of bacopa's active constituents.

2002
Bacopa is shown to improve recall of newly acquired information.

2008
Research shows bacopa has potential for enhancing cognition in the aging.

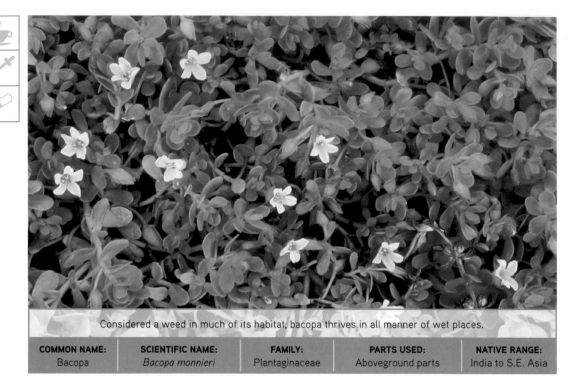

Considered a weed in much of its habitat, bacopa thrives in all manner of wet places.

COMMON NAME:	SCIENTIFIC NAME:	FAMILY:	PARTS USED:	NATIVE RANGE:
Bacopa	*Bacopa monnieri*	Plantaginaceae	Aboveground parts	India to S.E. Asia

Of the more than 50 species included in the genus *Bacopa, B. monnieri* is the most widespread, a weed found in wet areas in many parts of the world. Its variation in different regions of the world has led to much confusion among botanists, resulting in more than 30 botanical names being applied to the plant! Bacopa is a creeping, mat-forming, succulent annual. All parts of the plant are smooth (without hairs).

The opposite leaves are without stalks, oblong-oval, up to an inch long, and less than a half-inch wide. The tubular flowers range from blue to purplish or white, usually flowering from May through October.

Both bacopa and gotu kola share the names *brahmi* and *mandukaparni* in different parts of India, causing additional confusion. Typically, in Kerala, a state in southern India, bacopa is called brahmi. In north and west India, the name mandukaparni is applied to bacopa. Gotu kola is called brahmi in north and west India, and mandukaparni in south India.

Growing Habits

Bacopa is associated with wet habitats, growing in ditches and next to slow-moving steams, coastal estuaries, marshes, or sandy beaches. Found throughout tropical and subtropical areas of the world, bacopa is usually associated with Ayurvedic tradition as a medicinal plant of India. The plant is not generally associated with temperate climates; however, it is widely naturalized in the southern U.S. It occurs from Maryland south through the Carolinas, to Florida, westward through all of the states on the Gulf of Mexico to Texas, and Oklahoma, as well as southern Arizona, southernmost California, Puerto Rico, and Hawaii. Its wide range is a testament to the plant's ability to reproduce by seed or by spreading vegetatively in a variety of conditions. In the southeastern U.S., it occurs mostly in counties bordering coastal regions.

Cultivation and Harvesting

Bacopa is a wet-soil plant and can be grown as a semiaquatic. Although it grows mostly in the tropics, bacopa will grow in cool temperate climates, mostly as a seasonal annual, doing well if temperatures are at least 60°F. It does best if temperatures are 70°F or warmer, and it definitely will not survive a freeze. Bacopa is easily grown from seed or by planting a cutting with a node, which roots readily with plenty of moisture. It is sold at nurseries where aquatic plants or aquarium plants are sold. It can be grown near a pond—planted in muddy soil—to create a beautiful green carpet at water's edge. For an aquarium, plants can be grown in river sand with a little mud mixed in.

Most of the world's bacopa supply is wild-harvested in India, or planted near waterways for ease of harvesting. An **extract** is made from the whole plant and then sold to botanical markets throughout the world.

Therapeutic Uses

+ *Cognition*
+ *Memory*
+ *Antianxiety*

Bacopa may play a role in addressing what pharmaceuticals can only hope to do—namely, improving mental function or enhancing memory. In laboratory results, animal studies, and a few human trials, data are surfacing to support the long-standing traditional use of bacopa in India. Two **compounds** in a class called **saponins**, bacoside A and bacoside B, seem to help animals remember tasks and to reverse the memory loss that occurs with certain medications; whole bacopa can also help animals to learn tasks more quickly. It is possible that bacopa brings about these effects by acting as an **antioxidant** and by affecting levels and metabolism of acetylcholine, an important **neurotransmitter** in the brain and central nervous system.

When 2 150-mg capsules of bacopa extract were given to 23 healthy adults daily for three months, they scored better on a variety of mental tests than 23 people who took **placebo** capsules. After 3 months, the bacopa group had better memory, a more effective learning rate, less forgetting, less anxiety, and faster information processing.

Another interesting potential use of bacopa is in treating anxiety. Some preliminary animal research shows a decrease in anxiety with extracts of bacopa. This could be an interesting use of bacopa because many pharmaceutical antianxiety options can cause memory difficulties; bacopa, on the other hand, actually seems to enhance memory in some circumstances. Well-designed human clinical trials will help to further investigate this possible use.

How to Use

CAPSULES: Generally, 5 to 10 g per day of powdered bacopa.

TEA: Generally, 1 to 2 teaspoons of bacopa leaves steeped in 1 cup of water for 5 to 10 minutes, taken up to 3 times daily.

TINCTURE: Generally, 1 to 2 teaspoons of a **tincture** per day, or 2 tablespoons of the syrup daily; or per manufacturer's directions.

EXTRACT: Standardized extracts contain 20 to 55 percent bacosides; dosage is 150 mg twice daily.

Precautions

Some people taking bacopa experience dry mouth, nausea, and fatigue, but bacopa appears to be relatively free of adverse effects in most studies. Bacopa may increase drowsiness when used in combination with sedative medications, and it may interact with thyroid medications.

---

over the (kitchen) counter BACOPA CHUTNEY

In a saucepan, heat 1 tablespoon oil. Add 1 teaspoon urad dal (available at Indian markets). Sauté until golden brown. Add 3 stemmed red chilis, ½ cup chopped onion, 3 tablespoons grated coconut, and 2 cups bacopa leaves. Sauté 2 to 3 minutes. Cool. Stir in ½ teaspoon each of salt and tamarind pulp and a pinch of brown sugar. Blend until smooth in a food processor. This "brain food" is delicious on rice!

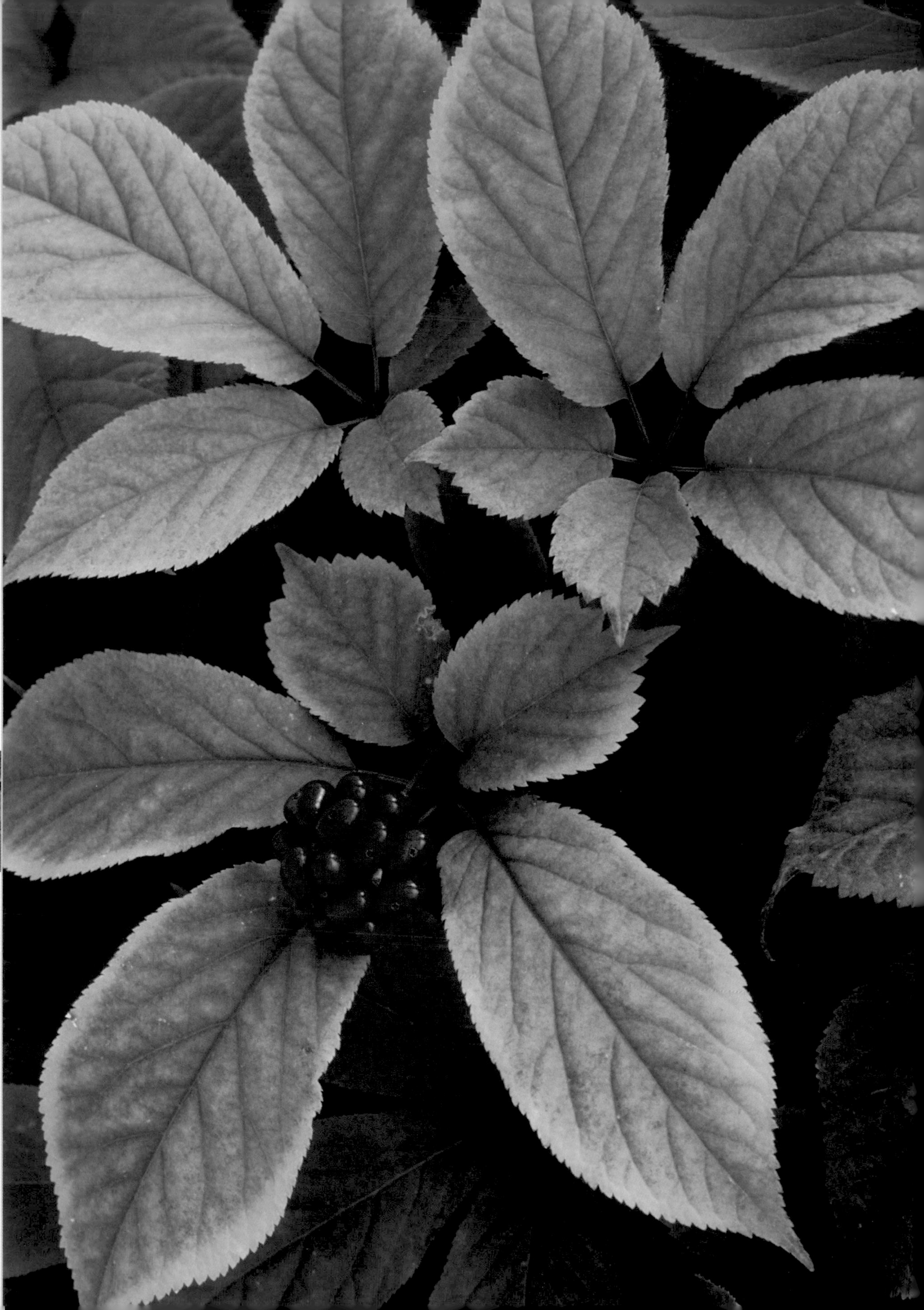

Ginseng

✺✺ *Panax ginseng, P. quinquefolius* ✺✺

Ginseng has been called the king of herbs, the root of heaven, and a wonder of the world. Used in China, Korea, and India for several thousand years, *Panax ginseng* is probably the most famous medicinal herb to have come out of Asia. Its North American counterpart, *Panax quinquefolius*, was discovered later but has similar effects and is prized almost as highly. Ancient Indian texts speak of ginseng as a life-giving plant with magical powers. Centuries ago, Koreans believed that ginseng's leaves gave off a glow on moonlit nights. Ginseng hunters scanned the woods for the eerie radiance, and shot arrows toward its source to mark the plant's location so its valuable roots could be collected the next day. Ginseng hunting was fraught with dangers, but the rewards were great. As a result, wild ginseng in China had been harvested nearly to extinction by the 1600s. The discovery of *Panax quinquefolius* in North America in the early 1700s set off a ginseng rush. Many pioneers made a living digging ginseng roots out of the damp soil of eastern woodlands. Several early American entrepreneurs and explorers, including John Jacob Astor and Daniel Boone, were involved in the profitable ginseng trade in which countless tons of American ginseng made its way to Asia.

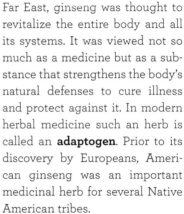

The **genus** name *Panax* is derived from the Greek *panakos*, meaning "cure-all." In the Far East, ginseng was thought to revitalize the entire body and all its systems. It was viewed not so much as a medicine but as a substance that strengthens the body's natural defenses to cure illness and protect against it. In modern herbal medicine such an herb is called an **adaptogen**. Prior to its discovery by Europeans, American ginseng was an important medicinal herb for several Native American tribes.

Western herbalists as well as traditional Asian practitioners today tout ginseng as an immune system-boosting tonic, especially for elderly patients. It is thought to strengthen the nervous system in people suffering from injury and disease, prolonged emotional stress, physical exertion, and fatigue. Ginseng may also help control diabetes, reduce cholesterol, promote mental clarity, and protect against certain types of cancer.

American ginseng roots, like those of its Asian cousin, are among the world's most highly prized medicinal herbs.

TIME LINE OF USAGE AND SPREAD

3000 B.C.	A.D. 1716	1842–1882	1993
The *Vedas*, ancient books of scripture from India, describe ginseng as a life-giving plant.	Jesuit missionary J.-F. Lafitau discovers wild American ginseng in Canada.	Ginseng is listed in the *United States Pharmacopeia*.	United States exports nearly 1.5 million pounds of ginseng.

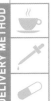
The most famous members of the ginseng family include about a dozen species in the genus *Panax*. American and Asian ginseng are closely related perennials having taproots and growing from 1 to 2 feet tall. They usually have compound leaves, dividing on the stem into groups of 2 to 5 branches. Each branch has smooth or sparsely hairy, oblong lance-shaped leaflets, up to 7 inches long and 3 inches wide. Tiny whitish green flowers are produced in a globe-shaped cluster. The unassuming flowers transform into bright red, shiny, 2-seeded berries.

In American ginseng the stalk on which the flower head sits is shorter than the primary leaflet stalks, sitting lower than the leaves. The leaflet margins have coarsely serrated or rounded teeth. In Asian ginseng the stalk holding the flower head is longer than the leaf stalk, rising above the plant's leaves, and the leaves have smaller, more sharply serrated teeth than those of American ginseng leaflets.

Growing Habits

Asian ginseng occurs in rich mountain slopes in the northeastern Chinese provinces of Heilongjiang, Jilin, and Liaoning, adjacent Korea and Russia, and the northern island of Hokkaido in Japan. Now extremely rare in the wild, the entire world's supply is cultivated, mostly in northeast China (Chinese ginseng) and South Korea (Korean ginseng).

American ginseng occurs on rich, rocky, deep-shaded, cool slopes, preferring sweet soils and ranging from Quebec to Manitoba, south to northern Florida, Alabama, and Oklahoma. It is abundant in the Cumberland Gap region of the southern Appalachians. Elsewhere it is relatively rare. While never a common plant in its range, American ginseng is found less frequently than it once was, considered rare, threatened, or in some areas endangered due to overharvesting.

The genus name, *Panax*, derives from Greek roots that emphasize the "panacea" nature of the root's healthful virtues. The "seng" in the **species** name *ginseng* is a term used by Chinese root diggers to refer to fleshy roots used as tonics in traditional Chinese medicine. It roughly translates into "essence of earth in the form of a man," referring to the humanlike shape of the roots. The species name *quinquefolius* means "five leaves."

Cultivation and Harvesting

Ginseng is a highly specialized crop requiring rich, moist, well-drained, friable soils, high in humus and needing at least 80 percent shade. Propagation is achieved only by seed, which is embryo-dormant, requiring a pregermination treatment to break dormancy. Seeds may take up to 2 years to germinate.

The root is usually harvested after the fourth or fifth year of growth. China and South Korea supply most of the world's Asian ginseng. Canada and the United States are major suppliers of American ginseng, which is now also produced in China.

Therapeutic Uses

+ *Tonic*
+ *Diabetes*
+ *Immune system function*

Ginseng is perhaps the most well known of the herbal tonics, or adaptogens, with possible

over the (kitchen) counter GINSENG TEA

In a saucepan, combine 3 cups water and 8 to 10 thin slices of high-quality dried ginseng root. Simmer covered for 15 to 20 minutes. Remove from heat and let cool. Strain into another container. Serve hot or chilled on ice to make ginseng iced tea. Hot or cold, adding a little honey or sugar will help mask the tea's slightly bitter aftertaste.

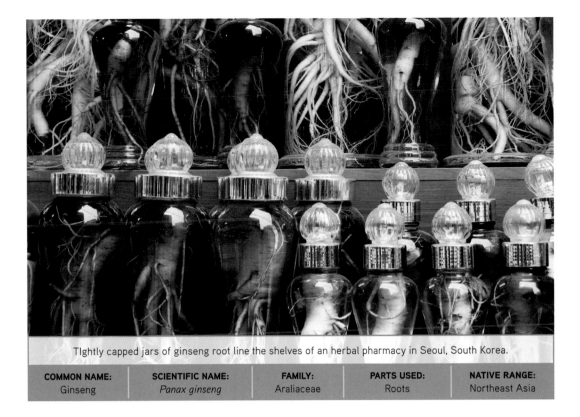

Tightly capped jars of ginseng root line the shelves of an herbal pharmacy in Seoul, South Korea.

COMMON NAME:	SCIENTIFIC NAME:	FAMILY:	PARTS USED:	NATIVE RANGE:
Ginseng	*Panax ginseng*	Araliaceae	Roots	Northeast Asia

benefits for many different medical conditions. Adaptogens are often used to help strengthen the body to resist disease or recover from illness. Each *Panax* species differs a bit from other species; **extracts** of roots of different ginsengs contain different **phytochemicals** and thus have different effects. Laboratory research shows extracts of both the whole root and isolated **compounds** act as **antioxidants**, affect immune system function, and combat **inflammation**.

Clinical research has been done mostly on Asian ginseng. While Asian ginseng doesn't control symptoms such as hot flashes in menopausal women, preliminary results suggest extracts may improve quality of life and lessen fatigue and psychological symptoms. For 36 people with type 2 non-insulin-dependent diabetes, both 100 and 200 mg of ginseng daily for 8 weeks helped with fasting glucose levels. Only those taking the larger dose had improvements in **hemoglobin** A1c tests, the standard tool for comparing blood sugar levels. Studies show that both ginseng species reduce blood sugar levels in people with type 2 diabetes.

Studies also show that American ginseng reduces blood glucose levels in type 1 diabetics. Both species of ginseng enhance immune function. In one study, a specific Asian ginseng extract boosted immune response to the flu vaccine and reduced the number of colds.

How to Use

EXTRACT: Standardized extracts of Asian ginseng containing 4 to 7 percent ginsenosides, dosed 100 to 200 mg daily.

TINCTURES: 1 to 2 ml, up to 3 times daily.

TEA: Simmer 3 to 6 teaspoons of the root for 45 minutes in 3 to 4 cups water. Strain, cool, and drink a cup 1 to 3 times daily.

CAPSULES: 500 to 1,000 mg dried powdered root, taken 1 to 2 times daily.

Precautions

Blood pressure should be monitored when taking ginseng. Caution is advised for diabetics because ginseng can lower blood sugar levels. Asian ginseng can act as a stimulant, causing insomnia or anxiety; some people experience mild stomach upset or headache.

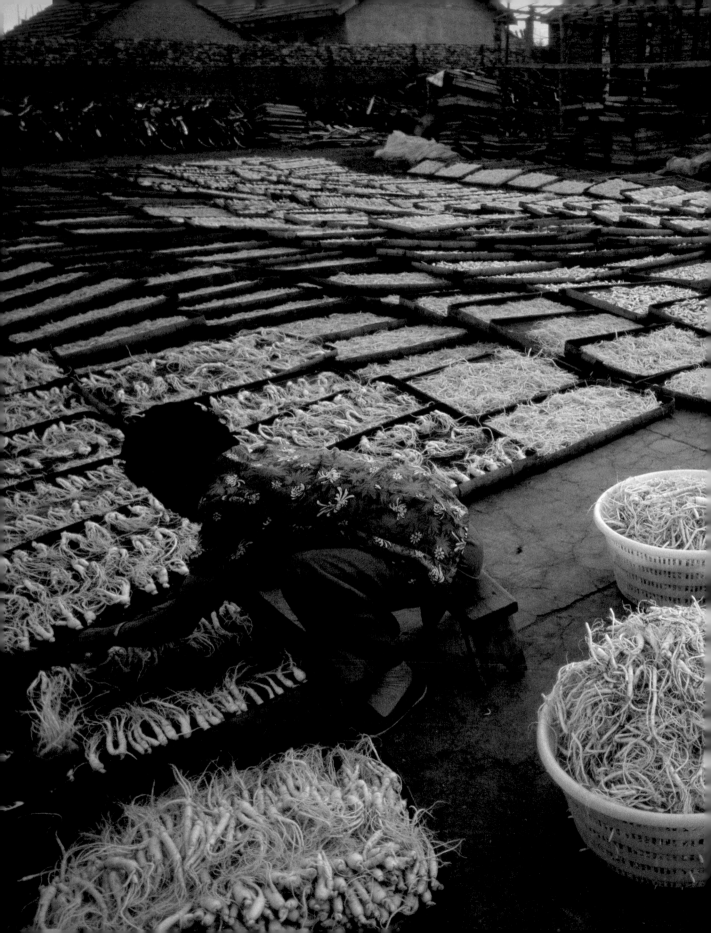

Ginseng Harvest

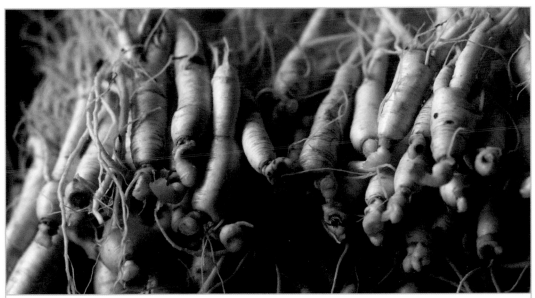

Because wild populations were exhausted centuries ago, essentially all Asian ginseng in the herbal marketplace is cultivated; China and South Korea are currently the world's largest producers. Ginseng cultivation requires considerable skill and training. Plants reach maturity between 4 and 6 years of age. In autumn, roots are carefully dug, gently washed, and dried (for white ginseng) or steamed and dried (for red ginseng). Chinese workers (opposite) arrange harvested ginseng roots in neat rows on drying racks laid out in the sun. After drying, the roots (above) are sorted, stored, or shipped. Chinese buyers (below) scrutinize roots that may be exported to the United States.

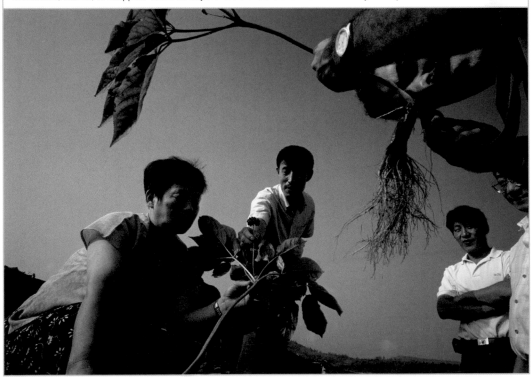

Goji

Lycium barbarum, L. chinense

Goji is the name for two closely related species of tall, woody shrubs traditionally grown in fertile Himalayan valleys of Tibet, Mongolia, and China, as well as in China's Xinjiang and Ningxia provinces. Both species produce bright red-orange berries, each about the size and shape of a Thompson's seedless grape. The berries are so delicate that instead of being hand-picked, they are gently shaken from the branches of the plants into trays. Their flavor is both faintly sweet and tart, sometimes likened to the taste of cranberries or a cross

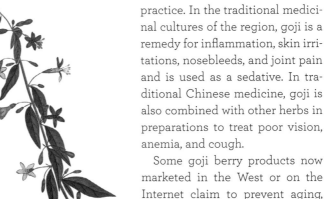

between a strawberry and a raspberry. Until recently, goji was relatively unknown in the West. Now, hundreds of goji products, ranging from dried berries and berry juices to goji berry crunch bars and capsules of berry **extract**, line the shelves of health food and specialty stores, often accompanied by extravagant claims of health benefits.

Goji has a long history in China and Tibet as both food and medicine. Tender young leaves and shoots are commonly eaten as vegetables. Fresh goji berry juice is very popular in areas where the plants are cultivated and is sometimes combined with tea to make a tonic. The dried berries are typically cooked and added to foods such as rice porridge and various tonic soups that may include other medicinal herbs. Boiling the berries to make tea is also a widespread

practice. In the traditional medicinal cultures of the region, goji is a remedy for inflammation, skin irritations, nosebleeds, and joint pain and is used as a sedative. In traditional Chinese medicine, goji is also combined with other herbs in preparations to treat poor vision, anemia, and cough.

Some goji berry products now marketed in the West or on the Internet claim to prevent aging, cure cancer, and improve sexual function. None of these claims are supported by solid scientific research. However, like many other fruits and vegetables, goji berries are rich in **antioxidants**, substances that have been shown to counter the effects of **free radicals**—chemicals that damage cells and may cause cancer. Goji juice may also be a mild **adaptogen.** Nevertheless, much more research is needed.

Despite a long history of use in Asia, goji berries are a recent addition to the Western herbal pharmacopoeia.

TIME LINE OF USAGE AND SPREAD

1400s
Goji is cultivated along China's Yellow River since at least this time.

1768
Scottish botanist Philip Miller describes *Lycium chinense* in *The Gardener's Dictionary.*

2004
China exports $120 million worth of goji berries and products.

2007
Anheuser-Busch markets energy drink 180 Red with Goji with goji berry juice.

Of the 80 species in the genus *Lycium*, or wolfberry, the most well known are the Chinese species *L. barbarum* and *L. chinense*, sources of what is sold in the America as goji berries. "Goji" is an English word coined to represent a truncated mispronunciation of the Chinese name *guo qi zi*. The center of diversity for *Lycium* is not China but western North America and South America, where more than 50 species of *Lycium* are found. In China, there are 7 species.

Lycium chinense is a vigorous, hardy, erect or sprawling **deciduous** shrub, with or without thorns, usually about 2 to 3 feet tall, sometimes reaching 6 feet in height. The alternate leaves are oval to somewhat triangular in shape and up to 3 inches long. The purple, tubular, lobed flowers are ½ inch or more across. The bright red-orange fruit, oval to oblong in shape, is about an inch long and half as wide. Fruiting is from June to September.

L. barbarum, very similar in appearance to *L. chinense*, grows from 2 to 6 feet tall. The linear to linear-oblong leaves are an inch long. The 5-part funnel-shaped purple flower differs from the flower of *L. chinense* in having a corolla tube longer than the flower lobes. The **genus** name *Lycium* comes from the Greek word *lycion*, referring to thorny shrubs of the ancient world.

Growing Habits

L. chinense is widespread in China, occurring on slopes, saline soils, and roadsides. Its range extends to Japan, Korea, Mongolia, Nepal, Pakistan, Thailand, Southwest Asia, and southern Europe. In North America, it is found in scattered locations from southern Maine to Georgia, west to Oklahoma and Kansas, and north to Ontario; it is also found in California.

L. barbarum is primarily restricted to its native habitats in Ningxia province in northern China, where much of the commercial supply is produced, though it is widely naturalized in China. *L. barbarum* is actually more widespread in North America than in China, naturalized in every one of the lower 48 states except Arizona and Mississippi. It also occurs in southeastern Europe, Iran, and North Africa.

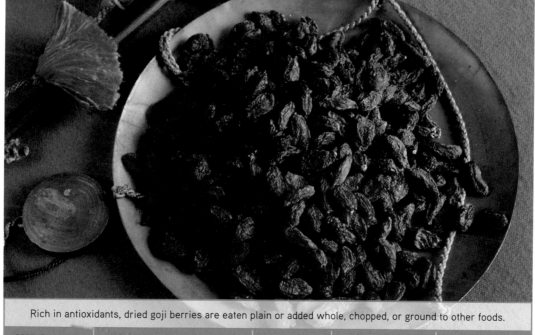

Rich in antioxidants, dried goji berries are eaten plain or added whole, chopped, or ground to other foods.

COMMON NAME:	SCIENTIFIC NAME:	FAMILY:	PARTS USED:	NATIVE RANGE:
Goji	*Lycium barbarum, L. chinense*	Solanaceae	Fruits ("berries")	Central China

over the (kitchen) counter GOJI-POM SMOOTHIE

Combine 2 tablespoons dried goji berries and ¼ cup water in a small bowl. Let the berries soften for about 20 minutes. Place the berries, along with 2 teaspoons ground flax seed, 6 medium-size strawberries, ½ banana, and 1 cup pomegranate juice, in a blender. Blend until smooth, adding more pomegranate juice if needed to achieve desired consistency.

Cultivation and Harvesting

Goji is generally a shrub of easy culture, propagated from seeds, which usually germinate in about 10 days, or by cuttings taken from new growth of the previous year. Goji prefers a relatively cool climate and a sandy, alkaline, moist but well-drained soil.

In commercial production regions in China, plants are pruned to create a rounded crown, facilitating easier harvest. Fruits are harvested when ripe in late summer or early autumn, then spread to dry on bamboo mats in shade. The fruits are not turned or handled during drying, as they may bruise and turn black. Most of the goji berry commercial supply sold in the U.S. is from China; goji is widely cultivated elsewhere for the fruits, found in bulk in every market in central and western Asia.

Therapeutic Uses

+ *General well-being*
+ *Antioxidant*

Looking like red raisins, goji berries are currently sold in every form marketers can devise as a "healthy" choice. The reddish orange berries, containing chemicals shown in laboratory testing to be rich in antioxidants, belong to a family of **compounds** called **carotenoids**, found in many fruits and vegetables that are bright red, orange, or yellow and well known for their antioxidant effects. Goji berries also contain beta-sitosterol, which may help balance cholesterol levels; **polysaccharides**, which probably account for boosts to the immune system; and many vitamins and minerals.

Two studies, partly financed by a company that produces goji berry juice, examined antioxidant effects as well as general well-being. In one study, in an examination of antioxidant effects, 25 people drank 60 ml of goji berry juice twice daily for a month.

Laboratory results were compared with those from a taste- and color-matched **placebo** drink. After a month, blood antioxidant levels in the goji berry group were 5 to 9 percent higher than they were in the placebo group.

The same research group also looked at the effects of the same goji berry juice on mental well-being. Seventeen people drank 120 ml of goji berry juice daily for 2 weeks. This group fared better in such areas as calmness, athletic performance, happiness, quality of sleep, and feelings of good health than the 18 people drinking a placebo juice. Nevertheless, despite a flurry of claims and products on the market, further solid research is necessary to draw any conclusions about goji's effectiveness.

How to Use

JUICE: Pressed from fresh and ripe goji berries, the juice is kept refrigerated until use. One clinical trial used 120 ml of the juice as a daily serving, considered a standard dose in traditional Chinese medicine.

TEA: In Chinese medicine, a water-based extract (the equivalent of 2 tablespoons of the dried root bark per ½ cup of water) is used daily for high blood pressure, while ⅓ to ½ that dose is used daily for diabetes.

CAPSULES: 500 mg, 1 to 3 times daily.

Precautions

Goji should be avoided by those undergoing chemotherapy or radiation therapy unless recommended by a health care provider. Due to goji's potential for lowering blood pressure and glucose levels, care should be taken by those taking high blood pressure or diabetes medicines. Goji may increase the activity of blood-thinning medications such as warfarin; avoid combining these.

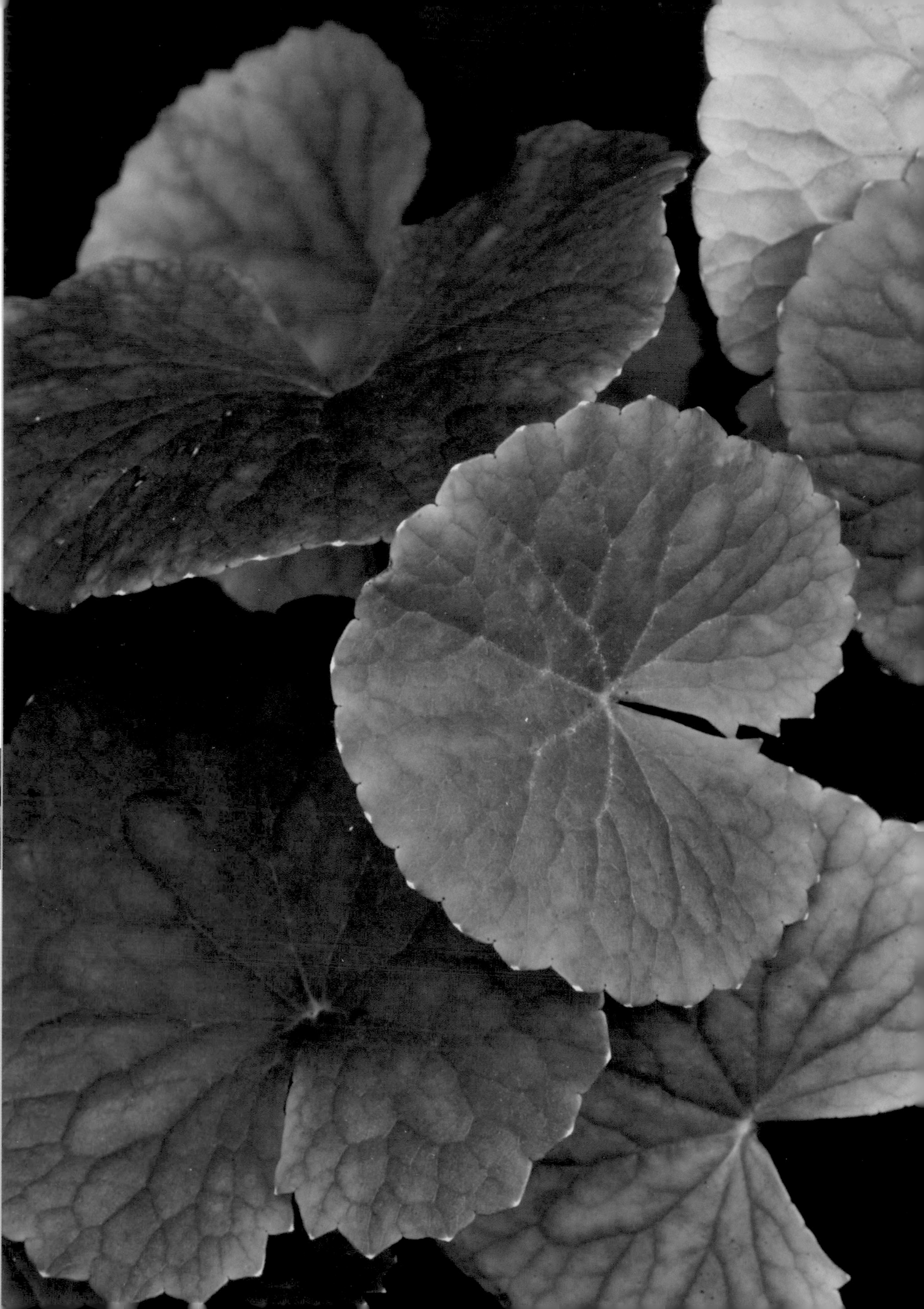

Gotu Kola

✺ *Centella asiatica* ✺

Native to India, Indonesia, China, and Southeast Asia, gotu kola thrives in and around swampy bodies of water, slowly spreading on slender stems that typically hug the ground or the water's surface. Its dainty, rounded leaves are about the size of an old British penny, hence one of its common English names, Indian pennywort. Although the leaves are relatively tasteless, gotu kola is a common salad green in Vietnamese, Thai, and Malay cuisines. In Sri Lanka, it is often prepared as a green vegetable to accompany curries. Gotu kola has been used medicinally for thousands of years where it occurs. Through the ages, it has gained a reputation for enhancing longevity. The Chinese name for gotu kola roughly translates as "fountain of youth."

In Indian **Ayurvedic** medicine, gotu kola is known by many names, including *brahmi*, which means "bringing the knowledge of Brahman." It was traditionally used to heal wounds and ulcerative skin diseases such as leprosy. Additionally, Ayurvedic practitioners prescribed it as a tonic to revitalize nerves and the brain, and in so doing, improve mental clarity and memory, especially in the elderly. The Chinese used gotu kola primarily to treat fever and respiratory ailments. American **Eclectic** physicians used a closely related **species** to treat skin problems during the 19th century. However, gotu kola was essentially unknown

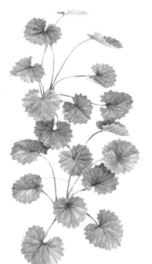

in the United States until after World War II, when a gotu kola-containing herbal tea—supposedly similar to one drunk by an ancient Chinese herbalist said to live to the age of 256—was marketed as a longevity booster. And gotu kola moved into the limelight.

Despite such unsubstantiated claims, research shows that gotu kola may aid memory and cognition. In modern integrative medicine, herbalists also recommend gotu kola to treat varicose veins and chronic venous insufficiency, in which blood tends to pool in the legs. The herb may relieve some symptoms of scleroderma, a disease characterized by joint pain and hardening of skin and connective tissue. Gotu kola is applied topically, in ointments, to help heal minor wounds and the red welts associated with psoriasis and to reduce scar tissue after surgery.

A mainstay in Ayurvedic medicine, gotu kola has distinctive leaves that may aid memory and enhance healing.

TIME LINE OF USAGE AND SPREAD

1754
First case of scleroderma—possibly relieved by gotu kola—is documented in Italy.

1880s
Gotu kola is accepted as an herbal medicine in France.

1940s
Researchers isolate many of gotu kola's active compounds.

1992
Studies indicating plant may improve memory spur popularity in U.S.

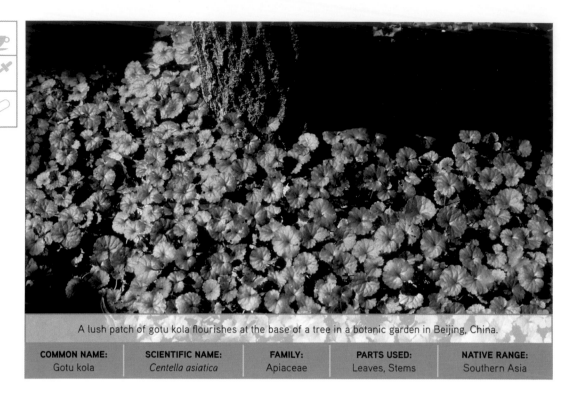

A lush patch of gotu kola flourishes at the base of a tree in a botanic garden in Beijing, China.

COMMON NAME:	SCIENTIFIC NAME:	FAMILY:	PARTS USED:	NATIVE RANGE:
Gotu kola	*Centella asiatica*	Apiaceae	Leaves, Stems	Southern Asia

Of the 50 species in the genus *Centella*, gotu kola is the most well known and the most widespread, a famous herb of Ayurvedic traditions from India. South Africa is the center of diversity for the genus *Centella*. A small, low-growing, herbaceous perennial, from 3 inches to nearly 12 inches in height, gotu kola is a slender-stemmed creeping plant, rooting at the nodes, often forming large patches. The leaves are round in outline, heart shaped at the base, and variable in size, up to 2 inches in diameter, with coarse, round-toothed margins. The leaf stalks are usually longer than the leaves. The upper and lower surface is usually smooth, though slightly hairy in some variations. The sparse groups of tiny whitish green or reddish flowers are inconspicuous and seldom noticed.

Growing Habits

Gotu kola is adaptable but usually found in shady, wet grasslands, waste places, forest margins, and ditches and along streams and rivers in tropical and subtropical countries worldwide. It is found throughout warmer parts of southern and eastern China, Bhutan, India, Indonesia, Japan, Korea, Laos, Malaysia, Myanmar, Nepal, Pakistan, Thailand, and Vietnam. In Asia it is used locally as a vegetable. In the Philippines it is one of the main plants worked by honeybees. Its weedlike, very common occurrence throughout warmer regions of Asia gives it a reputation comparable to that of dandelions in America. Gotu kola is also found in Central and South America, Africa, and the Middle East. Introduced by Asian immigrants, gotu kola is naturalized in Florida, Gulf Coast states, Hawaii, and Washington.

Cultivation and Harvesting

Centella is so common in wild habitats throughout much of warmer regions of the world that cultivating the herb for home use is considered a waste of garden space. Since it is essentially a weed in the tropics, suggesting to gardeners in those areas that they cultivate the plant might be met with skepticism. Instead, wild plants are harvested locally as a fresh vegetable or leaves are picked and dried for medicinal use.

In temperate areas, gotu kola can be grown as a container plant, provided it is watered frequently and given full sun. The plant is propagated from cuttings, using any piece of the stem with a node. It likes moist soils. Clumps can be divided and replanted. Once planted, it is of easy culture, requiring only occasional side-dressing with an organic fertilizer. It is sometimes available from nurseries specializing in aquatic plants and is commonly available from nurseries selling medicinal plants.

Indonesia produces more than 125 tons of the dried herb per year, though much of the world's supply comes from cultivation in Madagascar. The plant is also commercially grown in Sri Lanka and India for export markets. In Thailand, Vietnam, Laos, and Cambodia, the leaves are used to make a locally available soft drink product.

Therapeutic Uses

+ *Memory and cognition*
+ *Venous insufficiency*
+ *Wound healing*

Not to be confused with kola nut, gotu kola has been a revered plant for centuries, useful both topically and internally for many medical conditions. Recent focus in the United States has turned, in particular, to gotu kola's possibilities for enhancing learning—more well established in Asia. Various research studies have addressed the cognitive effects of gotu kola, showing improvements in learning and memory, as well as **antioxidant** effects.

One trial of 80 healthy elderly subjects used 250- to 750-mg capsules of a gotu kola water **extract**; over 3 months the participants demonstrated improved grip strength, leg strength, and overall satisfaction related to physical functioning. However, this result occurred only at the 750-mg dose and disappeared after the subjects stopped taking the gotu kola.

Applied topically, golu kola may help close up wounds by fostering the formation of **collagen** and by helping fibroblasts, the most common cells found in connective tissue, to heal the skin. Gotu kola's antioxidant effects on blood vessels also seem to help with circulatory troubles. Gotu kola extract standardized to **triterpenoid compounds** of 60 to 120 mg over 3 months can help to decrease leg swelling and symptoms caused by venous insufficiency. Gotu kola, both as standardized extract capsules and topically applied creams, is also used to help people with varicose veins.

The **triterpene** compounds in gotu kola are thought to provide many of its medicinal effects. Gotu kola also contains **flavonoids** such as quercetin and rutin, which are known to be **anti-inflammatory** and antioxidant, and **essential oils**, which may have various antibacterial effects.

How to Use

CAPSULES: Standardized extracts containing 30 mg of total triterpenoids per capsule, taken in 1 to 2 capsules twice daily. Total amount of dried leaves, stems, and flowers should equal 0.5 to 6 g daily.

TINCTURE: 2 to 4 teaspoons daily.

CREAMS: 1 percent gotu kola mixed into a cream, applied as per manufacturer's directions.

Precautions

Anyone with preexisting liver disease or taking medications that may cause liver problems should avoid taking gotu kola. Occasionally, stomach upset and nausea are reported by those taking gotu kola. If topical use of gotu kola causes a rash, use should be discontinued. Gotu kola should not be used during pregnancy.

---

over the (kitchen) counter GOTU KOLA SALAD OR STIR-FRY

Finely slice 2 cups rinsed gotu kola leaves. Toss together with ⅓ cup finely chopped onion, 1 fresh chili (seeded, stemmed, and sliced), ⅔ cup freshly grated coconut, 1 teaspoon fresh lime juice, ½ teaspoon sugar, and ⅛ teaspoon salt. Serve immediately. Alternatively, put all the ingredients in a wok with a tablespoon of water and sauté for about 1 minute over medium-high heat.

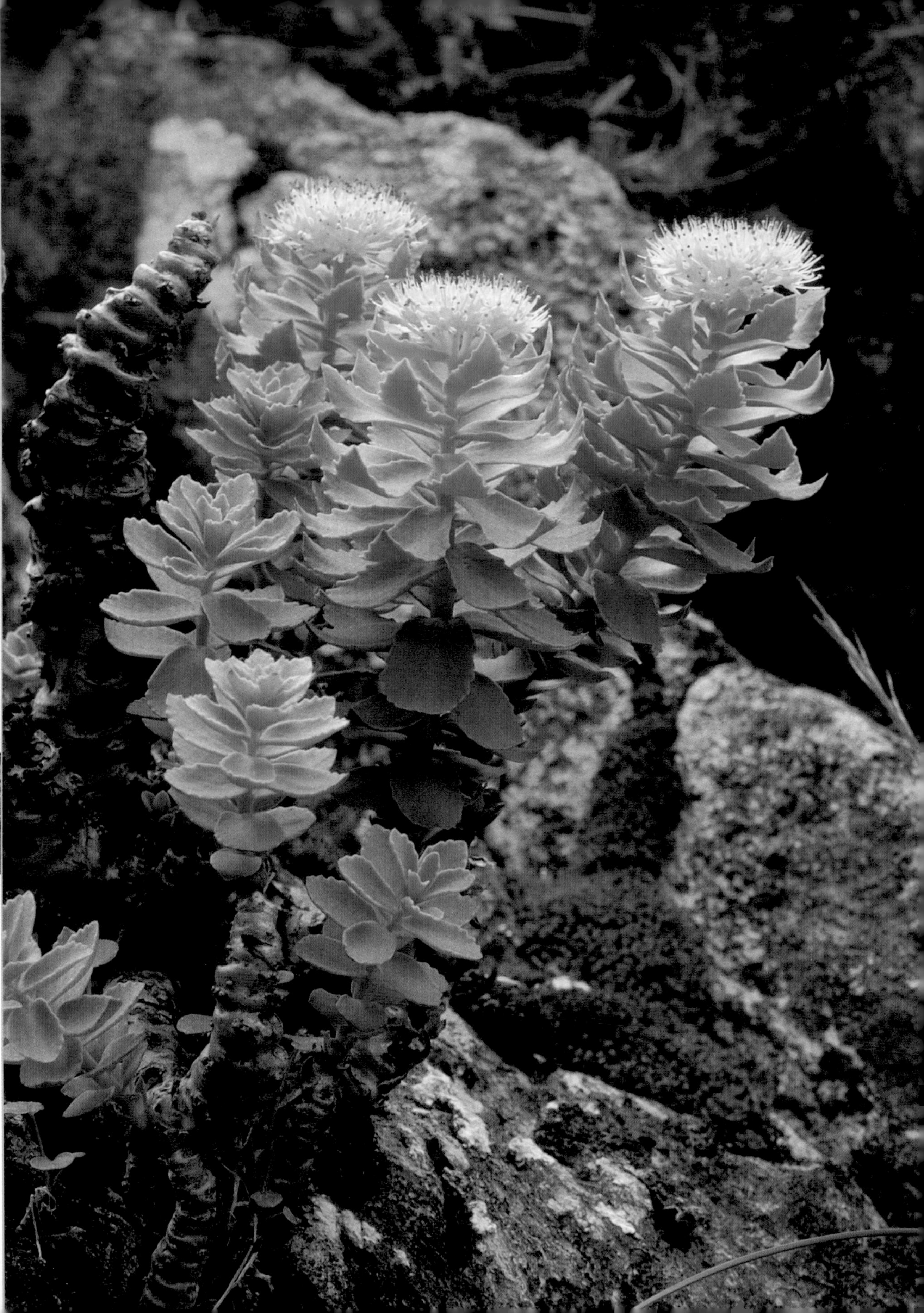

Rhodiola

❧ *Rhodiola rosea* ❧

C ommonly called golden root or rose root in English, and *hóng jǐng tiān* in traditional Chinese medicine, rhodiola is a thick-leaved, sedumlike plant that grows in cold Arctic and mountainous regions throughout the Northern Hemisphere. The English common names describe two characteristics of rhodiola's thick, tuberous roots—their fleshy interior is tinted a golden yellow color, and freshly cut, they give off a roselike aroma. The first-century Greek physician Dioscorides wrote about rhodiola in his medical reference text *De Materia Medica*. He called the plant *rodia riza*. Sixteen hundred years later, Swedish botanist and father of modern taxonomy Carolus Linnaeus renamed it *Rhodiola rosea*. For centuries, rhodiola has been part of traditional medicine in Russia, China, Scandinavia, and elsewhere.

The Vikings are thought to have used rhodiola to improve physical strength and endurance. In Siberia, rhodiola tea, prepared from the plant's fragrant roots, was a centuries-old effective remedy for colds and flu. The roots were considered so valuable that the location of wild rhodiola plants was often a well-guarded family secret. Chinese emperors were known to send expeditions into Siberia to bring back the roots for their own medicinal preparations. In some Siberian mountain villages, bouquets of rhodiola roots are still presented to marrying couples as a talisman to enhance fertility and ensure the health of children. By the 1700s, rhodiola was being used medicinally in a number of European countries, yet scientific analysis of the herb's medicinal actions was still in its infancy. It wasn't until the mid-1960s that intense research into rhodiola began, primarily in Russia and Scandinavia. **Extracts** of rhodiola root were found to contain a number of substances that have significant **adaptogenic** properties. By the mid-1970s, Russian physicians were prescribing an extract of rhodiola root as a **stimulant** to combat fatigue, increase stamina, and enhance attention span and memory.

Rhodiola is a relatively new herbal medicine in the United States. Herbalists consider it an adaptogen and typically suggest it to combat fatigue caused by stress and enhance work performance by increasing attention span and concentration.

Rhodiola has sweet-smelling roots that are the source of extracts used to increase stamina and fight fatigue.

TIME LINE OF USAGE AND SPREAD

50-70
Dioscorides notes medicinal applications of *rodia riza* in *De Materia Medica*.

1961
Botanist G. V. Krylov leads expedition to Siberia to retrieve samples of rhodiola.

1975
Large-scale production of rhodiola extract liquid begins in the Soviet Union.

1985
Sweden's medical community accepts rhodiola as stimulant and fatigue-fighting agent.

Rhodiola is a group of succulent plants, mostly found in mountain habitats or cooler regions of the Northern Hemisphere. A succulent perennial, rhodiola is erect or spreading, with pale green leaves, covered with a bluish film that rubs off between the fingers. In flower, the plant reaches up to a foot tall. The leaf blades are mostly in overlapping rosettes at the base of the plant. They are oval to oblong in shape, up to 2 inches long and about half as wide.

The margins are entire or round toothed. The flowers are in clustered groups, arising on a thick stem. The flowers are usually greenish yellow to pale yellow, often reddish at the tips. Up to 150 flowers crowd the flower heads. The plant is highly variable, especially in leaf structure and flower color. The root and the thick **rhizome**, with a pleasant roselike fragrance when cut, are the parts used in herbal medicine.

Growing Habits

Rhodiola is native to cooler areas of Eurasia and North America, growing on moist rock ledges, coastal cliffs, and north-facing rocky slopes. In Europe, rhodiola grows in rocky habitats, mostly in northern Europe, on mountains throughout central Europe and south to the Pyrenees, the southern Alps in Italy, eastward to Bulgaria. In China it grows in forested or grassy mountain slopes in the northern provinces, and is found in Japan, Kazakhstan, Korea, Mongolia, and much of Russia. As a medicinal plant it is associated with Russian traditions, adopted and developed as a widely used medicinal plant in the former Soviet Union. In North America, it is found in eastern Canada, Maine, Vermont, New York, Pennsylvania, and the mountains of western North Carolina and Alaska.

Cultivation and Harvesting

Rhodiola is suitable for alpine rock gardens in the northern U.S. and mountain regions. It is propagated by seeds or division of the rhizome.

Roots are harvested in the autumn of the second or third year of growth. Rhodiola is widespread in its native habitat, but increased demand—with rhodiola products now sold in more than 50 countries—has placed increased pressures on wild populations due to intensive collection, especially in the past 15 years. The plant is threatened in Russia due to overcollection and has seen pressure in Great Britain, the Czech Republic, Bosnia and Herzegovina, Slovakia, and Bulgaria, where it is endangered and collection is forbidden.

Commercial cultivation has succeeded in various countries, including China, Finland, Sweden, and Russia. Supported by Canadian and provincial government research, the province of Alberta also engages in successful large-scale production.

Therapeutic Uses

+ *Stress*
+ *Anxiety*
+ *Depression*
+ *Fatigue*

Researchers in Russia and Scandinavia have studied the effects of rhodiola for more than 40 years. Their research has confirmed that rhodiola does have broad and potent effects on health and well-being. Among many active **compounds** in rhodiola, the two that seem most powerful are rosavin and salidroside.

over the (kitchen) counter RHODIOLA ELIXIR

Grind 1 ounce of rhodiola root in coffee grinder and put in a 1-quart Mason jar. Chop up 1 ounce dried unsulfured apricots and put apricots and 1 cinnamon stick in jar. Add 6 to 8 ounces brandy and stir well. Close lid tightly and let sit covered for 14 days. Strain and put liquid in dark bottle. Take 1 teaspoon 1 to 2 times per day for its tonic effect. Delicious!

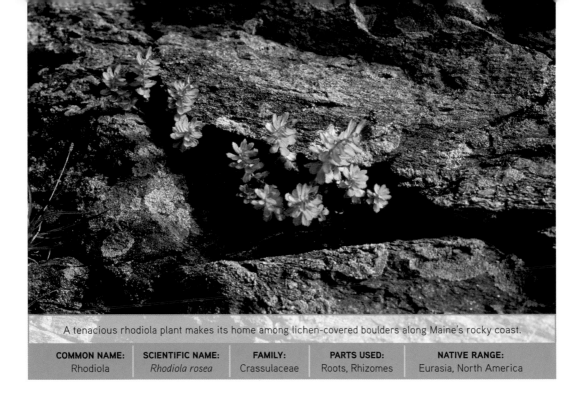

A tenacious rhodiola plant makes its home among lichen-covered boulders along Maine's rocky coast.

COMMON NAME:	SCIENTIFIC NAME:	FAMILY:	PARTS USED:	NATIVE RANGE:
Rhodiola	*Rhodiola rosea*	Crassulaceae	Roots, Rhizomes	Eurasia, North America

The role of rhodiola in the area of mental health is highly promising. A small pilot study conducted by the Department of Psychiatry at the University of California, Los Angeles, found that rhodiola significantly reduced anxiety in patients diagnosed with generalized anxiety disorder. The improvement was similar to that seen with prescription antianxiety medications, and no significant side effects were reported. Good news, given that anxiety disorders affect roughly 40 million American adults age 18 years and older in a given year.

Rhodiola appears not only to have a calming effect but also to ease depression. Animal studies have shown that **serotonin** levels increase in the brain under the administration of rhodiola. Serotonin reuptake inhibitors, such as Prozac and Zoloft, also alleviate depression. A study of patients with mild to moderate depression randomized them to receive 340 mg per day of rhodiola extract, 680 mg per day of rhodiola extract, or **placebo** for 6 weeks. Those taking either dose of rhodiola experienced an improvement in symptoms of overall depression, insomnia, and emotional instability compared with placebo.

Chronic fatigue syndrome is a condition characterized by persistent fatigue and weakness, as well as muscle and joint pain, headache, and inability to concentrate. A **double-blind** study of 60 people suffering from chronic fatigue syndrome randomized half to receive 575 mg daily of rhodiola or identical-looking **placebo** for 28 days. Researchers found that compared with placebo, rhodiola exerted an antifatigue effect that increased mental performance, particularly the ability to concentrate, and decreased cortisol response to stress. (Under stress, the body produces high levels of cortisol. Rhodiola reduced and normalized cortisol levels.)

How to Use

TEA: Steep 1 teaspoon rhodiola root in 1 cup hot water for 5 minutes. Strain. Drink 3 times a day.

TINCTURE: Generally, taken at 3 to 5 ml twice a day, or per manufacturer's recommendations.

EXTRACT: Daily dosage in studies ranged from 100 to 576 mg extract standardized to contain 3.6 percent rosavin and 1.6 percent salidroside.

Precautions

Rhodiola appears to be well tolerated; however, herb-drug interaction can occur when rhodiola is combined with antidepressant medications. Safety of rhodiola during pregnancy is not known. Those with a mental health condition should consult a health care professional before using rhodiola.

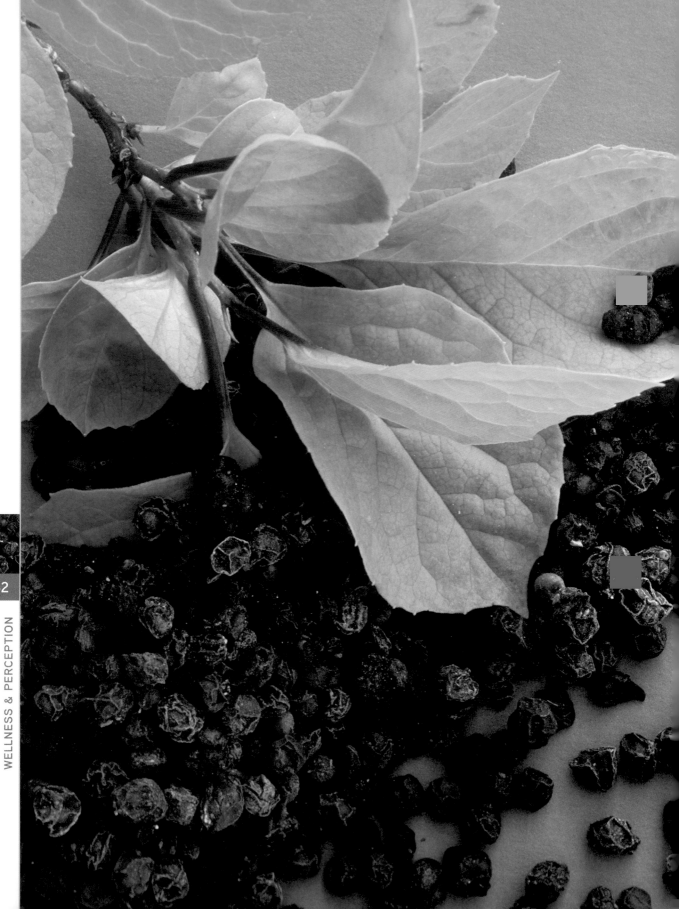

Schisandra

❧ *Schisandra chinensis* ❧

S hen Nong, legendary hero emperor of China who taught his people how to cultivate plants for food and medicine some 5,000 years ago, believed schisandra was a superior herb with the power to protect health and prolong life. A deciduous, woody vine, *Schisandra chinensis* is native to moist temperate forests of northern China, Korea, Japan, and the Russian Far East. It produces dense clusters of crimson berries that slightly resemble grapes. The Chinese name for the berries means "five flavor berry," because biting into them, one experiences sweet,

sour, bitter, and salty flavors, as well as a pungent heat, all at the same time. These 5 flavors correspond to the 5 elements of traditional Chinese medicine: sweet (earth), sour (wood), bitter (fire), salty (water), and acrid (metal). Rich in nutrients, the berries are eaten both raw and cooked. They are also dried and used as a nourishing, highly portable food on long journeys. Schisandra is considered one of the 50 fundamental herbs in traditional Chinese medicine. It is classified as a harmonizing tonic and has been used for centuries to treat diseases of the lungs, liver, kidneys, and heart, and to calm the heart and ease the mind.

Not until the 1960s, however, did schisandra gain recognition as an **adaptogen**, an herb that strengthens all the body's systems. This discovery came about largely as a result of many

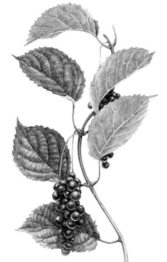

pharmacological and clinical studies carried out by Russian scientists during the 1940s and 1950s. Russian researchers were so impressed by schisandra's stress-protecting effects that the herb was incorporated into Russian conventional medicine. Pharmacological studies on animals have shown that schisandra increases physical stamina and affords a stress-protective effect. In particular, the herb appears to protect the liver against a variety of toxins.

In Western herbal medicine, schisandra is used primarily as an adaptogen to restore normal functioning in various body systems. Herbalists may specifically prescribe it to help enhance mental function, improve physical stamina and sexual performance, protect and detoxify the liver and kidneys, and treat insomnia.

Worldwide, herbalists use the leaves and dried berries of schisandra for increasing stamina and mental clarity.

TIME LINE OF USAGE AND SPREAD

3000 B.C.	**1850s**	**1947**	**1961**
Schisandra chinensis is already incorporated in Chinese herbal medicine.	*Schisandra chinensis* is imported to U.S. from Russia as ornamental plant.	Russian scientist N. Lazarev defines adaptogens as agents that help body counter stress.	Schisandra added to *Russian Pharmacopoeia* as an herb for conventional practice.

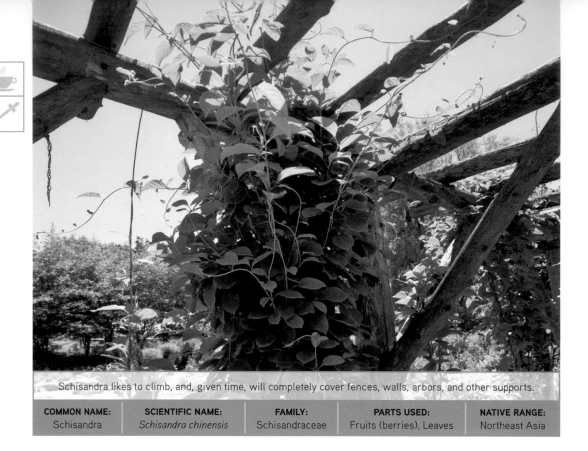

Schisandra likes to climb, and, given time, will completely cover fences, walls, arbors, and other supports.

COMMON NAME:	SCIENTIFIC NAME:	FAMILY:	PARTS USED:	NATIVE RANGE:
Schisandra	*Schisandra chinensis*	Schisandraceae	Fruits (berries), Leaves	Northeast Asia

There are about two dozen species of schisandra, all of which occur in China except one—southern magnolia vine *Schisandra glabra (S. coccinea),* a relatively rare plant at home in rich bottomlands in the southeastern United States. *Schisandra chinensis* is a climbing, deciduous, perennial vine growing up to 40 feet long. The alternate leaves are oblong-ovate to rounded, 3 inches long and about half as wide, with wavy teeth along the margin. The nodding, solitary, creamy white flowers are in lower **axils** of younger leaf shoots. Male and female flowers grow on separate plants, and both male and female plants must be present to produce schisandra fruits. The small, smooth scarlet fruits hang in grapelike bunches. Dried fruits are about the size of peppercorns.

Growing Habits

Schisandra grows in mixed **deciduous** forests, slopes, and river ravines from the mountains of northeastern China in Heilongjiang, Jilin, and Liaoning provinces, south through the mountains of central China to Hubei, Sichuan, and Yunnan provinces. It is also found in mountain habitats on the islands of Hokkaido and Honshu in Japan, in Korea, Sakhalin, and adjacent regions of Russia. Outside of its native home in northeastern Asia, it is grown as a horticultural specimen plant. A closely related **species**, *S. sphenanthera,* is also widespread in southern China. In Chinese markets, the fruits of *S. sphenanthera* are designated *nan wei zi* (southern wei zi); the fruits of *S. chinensis* are called *bei wei zi* (northern wei zi).

The **genus** name *Schisandra* is from the Greek *schizein,* meaning "to cleave" and *andros* ("man"), referring to the anther cells on the stamens. The Chinese name, wei zi, calls attention to the remarkable combination of flavor sensations that the fruits deliver.

Cultivation and Harvesting

Schisandra is a relatively rare plant in American horticulture, suitable for cooler climates, where it is grown along walls for its beautiful fall-ripening fruit. In commercial production systems it is trellised. Schisandra likes moist rich, shady conditions and is very hardy. In the northern U.S., it can be grown in full sun; in the South it needs shade. Schisandra is propagated by seeds, layering, or softwood cuttings. Seeds are planted in autumn, soon after ripening, or saved for planting in spring. The vine does best in a rich, friable, well-drained, deep, sandy soil.

Fruits are harvested in September through November and dried in the sun, allowing plenty of ventilation to avoid spoilage. Much of the world's supply comes from China. It is also grown in Russia but is not a significant export. It was formerly grown in several East European countries for the Russian market.

Therapeutic Uses

+ *Adaptogen*
+ *Hepatitis*

The bunches of little red berries growing on the schisandra vine can be eaten dried, like raisins, or ground into a powder. The herb's berries and its leaves are used to treat many medical conditions, but one of the most intriguing uses is as a tonic, or adaptogen, for fighting stress and enhancing physical and mental performance. For those recovering from illness, suffering from physical or mental fatigue, or regularly getting sick in winter, adaptogens like schisandra may play an important role.

Much of the original research on schisandra was initiated in Russia and China. Schisandra fruits contain 3 main types of medicinal **compounds** that may be responsible for the herb's tonic effects: a fatty oil, ether oils, and organic acids. Schisandrin, the compound most likely responsible for many of the cognitive effects, is contained in the ether oils.

Animal studies of schisandra have demonstrated increased abilities to do physical activity and increased resistance to various stressors, hallmarks of an effective adaptogen. How schisandra achieves this is still being investigated, but some initial research shows that **extracts** seem to fight oxidation and inflammation; affect the hypothalamus, pituitary, and adrenal glands, which affect many body systems and processes; and lead to changes in the **neurotransmitter** acetylcholine, important for many brain activities. Overall, schisandra seems to work as a gentle **stimulant**, helping the body to mobilize energy for physical or mental work.

Schisandra is often used by herbal experts in the treatment of liver diseases. It is thought of as a liver protectant, an enhancer of liver function; additionally, it may help with detoxification, boosting the liver's ability to process toxins both from food or alcohol and from the everyday environment.

How to Use

TINCTURE: Generally, 1 to 2 ml, 3 times a day.

TEA: Bring 1 cup water to a boil and reduce to a simmer. Add 1 to 2 teaspoons of the dried fruits for 10 minutes. Strain, cool, and drink, 1 to 3 times per day.

EXTRACT: Follow the manufacturer's dosage guidelines for extracts standardized for schisandrins.

Precautions

Schisandra is a stimulant that can affect many body systems, so caution is advised for diabetics and those with high blood pressure. Those sensitive to mildly stimulating herbs or who take medicine for psychological conditions should take care at onset of schisandra therapy.

---

over the (kitchen) counter SCHISANDRA BERRY TEA

Place 2 tablespoons of dried schisandra berries in an infuser or steeping bag (available at most health food stores). Bring 2 cups water to boil in a saucepan with a tight-fitting lid. Drop the infuser, or bag, into the boiling water. Reduce heat and simmer, covered, for 15 minutes. Remove the berries and pour yourself a cup of tea. Sweeten with honey, if desired.

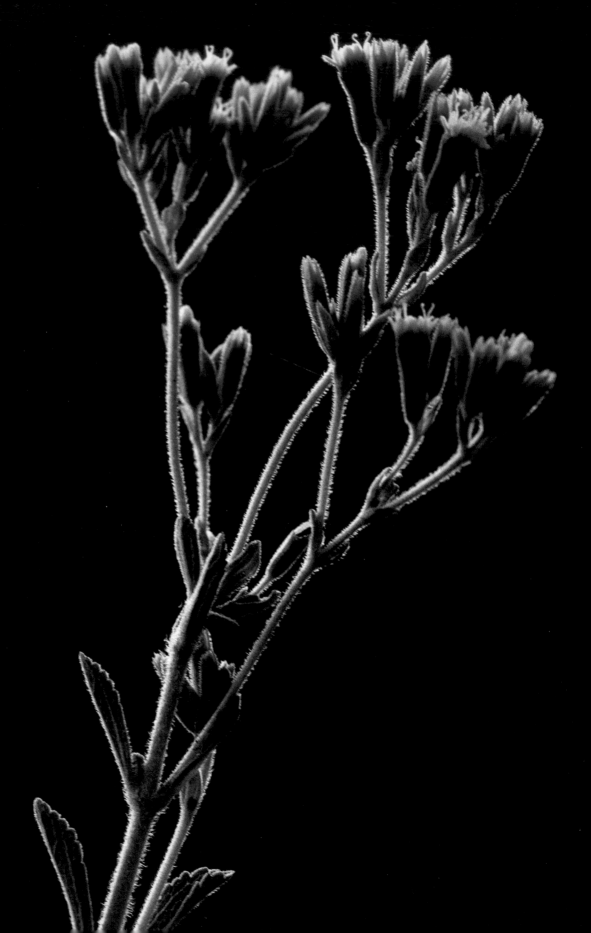

Stevia

✿ *Stevia rebaudiana* ✿

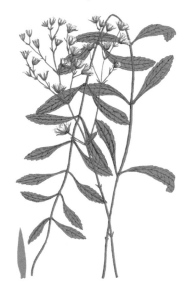

Commonly known as sugar leaf, honey leaf, or sweet leaf of Paraguay, stevia is a small South American shrub whose narrow leaves are nearly 50 times as sweet as ordinary table sugar. The Guarani Indians of Paraguay called the herb *ka'a he'ê*, meaning "sweet herb." The Guarani used stevia leaves to sweeten bitter yerba maté and other beverages and to improve the taste of herbal medicines. They also employed the herb medicinally as a tonic for the heart and to help lower high blood pressure, relieve heartburn and kidney ailments, and dull cravings for sweets.

Spanish explorers noted how **indigenous** tribes used stevia, and by the 1800s, European settlers in Paraguay, Brazil, and Argentina were also consuming the herb, primarily as a sweetener for teas. In 1899 Swiss botanist Moisés Bertoni, then director of an agriculture college in Asunción, Paraguay, published the first description of the plant. He named it *S. rebaudiana* to honor Paraguayan chemist Ovidio Rebaudi, who conducted the first analysis of stevia's chemical components. The **genus** name, *Stevia*, honors Peter James Esteve, a 16th-century Spanish professor of botany. Stevia is still called *estévia* in most Spanish-speaking countries.

Western interest in stevia had its start in the early 1900s, when word of this uniquely sweet herb spread and the prospect of developing an alternative to sugar—one safe for diabetics—seemed a viable commercial possibility. The idea met with strong opposition from sugar producers, however, and plans for developing a stevia industry faltered. In the 1930s, two of the key **compounds** responsible for stevia's sweetness—stevioside and rebaudioside—were isolated and found to be at least 250 times sweeter than sugar. Within 30 years, the Japanese had embraced stevia **extract** as a safe and natural alternative to sugar. Acceptance of the natural sweetener in North America and Europe, however, has been much slower. Initially banned in the United States, stevia became commercially available as a sweetener only in 2008.

Stevia's leaves are the source of an extract that is hundreds of times sweeter than sugar, yet has no calories.

TIME LINE OF USAGE AND SPREAD

1887
Swiss botanist Moisés Santiago Bertoni first learns of stevia from Indian guides

1931
Two French chemists isolate stevioside and rebaudioside.

1971
Japanese firm Morita Kagaku Kogyo Co., Ltd. produces the first commercial stevia.

2006
World Health Organization approves stevia as a safe sweetener.

Stevia is an herbaceous perennial growing from 12 to 30 inches in height. The leaves are opposite, toothed, oblong-oval, without stalks, and conspicuously veined. The leaves are about an inch in length and half as wide. Flowers are in a loose head, with disk flowers that are white or pale purple, tubular, and 5-lobed, with glandular hairs on the outer surface. The ribbed seeds (fruits) have bristly hairs at the top. The plant often produces sucker shoots at the base.

The most remarkable feature of stevia, however, is not seen but tasted. There is not a single plant that produces such a striking sweetness from just a tiny part of its leaf. Of great promise as a sweetener for decades, it was only in 2008 that the sweet constituents of the leaf became available as a flavoring for foods in the United States. Despite the absence of regulatory approval up until now, the dried leaf has been available wherever herbs are sold.

Growing Habits

There are about 230 **species** in the genus *Stevia*, the vast majority native to drier regions of South America and western North America. Stevia is native to the highlands of the Amambay and Iguaçu districts on the border region of Brazil and Paraguay. The natural range is very limited, and stevia is believed to be **endemic** only to Paraguay. It grows in a region with a subtropical humid climate with little rainfall in winter. Stevia is now rare in the wild; when Paraguay immigrant and botanist Moisés Santiago Bertoni first described it in 1899 (and again in 1905), he noted its scarcity even then. An herbalist from northeastern Paraguay had described to him a plant with sweet leaves that he used to sweeten yerba maté (*Ilex paraguariensis*). In the 1960s and 1970s, publicity about stevia's potential as a sweetener placed additional pressure on the plant in Paraguay, leading to loss of natural populations.

Cultivation and Harvesting

In most of the United States, stevia is grown as a container plant or in greenhouses. Optimal growing conditions in a greenhouse require a temperature range of 50°F to 80°F. The plant is not hardy and will not survive temperatures below 30°F. It likes dry soil, especially when

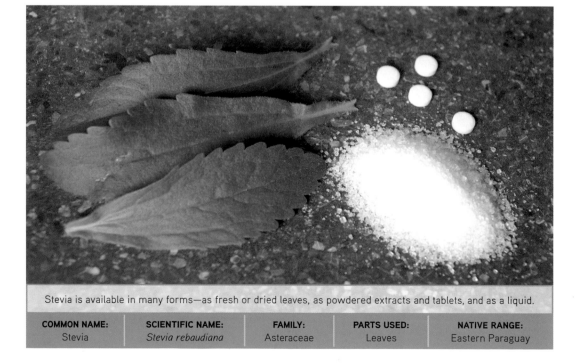

Stevia is available in many forms—as fresh or dried leaves, as powdered extracts and tablets, and as a liquid.

COMMON NAME:	SCIENTIFIC NAME:	FAMILY:	PARTS USED:	NATIVE RANGE:
Stevia	*Stevia rebaudiana*	Asteraceae	Leaves	Eastern Paraguay

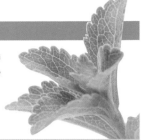
Harvest fresh stevia leaves and dry them thoroughly in the sun or a home dehydrator. Finely crush enough of the dried leaves to make ¼ cup. Add the dried, crushed stevia leaf to 1 cup warm water. Stir, cover, and steep for 24 hours. Strain the mixture through fine cheesecloth and refrigerate the liquid. Use to taste as a sugar substitute in drinks.

dormant, but responds with luxuriant leaf growth to feeding with a liquid fertilizer and moisture. Propagation is usually by cuttings.

Commercial operations in temperate climates are mostly greenhouse based. Countries with commercial production for export include Brazil, Canada, China, Japan, Paraguay, South Korea, and Thailand. In recent years, much of the Asian production has been exported to Japan, the first country to allow stevia's widespread use as a sugar substitute.

Therapeutic Uses

+ *Diabetes*
+ *Insulin resistance (prediabetes)*
+ *High blood pressure*

Stevia could have a brilliant future. A powerful sweetener with no calories, stevia could be a dietary phenomenon, especially for people watching calories and carbs. If this noncaloric sweetener should take the place of high-glycemic white sugar, the quality of carbohydrates in the diet would improve—with benefits for teeth, blood sugar, and digestion. Further, stevia may directly affect the hormones and mechanisms involved with elevated blood sugar in diabetics, helping to lower sugar levels and protect against the effects of high sugars.

Most of the benefits of stevia come from a compound called stevioside, which occurs primarily in the leaves, accounting for from 4 to 20 percent of the weight of the dry leaves. A compound similar in structure to stevioside and thought to have some physiological effects is rebaudioside A. Some animal studies show that stevia does not affect glucose absorption, though it may promote **insulin** release from the pancreas, increase sensitivity to insulin throughout the body, and slow glucose production in the liver. In humans, one study involved

12 people with type 2 diabetes. Researchers examined the use of 1 g of an extract (consisting of 91 percent stevioside and 4 percent rebaudoside A) or **placebo** with a meal. Those receiving the stevia extract had a lower glucose level after the meal than the placebo group, possibly as a result of increased insulin secretion (which would bring down blood sugar).

The blood pressure-lowering effects of stevioside and rebaudoside A also have been studied, and results have been mixed. Some clinical trials demonstrated a decrease in both systolic and diastolic blood pressure with these compounds, while other trials disputed these results. This effect needs further study.

How to Use

POWDER: Stevia leaf, in powder form, can simply be used as a sugar substitute in various ways, such as sprinkling as a sweetener on food, in hot beverages, or in most recipes.

LIQUID EXTRACT: Glycerin extracts are available, often standardized to the primary component of stevia leaf, stevioside. Several drops of these extracts can be added to food as a sweetener.

> **NOTE:** Stevia is 300 times sweeter than sucrose, or table sugar, yet has none of the calories of table sugar.

Precautions

The safety of the chemical compound stevioside and of whole stevia leaf has been evaluated extensively in laboratory tests looking at possible toxic, genetic, or cancer-causing effects. Both have been determined to be safe when used as a sweetener. Care should be taken when stevia is used in combination with medications that also lower blood sugar. Uncommonly, stevia can cause stomach upset.

Index *of* Therapeutic Uses

This index links medicinal plants with their potential therapeutic effects. The lefthand column names conditions of concern. The middle column lists the pages in this book that refer to how those conditions might be treated. The righthand column lists additional sources of information that may help with the condition, as described in National Geographic's volume *Desk Reference to Nature's Medicine*. However, this index is not in any way intended as a therapeutic guide. Readers should consult a licensed health care professional before using any medicinal plants listed on this index.

CONDITION OR BENEFIT	HERBS *GUIDE TO MEDICINAL HERBS*	ADDITIONAL HERBS FOUND IN *DESK REFERENCE TO* *NATURE'S MEDICINE* (NGS, 2006)
Acne	Slippery Elm, *p. 179* Tea Tree, *p. 225*	Arnica, *p. 20* Chaparral, *p 96* Chaste Tree, *p. 98* Dandelion, *p. 130* Patchouli, *p. 282* Yellow Dock, *p. 378*
Alzheimer's	Ginkgo, *p. 115* Lemon Balm, *p. 35* Turmeric, *p. 183*	Calabar Bean, *p. 70* Clubmoss, *p. 110* Sage, *p. 318*
Antioxidant	Bilberry, *p. 103* Chocolate, *p. 107* Ginkgo, *p. 115* Goji, *p. 331* Grapes, Grape Seed, *p. 119* Hibiscus, *p. 127* Pomegranate, *p. 249* Rosemary, *p. 221* Tea, *p. 135* Willow Bark, *p. 229*	
Arthritis *(osteoarthritis and/or* *rheumatoid arthritis)*	Black Cohosh, *p. 279* Cat's Claw, *p. 205* Cayenne, *p. 209* Devil's Claw, *p. 217* Ginger, *p. 159* Stinging Nettle, *p. 263* Turmeric, *p. 183* Willow Bark, *p. 229*	Arnica, *p. 20* Ashwagandha, *p. 22* Brazil Nut, *p. 64* Catnip, *p. 88* European Elder, *p. 150* Juniper, *p. 220* Kelp, *p. 224* Licorice, *p. 230* Noni, *p. 260* Parsley, *p. 268* Rosemary, *p. 316* White Willow, *p. 366*

CONDITION OR BENEFIT	HERBS GUIDE TO MEDICINAL HERBS	ADDITIONAL HERBS DESK REFERENCE TO NATURE'S MEDICINE
Asthma	Eucalyptus, *p. 75*	Ashwagandha, *p. 22* Black Cohosh, *p. 54* Black Haw, *p. 56* Butterbur, *p. 68* Echinacea, *p. 138* Evening Primrose, *p. 154* Forskohlii, *p. 172* Hops, *p. 212* Licorice, *p. 230* Marshmallow, *p. 244* Mullein, *p. 254* Myrrh, *p. 256* Parsley, *p. 268* Schisandra, *p. 324* Spikenard, *p. 336* Stinging Nettle, *p. 340* Turmeric, *p. 360*
Back pain	Devil's Claw, *p. 217* Willow Bark, *p. 229*	
Benign prostatic hyperplasia	Pygeum, *p. 253* Saw Palmetto, *p. 257* Stinging Nettle, *p. 263*	Pumpkin, *p. 296*
Bladder health	Cranberry, *p. 291*	Alfalfa, *p. 12* Forskohlii, *p. 172* Licorice, *p. 230* Parsley, *p. 268* Pumpkin, *p. 296* Queen Anne's Lace, *p. 300* St. John's Wort, *p. 338*
Breast tenderness	Chaste Tree, *p. 98*	
Bronchitis	Butterbur, *p. 19* Juniper, *p. 241* Mullein, *p. 83* Pelargonium, *p. 87* Rosemary, *p. 221*	Ashwagandha, *p. 22* Black Cherry, *p. 52* Eucalyptus, *p. 148* Flax, *p. 170* Marshmallow, *p. 244* Myrrh, *p. 356* Schisandra, *p. 324*
Bruises	Arnica, *p. 197*	Bilberry, *p. 40* Calendula, *p. 74* Comfrey, *p. 114* Eucalyptus, *p. 148* Heal All, *p. 206* Witch Hazel, *p. 372*

CONDITION OR BENEFIT	HERBS *GUIDE TO MEDICINAL HERBS*	ADDITIONAL HERBS *DESK REFERENCE TO NATURE'S MEDICINE*
Burns	Aloe, *p. 191*	Chinese Rhubarb, *p. 104* Chocolate, *p. 106* English Lavender, *p. 144* Gotu Kola, *p. 188* Heal All, *p. 206* Tea Tree, *p. 354* Yellow Dock, *p. 378*
Cholesterol management	Cacao, Chocolate, *p. 107* Grapes, Grape Seed, *p. 119* Tea, *p. 135*	Alfalfa, *p. 12* Psyllium, *p. 292* Soy Bean, *p. 334* Turmeric, *p. 360*
Chronic venous insufficiency	Horse Chestnut, *p. 131*	
Circulation	Ginkgo, *p. 115* Rosemary, *p. 221*	Guaiacum, *p. 190* Soy Bean, *p. 334* Stinging Nettle, *p. 340* Turmeric, *p. 360* Yarrow, *p. 376*
Cognition	Bacopa, *p. 321* Gotu Kola, *p. 335* Rosemary, *p. 221*	Asian Ginseng, *p. 24* Ginkgo, *p. 182* Guarana, *p. 192* Schisandra, *p. 324*
Colds, flus	Astragalus, *p. 61* Echinacea, *p. 65* Elder, *p. 71* Eucalyptus, *p. 75* Fennel, *p. 149* Garlic, *p. 153* Ginger, *p. 159* Hibiscus, *p. 127* Mullein, *p. 83* Pelargonium, *p. 87* Peppermint, *p. 171* Sage, *p. 91* Thyme, *p. 95*	Buchu, *p. 66* Catnip, *p. 88* Dog Rose, *p. 134* Lemongrass, *p. 228* Marshmallow, *p. 244* Yarrow, *p. 376*
Colic	Chamomile, *p. 145* Fennel, *p. 149* Lemon Balm, *p. 35*	Black Haw, *p. 56* Blue Cohosh, *p. 60* Buchu, *p. 66* Catnip, *p. 88* Wintergreen, *p. 370*
Constipation	Psyllium, *p. 175*	Flax, *p. 170*
Contusions	Arnica, *p. 197*	

CONDITION OR BENEFIT	HERBS *GUIDE TO MEDICINAL HERBS*	ADDITIONAL HERBS *DESK REFERENCE TO NATURE'S MEDICINE*
Eczema continued		Patchouli, *p. 282* Stinging Nettle, *p. 340* Tea Tree, *p. 354* Thuja, *p. 356* Turmeric, *p. 360* Yellow Dock, *p. 378*
Excessive sweating	Sage, *p. 91*	Astragalus, *p. 28*
Eye health	Bilberry, *p. 103*	
Fatigue	Rhodiola, *p. 339* Schisandra, *p. 343*	Ashwagandha, *p. 22* Asian Ginseng, *p. 24* Eleuthero, *p. 142* Evening Primrose, *p. 154* Guarana, *p. 192* Rosemary, *p. 316* Sage, *p. 318* Valerian, *p. 362*
Fever blisters	Lemon Balm, *p. 35* St. John's Wort, *p. 49*	
Gastritis	Licorice, *p. 79*	Cat's Claw, *p. 90* Slippery Elm, *p. 332*
Gingivitis	Tea Tree, *p. 225*	
Heartburn	Chamomile, *p. 145* Licorice, *p. 79* Slippery Elm, *p. 179*	Dandelion, *p. 130* Juniper, *p. 220* Peppermint, *p. 286*
Heart health	Chocolate, *p. 107* Garlic, *p. 153* Grapes, Grape Seed, *p. 119* Hawthorn, *p. 123* Hibiscus, *p. 127* Pomegranate, *p. 249* Psyllium, *p. 175* Soy, *p. 309* Tea, *p. 135*	Ginkgo, *p. 182* Rhodiola, *p. 306* Schisandra, *p. 324*
Hemorrhoids	Horse Chestnut, *p. 131* Witch Hazel, *p. 233*	Bilberry, *p. 40* Catnip, *p. 88* Coca, *p. 112* Ginkgo, *p. 182* Heal All, *p. 206* Psyllium, *p. 292* Sage, *p. 318* Tea Tree, *p. 354* Yellow Dock, *p. 378*

CONDITION OR BENEFIT	HERBS *GUIDE TO MEDICINAL HERBS*	ADDITIONAL HERBS *DESK REFERENCE TO NATURE'S MEDICINE*
High blood pressure	Grapes, Grape Seed, *p. 119* Parsley, *p. 245* Stevia, *p. 347*	Black Haw, *p. 56* Buchu, *p. 66* Chocolate, *p. 106* Dandelion, *p. 130* Evening Primrose, *p. 154* Gotu Kola, *p. 188* Hawthorn, *p. 204* Kelp, *p. 224* Psyllium, *p. 292* Yarrow, *p. 376*
Immune support	Astragalus, *p. 61* Cat's Claw, *p. 205* Ginseng, *p. 325*	Asian Ginseng, *p. 24* Echinacea, *p. 138* Eleuthero, *p. 142* European Elder, *p. 150* Goldenseal, *p. 186* Sage, *p. 318*
Indigestion	Chamomile, *p. 145* Devil's Claw, *p. 217* Fennel, *p. 149* Goldenseal, *p. 163* Hops, *p. 27* Juniper, *p. 241* Lemon Balm, *p. 35* Peppermint, *p. 171* Shatavari, *p. 305*	Alfalfa, *p. 12* Black Cherry, *p. 52* Chicory, *p. 102* English Lavender, *p. 144* Ginger, *p. 180* Lemongrass, *p. 228* Parsley, *p. 268* Queen Anne's Lace, *p. 300* Rosemary, *p. 316* Turmeric, *p. 360*
Inflammation	Ashwagandha, *p. 317* Calendula, *p. 201* Chocolate, *p. 107* Comfrey, *p. 213* Ginger, *p. 159* Tea, *p. 135* Turmeric, *p. 183* Witch Hazel, *p. 233*	Cat's Claw, *p. 90* Cinnamon, *p. 108* Hops, *p. 212* Myrrh, *p. 256* St. John's Wort, *p. 338*
Inflammatory bowel disease	Turmeric, *p. 183*	Chinese Rhubarb, *p. 104* Marshmallow, *p. 244* Psyllium, *p. 292*
Insomnia	Hops, *p. 27* Lemon Balm, *p. 35* Passionflower, *p. 39* Skullcap, *p. 45* Valerian, *p. 53*	Ashwagandha, *p. 22* Chamomile, *p. 94* English Lavender, *p. 144* Gotu Kola, *p. 188* Hawthorn, *p. 204* Kava, *p. 222* Mullein, *p. 254* Sage, *p. 319* Schisandra, *p. 324* St. John's Wort, *p. 338*

CONDITION OR BENEFIT	HERBS	ADDITIONAL HERBS
Intestinal cramps	Black Haw, *p. 283*	
Irritable bowel syndrome	Peppermint, *p. 171*	Chamomile, *p. 94* Psyllium, *p. 292*
Itchy/inflamed skin	Slippery Elm, *p. 179*	
Joint pain	Arnica, *p. 197* Butterbur, *p. 19* Comfrey, *p. 213* Rosemary, *p. 221* Turmeric, *p. 183*	Dandelion, *p. 130* Tea Tree, *p. 354* Wintergreen, *p. 370*
Kidney stones	Parsley, *p. 245*	Bearberry, *p. 32* Cranberry, *p. 126* Stinging Nettle, *p. 340*
Liver Protection	Milk Thistle, *p.167* Schisandra, *p. 343*	Dandelion, *p. 130* Soy Bean, *p. 334*
Memory loss	Bacopa, *p. 321* Gotu Kola, *p. 335* Rosemary, *p. 221* Sage, *p. 91*	Eleuthero, *p. 142* Ginkgo, *p. 182*
Menopause	Black Cohosh, *p. 279* Dong Quai, *p. 297* Hops, *p. 27* Kava, *p. 31* Sage, *p. 91* Shatavari, *p. 305*	Asian Ginseng, *p. 24* Black Haw, *p. 56* Chaste Tree, *p. 98* Red Clover, *p. 304* Soy Bean, *p. 334* St. John's Wort, *p. 338*
Menstrual cramps	Black Cohosh, *p. 279* Black Haw, *p. 203* Dong Quai, *p. 297* Fennel, *p. 149* Shatavari, *p. 305*	Angelica, *p. 18* Bee Balm, *p. 34* Chamomile, *p. 94* Hops, *p. 212* Noni, *p. 260* Wild Yam, *p. 368*
Migraine headaches	Butterbur, *p. 19* Feverfew, *p. 23*	Chaste Tree, *p. 98* English Lavender, *p. 144* Guarana, *p. 192* Hemp, *p. 208*
Minor depression	Black Cohosh, *p. 279* Rhodiola, *p. 339* St. John's Wort, *p. 49*	
Morning sickness	Ginger, *p. 159*	Black Haw, *p. 56* Turmeric, *p. 360* Wild Yam, *p. 368*

INDEX OF THERAPEUTIC USES

Contributors

REBECCA L. JOHNSON is an award-winning science writer and the author of more than 75 books for adults, young adults, and children on diverse subjects ranging from climate change and polar exploration to carnivorous plants. To gather firsthand information for her books, she has worked with scientists around the world, including in Antarctica, Australia, and New Zealand. Her books have received national awards from *Scientific American*, the National Science Teachers Association, and the Children's Book Council. Johnson wrote, with Steven Foster, the National Geographic Society's best-selling *Desk Reference to Nature's Medicine*, named a 2007 New York Public Library Best of Reference. She is an avid herb gardener and makes her home in Sioux Falls, South Dakota.

STEVEN FOSTER is internationally respected for his work in the field of herbs and botanical photography. For 35 years he has photographed and researched herbs from the Amazon rain forest to the highlands of Vietnam. He has written and photo-illustrated more than 800 articles. He serves as board chairman of the American Botanical Council (ABC) and associate editor of ABC's journal, *HerbalGram*. Foster is the author of six books, including, with Rebecca L. Johnson, National Geographic's *Desk Reference to Nature's Medicine*. He is senior author of three Peterson Field Guides, including *A Field Guide to Medicinal Plants and Herbs* (with Dr. James A. Duke, 2nd edition); *A Field Guide to Western Medicinal Plants and Herbs* (with Christopher Hobbs); and *A Field Guide to Venomous Animals and Poisonous Plants of North America* (with Roger Caras). He is president of Steven Foster Group, Inc., a consulting and stock photography firm: *www.stevenfoster.com*. He makes his home in Eureka Springs, Arkansas.

TIERAONA LOW DOG is a physician, associate professor, and director of the fellowship for the Arizona Center for Integrative Medicine at the University of Arizona. She was appointed by President Bill Clinton to the White House Commission on Complementary and Alternative Medicine. She has served on the advisory board for the National Institutes of Health National Center for Complementary and Alternative Medicine and, since 2000, has been the elected chair of the U.S. Pharmacopeia Dietary Supplements–Botanicals Expert Committee. Before attending medical school, Low Dog was a respected herbalist with training in midwifery, massage, and martial arts. She has lectured at 350 conferences and written more than 35 peer-reviewed articles and textbook chapters. She is an internationally known voice in the fields of women's health and herbal medicine and in the growing field of integrative medicine.

DAVID KIEFER is a board-certified family physician with licenses in Washington, Arizona, and Wisconsin. In Seattle, he teaches naturopathic medicine at Bastyr University and recently supervised family medicine residents at a homeless youth clinic. He is assistant clinical professor of medicine at the Arizona Center for Integrative Medicine at the University of Arizona. His research and teaching interests include ethnobotany and the clinical applications of evidence-based herbal medicine.

LINDA B. WHITE (medical consultant) is a physician and assistant professor in the Integrative Therapeutic Practices program at The Metropolitan State College of Denver, where she teaches botanical medicine and other classes. For more than 20 years she has lectured and written on natural health. She is the co-author of *Kids, Herbs, and Health* and *The Herbal Drugstore* and is a regular contributor to *Mother Earth News* and *The Herb Companion*. Her articles have also appeared in *Mothering, Herbs for Health, Runner's World, Natural Home*, and *Natural Pharmacy*. She has appeared on CNN and *Good Morning America*, as well as local radio and TV news shows.

ROBERT WOODING (herbal consultant) grew up in southern Virginia, where he learned the importance of land stewardship as well as farming, gardening, and timberland conservation. He began working with medicinal herbs in 1976 and has worked as an herbalist for more than 30 years, growing and harvesting medicinal plants for use in herbal products. He is an enthusiastic holistic healing educator, a chartered herbalist, and a registered nurse.

Glossary

ABORTIFACIENT A substance that causes or promotes abortion.

ACETAMINOPHEN A white crystalline compound that reduces pain and fever but not inflammation, sold under brand names such as Tylenol, Datril, and others.

ADAPTOGEN An herb that acts in a nonspecific way to strengthen the body and increase resistance to disease and stress with few side effects.

ALKALOID Any of numerous usually colorless, complex, and bitter organic bases (such as morphine or codeine) containing nitrogen and usually oxygen that occur especially in seed plants. An alkaloid is a basic organic compound with alkaline properties and generally a marked physiological effect on the nervous and circulatory systems. Alkaloids show varying pharmacological effects; for example, they can act as analgesics, local anesthetics, tranquilizers, vasoconstrictors, antispasmodics, and hallucinatory agents.

AMINO ACID Any of a class of 20 molecules that are combined to form proteins in living organisms. The sequence of amino acids in a protein—and hence protein function—is determined by the genetic code.

ANALGESIC A medication used to relieve pain.

ANTHOCYANIDIN OR ANTHOCYANIN OR ANTHOCYANOSIDE Any of many water-soluble red to violet plant pigments in the flavonoid family that act as powerful antioxidants in the body.

ANTHRANOID GLYCOSIDE (Also known as anthraquinone glycoside or anthraquinone) Any one of a number of plant-produced glycosides that tend to exert laxative effects in the body; they are present in many plants, including aloes, senna, and rhubarb.

ANTHRAQUINONE An aromatic organic compound that has a strong laxative effect.

ANTHRAQUINONE GLYCOSIDE A glycoside that contains a glycone group that is a derivative of anthraquinone. Glycosides are present in senna, rhubarb, and aloe and have a laxative effect.

ANTIBODY A protein produced by the body's immune system in response to a foreign substance (antigen). An antibody inactivates the antigen that triggered its formation.

ANTIHISTAMINE A drug that blocks histamine, typically used to treat allergic reactions.

ANTI-INFLAMMATORY An agent that reduces the heat, redness, and swelling of inflammation.

ANTIOXIDANT A chemical compound that protects against cell damage from molecules called oxygen-free radicals, which are major causes of disease and aging.

ANTISEPTIC A substance that discourages the growth of microorganisms.

ATHEROSCLEROSIS A type of arteriosclerosis; a disease in which the arteries become inelastic and narrowed by fatty deposits that accumulate within the arterial walls.

ASTRINGENT An agent that causes contraction or shrinkage of tissues; it is used to decrease secretions or control bleeding.

AXIL The point of divergence between the upper side of a leaf and the stem or branch from which it springs.

AYURVEDIC MEDICINE The ancient Indian medical system of sustaining health and fighting disease based on equilibrium with nature. Ayurvedic medicine uses thousands of plants.

BENZODIAZEPINE A class of medications that act upon the central nervous system to reduce communication among certain neurons, lowering the level of activity in the brain. Benzodiazepines are effective in reducing anxiety, promoting sleep, and relaxing muscles.

BETA AMYLOID A sticky protein whose formation is accelerated by high cholesterol levels and that can lead to a greatly increased risk of late onset Alzheimer's. This protein creates plaques in the tiny spaces between nerve cells in the brain, thus interfering with their function.

BIENNIAL A plant whose life cycle extends over two growing seasons.

BULBIL A small bulb that is produced on the aboveground parts of plants.

CARMINATIVE An agent that relieves and removes gas from the digestive system.

CAROTENOID Natural, fat-soluble pigments found in certain plants that provide the bright red, orange, or yellow coloration of many fruits and vegetables.

CATECHINS The most important component in the polyphenol family; catechins are found in green tea and have powerful antioxidant and disease-fighting properties.

CIPROFLOXACIN A synthetic antibiotic used for the treatment of severe and life-threatening bacterial infections.

COLLAGEN An insoluble, fibrous protein that is the main component of connective tissues in the body.

COMPOUND A substance formed by the chemical union of two or more elements.

COUMARIN A vanilla-scented plant constituent, used in perfumes and flavorings and in remedies to reduce blood clotting.

CURCUMIN An antioxidant found in turmeric. It is known for its antitumor and anti-inflammatory properties. It may also be effective in treating cancer and HIV infection.

DECIDUOUS Shedding leaves annually.

DECOCTION A preparation made by simmering tough plant parts in water.

DIURETIC A substance that increases the flow of urine from the body.

DOPAMINE A neurotransmitter associated with movement, attention, learning, and the brain's pleasure system.

DOUBLE-BLIND A clinical trial in which neither the doctor nor the patient knows whether the patient is being administered a placebo or the test drug.

ECLECTIC Referring to a medical movement that flourished in the United States from 1850 to 1940. Physicians who used the Eclectic approach relied heavily on American medicinal plants. Eclectic physicians introduced echinacea and black cohosh and other botanical remedies.

EDEMA Swelling caused by fluid retention in the tissues of the body.

ENDEMIC Occurring naturally only in a single geographic area.

ENZYME A protein that accelerates chemical reactions.

ESSENTIAL OIL (Also called volatile oil) A hydrophobid, aromatic volatile oil found in specialized glands of plants (as in the mint family). Many plants containing essential oils are known for their fragrance and cultivated for the food and perfume industries.

ESTROGEN A group of hormones produced mainly in the mammalian ovaries that are necessary for female sexual development and reproductive functioning.

ESTROGENIC A substance that induces female hormonal activity.

EXPECTORANT A substance that stimulates removal of mucus from the lungs.

EXTRACT A concentrated active constituent that is obtained from a plant using a solvent, such as ethanol or water.

FAMILY A level of classification in the plant kingdom above genus and species, with technical family names usually ending in the suffix "-aceae."

FLAVONOID A group of chemical compounds—low-molecular-weight phenylbenzopyrones—occurring in all vascular plants. In the diet, flavonoids are found in many fruits, vegetables, teas, wines, nuts, seeds, and roots. Many of the medicinal actions of foods, juices, and herbs are directly related to their flavonoid content. They exhibit antioxidant properties and other effects. Flavonoids include anthocyanins and tannins.

FORMULARY A book containing a list of pharmaceutical substances as well as their formulas, uses, and methods of preparation.

FREE RADICAL A chemical that is highly reactive and can oxidize other molecules. When produced within cells, free radicals can react with membranes and genetic material to damage or destroy cells and tissues.

GENUS A level of classification in the plant kingdom below family; the first word of the two-name Latin binomial, which is always capitalized.

GLYCOPROTEIN A protein coated with sugars that plays essential roles in the body. For instance, in the immune system almost all of the key molecules involved in the immune response are glycoproteins.

GLYCOSIDE A product of secondary metabolism in plants. Glycosides break down into two parts—the glycone component, or sugar, and the nonsugar, or aglycone component. The therapeutically active constituent is the aglycone, which can selectively affect a particular organ in the body. Glycosides include some of the most effective plant drugs, but some plants containing them are highly toxic.

HEMOGLOBIN A type of protein in the red blood cells; it carries oxygen to the tissues of the body.

HERBACEOUS A type of plant with little or no woody tissue, usually living a single season.

HIGH-DENSITY LIPOPROTEIN (HDL) Lipoprotein that contains a small amount of cholesterol and carries cholesterol away from body cells and tissues to the liver for excretion from the body. Lower levels of HDL increase the risk of heart disease, so the higher the level of HDL in the bloodstream, the better. The HDL component normally contains 20 to 30 percent of total cholesterol.

HOMEOPATHY A form of alternative medicine that treats patients using preparations containing infinitesimal doses of a substance that, in normal doses, would produce symptoms of the disease it is intended to treat.

INDIGENOUS Native to a particular area.

INFLAMMATION OR INFLAMMATORY RESPONSE The immune system's response to tissue injury or harmful stimulation caused by physical or chemical substances. Release of inflammatory chemicals and increased blood flow to affected areas results in swelling, redness, and pain.

INFLORESCENCE Group or cluster forming the flowering part of a plant.

INFUSED OIL The result of an herb or plant part being soaked or macerated in oil and heated. The infused oil is then strained out.

INFUSION Tea made by steeping an herb in hot water.

INSULIN A hormone that is needed to convert sugar, starches, and other food into glucose (blood sugar); excessively high blood glucose levels could lead to diabetes.

INTERFERON A protein made and released by the cells of most vertebrates in response to the presence of pathogens such as viruses; interferons allow communication between cells to trigger the protective defenses of the immune system that eradicate pathogens or tumors.

ISOFLAVONE A compound found in soy and other plants that has been shown to significantly reduce serum cholesterol levels—the leading risk factor for heart disease—as well as alleviate menopausal symptoms in women and assist in combating numerous other serious health risks.

LACTONE A chemical compound derived from a hydroxy acid.

LECTIN A protein found in plants and animals. Lectins have properties that make them resemble antibodies; they have agglutinating and precipitating effects on microorganisms.

LIGNAN A diverse group of plant-derived compounds that form the building blocks for plant cell walls. Lignans can influence hormonal metabolism and may also be anticarcinogenic.

LINIMENT A thin medicinal fluid rubbed on the skin to reduce pain.

LOW-DENISITY LIPOPROTEIN (LDL) The major cholesterol carrier in the blood. LDL transports cholesterol from the liver and intestines to various tissues. LDL is known as bad cholesterol because high levels are linked to coronary artery disease.

MUCILAGE A gelatinous substance produced by some plants that is often used in herbal medicine as a soothing agent.

MUCOPOLYSACCHARIDE Complex polysaccharides containing an amino group that occur chiefly as components of connective tissue, such as the bladder lining.

NATUROPATHY A system of therapy that avoids drugs and surgery and emphasizes the use of natural remedies.

NEUROTRANSMITTER A chemical compound that transmits nerve impulses across synapses between nerve cells and between nerve and muscle or gland cells.

NOREPINEPHRINE A neurotransmitter found mainly in areas of the nervous system involved in arousal, alertness, and the fight or flight response; activation increases the respiratory rate, heart rate, blood pressure, and blood sugar.

PECTIN A polysaccharide extracted from the cell walls of plants, used in making jellies and jams.

PHARMACOPOEIA A book containing an official list of medicinal drugs together with articles on their preparation, usually produced by legislative authority.

PHENOLICS OR POLYPHENOLS A large group of chemicals derived from phenol (a benzene ring with one hydroxyl group attached) that contribute to the color, taste, flavor, and medicinal actions of many plants. In wine grapes, phenolics are found widely in the skin, stems, and seeds. (Many of the plants listed in this book—willow, uva ursi, black haw, cayenne, black cohosh, aloe—contain polyphenols.)

PHEROMONE A chemical released by one organism that influences the behavior of another organism of the same species.

PHYTOCHEMICAL A chemical found naturally in plants that has metabolically active qualities.

PHYTOESTROGEN A diverse group of naturally occurring, nonsteroidal compounds that cause estrogen-like effects in the body.

PHYTOMEDICINE A medicine based on active ingredients within an herbal base, sometimes used to describe all plant-based medicines.

PHYTOSTEROLS A group of steroid alcohols; phytochemicals occurring naturally in plants that lower cholesterol in humans.

PLACEBO An inactive pill, liquid, or powder that has no treatment value but is used in tests to determine whether the effects of a drug are real or brought on by the patient's desire to be cured.

PLATELET One of the main components of the blood that forms clots, sealing up injured areas and preventing hemorrhage.

PLATELET AGGREGATION The process of platelets clumping together in the blood; also known as clotting.

POLYSACCHARIDE Any of a class of carbohydrates consisting of chains of simple sugars; often found in cell walls of living organisms.

POULTICE A preparation of fresh, moistened, or crushed dried herbs, applied externally.

PROANTHOCYANIDIN The principal vasoactive polyphenol in red wine (also hawthorn, ginkgo, green tea, cranberry), which is linked to a reduced risk of coronary heart disease and to lower overall mortality.

PROGESTERONE A steroid hormone produced in the ovary that prepares and maintains the uterus for pregnancy.

PROPHYLACTIC A medical procedure designed to prevent, rather than treat or cure, a disease.

PROSTAGLANDINS Compounds made in the body from fatty acids, with a range of effects, including inhibition or stimulation of smooth muscle contractions.

PURGATIVE (Also called cathartic) Agent used to relieve severe constipation, often with intense effects.

RHIZOME A somewhat elongated, usually horizontal, subterranean plant stem, often thickened by deposits of reserve food material, that produces shoots above and roots below; distinguished from a true root in having buds, nodes, and usually scalelike leaves.

SALICIN A type of polyphenol (phenolic compound) contained in willow bark, meadowsweet, black haw root bark, and other plants. After it is ingested, it is converted by the human body to salicylic acid, the compound from which aspirin is derived. It is analgesic, anti-inflammatory, and fever reducing.

SAPONIN Any of several glycosides in plants that make a soapy lather if mixed with water.

SEROTONIN A neurotransmitter involved in many functions, including emotion, behavior, and thought.

SERUM ALBUMIN The most abundant plasma protein in humans and other mammals, it is essential for maintaining the osmotic pressure needed for proper distribution of body fluids.

SESQUITERPENE A terpene-based compound that, when taken from a plant, can stimulate glands in the liver. Sesquiterpenes may have antiallergenic, antispasmodic, and anti-inflammatory properties.

SESQUITERPENE LACTONE A class of chemicals found in many plants that can cause allergic reactions and toxicity if overdosed, particularly in grazing livestock. In moderate amounts, such chemicals can have anti-inflammatory, antibacterial, antiparasitic, anticancer, and antispasmodic properties.

SILYMARIN A chemical complex found in milk thistle that may protect liver cells against toxins.

SPECIES A level of classification in the plant kingdom below genus; second name in the Latin binomial, designating organisms in a genus.

STEROID A chemical class whose members share a similar ringlike structure. The group includes cholesterol, estrogen, progesterone, testosterone, cortisone, and vitamin D. These chemicals have widespread effects in the body.

SUBSPECIES A level of classification in the plant kingdom below species, recognizing differences in a species not great enough to warrant classification as a species; designated, following the species name, by the abbreviation subsp.

SYNAPSE The gap between two neurons over which impulses travel; specialized junctions through which cells of the nervous system signal to one another and to nonneuronal cells such as muscles or glands.

TANNIN A group of simple and complex phenol, polyphenol, and flavonoid compounds bound with starches. Aside from their astringent, mouth-puckering properties, these chemicals can help stanch bleeding from small wounds, slow uterine bleeding, reduce inflammation and swelling, dry out weepy mucous membranes, and relieve diarrhea.

TAPROOT A somewhat straight tapering root that grows vertically downward. It forms a center from which other roots sprout laterally.

TERPENE A class of hydrocarbon compounds produced by a wide variety of plants; terpenes, along with closely related compounds called terpenoids, are major constituents of many essential oils in plants.

TERPENE LACTONES Active constituents associated with increased circulation to the brain and other parts of the body, terpene lactones may exert a protective action on the nerve cells.

TINCTURE A plant medicine prepared by soaking an herb in water and ethanol (never isopropyl alcohol); traditional herbal preparations are dispensed as alcohol-based liquid medicines.

TRITERPENE GLYCOSIDE A glycoside that has a 30-carbon structure as part of its chemical composition.

TRITERPINOID A terpene-based compound.

U.S. PHARMACOPEIA Not-for-profit organization of scientists, physicians, pharmacists, and others that produces the *Pharmacopeia of the United States*.

VARIETY A level of classification in the plant kingdom below species and subspecies noting minor differences within a species, such as variations in flower color; designated, following the species and subspecies name, by the abbreviation var.

Plant Index

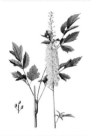

Actaea racemosa
Black cohosh
page 279

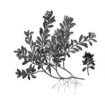

Arctostaphylos uva-ursi
Uva ursi
page 271

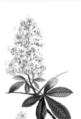

Aesculus hippocastanum
Horse chestnut
page 131

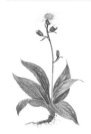

Arnica montana
Arnica
page 197

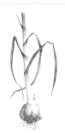

Allium sativum
Garlic
page 153

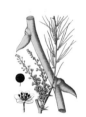

Asparagus racemosus
Shatavari
page 305

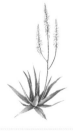

Aloe vera
Aloe
page 191

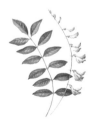

Astragalus membranaceus
Astragalus
page 61

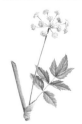

Angelica sinensis
Dong quai
page 297

Bacopa monnieri
Bacopa
page 321

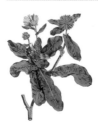

Calendula officinalis
Calendula
page 201

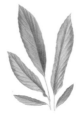

Curcuma longa
Turmeric
page 183

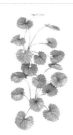

Camellia sinensis
Tea
page 135

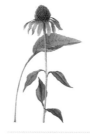

Echinacea purpurea
Echinacea
page 65

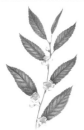

Capsicum annuum
Cayenne
page 209

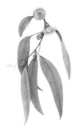

Eucalyptus globulus
Eucalyptus
page 75

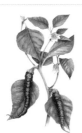

Centella asiatica
Gotu kola
page 335

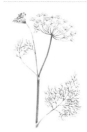

Foeniculum vulgare
Fennel
page 149

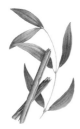

Cinnamonum verum
Cinnamon
page 111

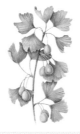

Ginkgo biloba
Ginkgo
page 115

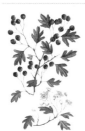

Crataegus laevigata
Hawthorn
page 123

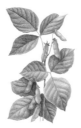

Glycine max
Soy
page 309

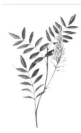

Glycyrrhiza glabra
Licorice
page 79

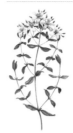

Hypericum perforatum
St. John's wort
page 49

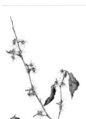

Hamamelis virginiana
Witch hazel
page 233

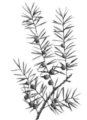

Juniperus communis
Juniper
page 241

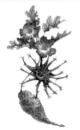

Harpagophytum procumbens
Devil's claw
page 217

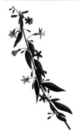

Lycium barbarum
Goji
page 331

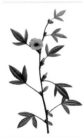

Hibiscus sabdariffa
Hibiscus
page 127

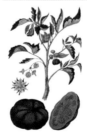

Lycopersicon esculentum
Tomato
page 267

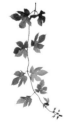

Humulus lupulus
Hops
page 27

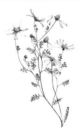

Matricaria recutita
Chamomile
page 145

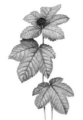

Hydrastis canadensis
Goldenseal
page 163

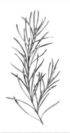

Melaleuca alternifolia
Tea tree
page 225

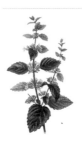

Melissa officinalis
Lemon balm
page 35

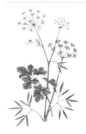

Petroselinum crispum
Parsley
page 245

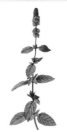

Mentha x piperita
Peppermint
page 171

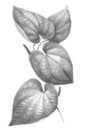

Piper methysticum
Kava
page 31

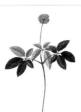

**Panax ginseng
& P. quinquefolius**
Ginseng
page 325

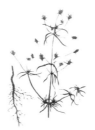

Plantago ovata
Psyllium
page 175

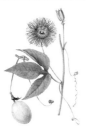

Passiflora incarnata
Passionflower
page 39

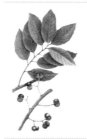

Prunus africana
Pygeum
page 253

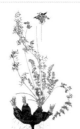

Pelargonium sidoides
Pelargonium
page 87

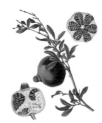

Punica granatum
Pomegranate
page 249

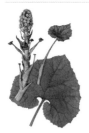

Petasites hybridus
Butterbur
page 19

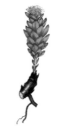

Rhodiola rosea
Rhodiola
page 339

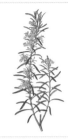

Rosmarinus officinalis
Rosemary
page 221

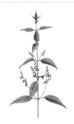

Scutellaria lateriflora
Skullcap
page 45

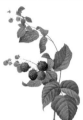

Rubus idaeus
Raspberry leaf
page 301

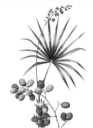

Serenoa repens
Saw palmetto
page 257

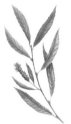

Salix alba
Willow bark
page 229

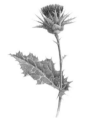

Silybum marianum
Milk thistle
page 167

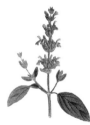

Salvia officinalis
Sage
page 91

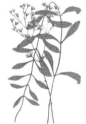

Stevia rebaudiana
Stevia
page 347

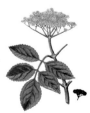

Sambucus nigra
Elder
page 71

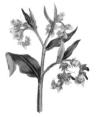

Symphytum officinale
Comfrey
page 213

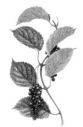

Schisandra chinensis
Schisandra
page 343

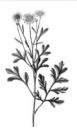

Tanacetum parthenium
Feverfew
page 23

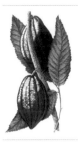

Theobroma cacao
Cacao, Chocolate
page 107

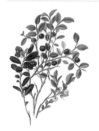

Vaccinium myrtillus
Bilberry
page 103

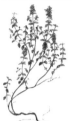

Thymus vulgaris
Thyme
page 95

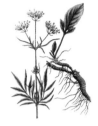

Valeriana officinalis
Valerian
page 53

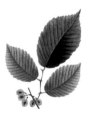

Ulmus rubra
Slippery elm
page 179

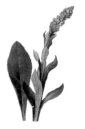

Verbascum thapsus
Mullein
page 83

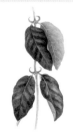

Uncaria tomentosa
Cat's claw
page 205

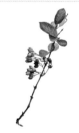

Viburnum prunifolium
Black haw
page 283

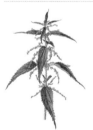

Urtica dioica
Stinging nettle
page 263

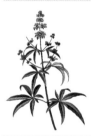

Vitex agnus-castus
Chaste tree
page 287

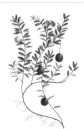

Vaccinium macrocarpon
Cranberry
page 291

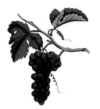

Vitis vinifera
Grapes, grape seed
page 119

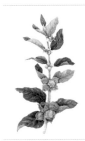

Withania somnifera
Ashwagandha
page 317

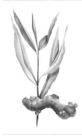

Zingiber officinale
Ginger
page 159

Illustration Credits

All images are © Steven Foster, Steven Foster Group, Inc. except for the following: 1, Waldemar Boniecki/Shutterstock; 6, Lynn Johnson; 9, Tania Midgley/CORBIS; 10, Emma Shervington/CORBIS; 11, Lynn Johnson/NationalGeographicStock.com; 17, Missouri Botanical Garden; 19, Mary E. Eaton; 20, Ken Wilson/CORBIS; 21, jo unruh/iStockphoto.com; 23, Missouri Botanical Garden; 24, Sandra Caldwell/Shutterstock; 27, Michaela Stejskalova/Shutterstock; 29 (LO LE), Mary E. Eaton; 29 (UP), Kletr/Shutterstock; 31, Jane Watkins; 33, Tammy Peluso/iStockphoto.com; 35, Courtesy of Hunt Institute for Botanical Documentation, Carnegie Mellon University, Pittsburgh, PA; 37, Lilyana Vynogradova/Shutterstock; 39, Mary E. Eaton; 45, Mary E. Eaton; 47, Colour/Shutterstock; 49, Jane Watkins; 53, Missouri Botanical Garden; 55, Mona Makela/Shutterstock; 59, Missouri Botanical Garden; 61, Jane Watkins; 63, Jane Watkins; 65, Mary E. Eaton; 66, LianeM/Shutterstock; 71, Missouri Botanical Garden; 75, Jane Watkins; 79, Jane Watkins; 81, Jane Watkins; 83, Mary E. Eaton; 87, Missouri Botanical Garden; 89, Maksym Protsenko/Shutterstock; 91, Courtesy of Hunt Institute for Botanical Documentation, Carnegie Mellon University, Pittsburgh, PA; 95, Jane Watkins; 97, Lilyana Vynogradova/Shutterstock; 101, Missouri Botanical Garden; 103, Courtesy of Hunt Institute for Botanical Documentation, Carnegie Mellon University, Pittsburgh, PA; 106, Dr. Morley Read/Shutterstock; 107, Jane Watkins; 109, Alex Staroseltsev/Shutterstock; 111, Jane Watkins; 113, Carolina Garcia Aranda/iStockphoto.com; 115, Jane Watkins; 119, Missouri Botanical Garden; 121, matka_Wariatka/Shutterstock; 123, Jane Watkins; 125, Danny Smythe/Shutterstock; 127, Missouri Botanical Garden; 128, Alexander Maksimenko/Shutterstock; 131, Courtesy of Hunt Institute for Botanical Documentation, Carnegie Mellon University, Pittsburgh, PA; 133, Olan/Shutterstock; 135, Jane Watkins; 136, polat/Shutterstock; 138, Frans Lanting; 139 (UP), Palani Mohan; 139 (LO), Priit Vesilind/NationalGeographicStock.com; 143, Missouri Botanical Garden; 145, Jane Watkins; 147, Nanka (Kucherenko Olena)/Shutterstock; 149, Jane Watkins; 153, Jane Watkins; 154, Fortish/Shutterstock; 156-157, Lynn Johnson; 159, Jane Watkins; 161, Corbis Premium RF/Alamy; 163, Jane Watkins; 167, Jane Watkins; 168, iStockphoto.com; 171, Mary E. Eaton; 175, Courtesy of Hunt Institute for Botanical Documentation, Carnegie Mellon University, Pittsburgh, PA; 177, Bildagentur-online/Alamy; 179, Courtesy of Hunt Institute for Botanical Documentation, Carnegie Mellon University, Pittsburgh, PA; 180, Janet Faye Hastings/Shutterstock; 181, Pat Crowe II/Getty Images; 183, Jane Watkins; 185, matin/Shutterstock; 189, Missouri Botanical Garden; 191, Jane Watkins; 193, Smit/Shutterstock; 194-195, Joel Sartore/NationalGeographicStock.com; 197, Jane Watkins; 199, SPbPhoto/Shutterstock; 201, Courtesy of Hunt Institute for Botanical Documentation, Carnegie Mellon University, Pittsburgh, PA; 205, Jane Watkins; 207, Pindyurin Vasily/Shutterstock; 209, Jane Watkins; 211, omkar.a.v/Shutterstock; 213, Mary E. Eaton; 215, TH Foto/Alamy; 217, Jane Watkins; 219, WILDLIFE GmbH/Alamy; 221, Courtesy of Hunt Institute for Botanical Documentation, Carnegie Mellon University, Pittsburgh, PA; 223, Krzysztof Slusarczyk/iStockphoto.com; 224, Robert Harding Picture Library Ltd/Alamy; 225, Jane Watkins; 227, Marilyn Barbone/Shutterstock; 229, Jane Watkins; 230, Lynn Johnson; 233, Mary E. Eaton; 234, Arunas Gabalis/Shutterstock; 239, Missouri Botanical Garden; 241, Jane Watkins; 243, Richard Peterson/Shutterstock; 245, Jane Watkins; 249, Missouri Botanical Garden; 252, www.FloraoftheWorld.com; 253, Jane Watkins; 254, www.FloraoftheWorld.com; 257, Jane Watkins; 263, Mary E. Eaton; 264, iStockphoto.com; 266, Tereza Dvorak/Shutterstock; 267, Missouri Botanical Garden; 268, Chris Price/iStockphoto.com; 269, T.W./Shutterstock; 271, Missouri Botanical Garden; 273, Lorraine Kourafas/Shutterstock; 277, Missouri Botanical Garden; 279, Mary E. Eaton; 283, Mary E. Eaton; 285 (UP), Trykster/Shutterstock; 285 (LO), Geoffrey Kidd/Alamy; 287, Courtesy of Hunt Institute for Botanical Documentation, Carnegie Mellon University, Pittsburgh, PA; 289, Bildagentur-online/TH Foto-Werbung/Photo Researchers, Inc.; 291, Jane Watkins; 292, Nigel Paul Monckton/Shutterstock; 293, Bill Curtsinger; 294-295, James P. Blair; 295, Lynn Johnson/NationalGeographicStock.com; 297, Jane Watkins; 299, Leian/Shutterstock; 301, Missouri Botanical Garden; 302, Peter Dennen/Aurora Photos/CORBIS; 303, Maksymilian Skolik/Shutterstock; 304, Hornbil Images/Alamy; 305, Missouri Botanical Garden; 307, ephotocorp/Alamy; 308, John Sommers II/Reuters/CORBIS; 309, Jane Watkins; 310, Chris Johns; 311, Dennis DeSilva/iStockphoto.com; 315, Missouri Botanical Garden; 317, Jane Watkins; 319, Geoffrey Kidd/Alamy; 321, Missouri Botanical Garden; 322, Hal Horwitz/CORBIS; 323, Robert Asento/Shutterstock; 325, Courtesy of Hunt Institute for Botanical Documentation, Carnegie Mellon University, Pittsburgh, PA; 326, cllakay/Shutterstock; 327, Amy Nichole Harris/Shutterstock; 328, Lynn Johnson/NationalGeographicStock.com; 329, Lynn Johnson/NationalGeographicStock.com; 331, Missouri Botanical Garden; 333, svry/Shutterstock; 335, Jane Watkins; 338, FloralImages/Alamy; 339, Courtesy of Hunt Institute for Botanical Documentation, Carnegie Mellon University, Pittsburgh, PA; 340, Bartosz Koszowski/Shutterstock; 343, Jane Watkins; 345, iStockphoto.com; 347, Missouri Botanical Garden; 348, iStockphoto.com; 349, Olivier Le Moal/Shutterstock.

General Index

NATIONAL GEOGRAPHIC GUIDE TO
Medicinal Herbs

Rebecca L. Johnson, Steven Foster,
Tieraona Low Dog, and David Kiefer

PUBLISHED BY THE NATIONAL GEOGRAPHIC SOCIETY

John M. Fahey, Jr., *President and Chief Executive Officer*

Gilbert M. Grosvenor, *Chairman of the Board*

Tim T. Kelly, *President, Global Media Group*

John Q. Griffin, *Executive Vice President; President, Publishing*

Nina D. Hoffman, *Executive Vice President; President, Book Publishing Group*

PREPARED BY THE BOOK DIVISION

Barbara Brownell Grogan, *Vice President and Editor in Chief*

Marianne R. Koszorus, *Director of Design*

Susan Tyler Hitchcock, *Senior Editor*

Carl Mehler, *Director of Maps*

R. Gary Colbert, *Production Director*

Jennifer A. Thornton, *Managing Editor*

Meredith C. Wilcox, *Administrative Director, Illustrations*

STAFF FOR THIS BOOK

Barbara H. Seeber, *Editor*

Jane Menyawi, *Illustrations Editor*

Melissa Farris, *Art Director*

Al Morrow, *Designer*

Linda White, M.D., *Medical Consultant*

Robert Wooding, *Herbal Consultant*

Lisa A. Walker, *Production Project Manager*

Marshall Kiker, *Illustrations Specialist*

Jennifer Tchinnosian, *Editorial Intern*

Allison Gaffney, *Design Intern*

Susan Blair, *Consulting Editor*

MANUFACTURING AND QUALITY MANAGEMENT

Christopher A. Liedel, *Chief Financial Officer*

Phillip L. Schlosser, *Vice President*

Chris Brown, *Technical Director*

Nicole Elliott, *Manager*

Rachel Faulise, *Manager*

Library of Congress Cataloging-in-Publication Data

Johnson, Rebecca L.
 National Geographic guide to medicinal herbs : the world's most effective healing plants / Rebecca L. Johnson & Steven Foster, Tieraona Low Dog ; foreword by Andrew Weil.
  p. cm.
 Includes indexes.
 ISBN 978-1-4262-0700-6 -- ISBN 978-1-4262-0701-3 (deluxe ed.)
 1. Herbs--Therapeutic use. 2. Materia medica, Vegetable.
I. Foster, Steven, 1957- II. Low Dog, Tieraona. III. National Geographic Society (U.S.) IV. Title. V. Title: Guide to medicinal herbs.
 RM666.H33J644 2010
 615'.321--dc22
                2010008723

The National Geographic Society is one of the world's largest nonprofit scientific and educational organizations. Founded in 1888 to "increase and diffuse geographic knowledge," the Society works to inspire people to care about the planet. It reaches more than 325 million people worldwide each month through its official journal, *National Geographic*, and other magazines; National Geographic Channel; television documentaries; music; radio; films; books; DVDs; maps; exhibitions; school publishing programs; interactive media; and merchandise. National Geographic has funded more than 9,000 scientific research, conservation and exploration projects and supports an education program combating geographic illiteracy. For more information, visit nationalgeographic.com.

For more information, please call 1-800-NGS LINE (647-5463) or write to the following address:

National Geographic Society
1145 17th Street N.W.
Washington, D.C. 20036-4688 U.S.A.

Visit us online at www.nationalgeographic.com

For information about special discounts for bulk purchases, please contact National Geographic Books Special Sales: ngspecsales@ngs.org

For rights or permissions inquiries, please contact National Geographic Books Subsidiary Rights: ngbookrights@ngs.org

First trade printing 2012

ISBN: 978-1-4262-0700-6
ISBN: 978-1-4262-0701-3 (deluxe)

Printed in China

11/CCOS/2

Important Note to Readers

This book is meant to increase your knowledge about medicinal herbs and the latest developments in the use of plants and herbal dietary supplements for medicinal purposes, and to the best of our knowledge the information provided is accurate at the time of its publication. It is not intended as a medical manual, and neither the authors nor the publisher is engaged in rendering medical or other professional advice to the individual reader. You should not use the information contained in this book as a substitute for the advice of a licensed health care professional. Because everyone is different, we urge you to see a licensed health care professional to diagnose problems and supervise the use of herbs and dietary supplements to treat individual conditions.

The botanical illustrations and descriptions of the physical characteristics of plants in this book are for general informational purposes, and they are not intended to be used to identify and gather plants in the field.

The authors and publisher disclaim any liability whatsoever with respect to any loss, injury, or damage arising directly or indirectly from the use of this book.